AṢṬADAḶA YOGAMĀLĀ

AṢṬADAḶA YOGAMĀLĀ

(COLLECTED WORKS)

B.K.S. IYENGAR

Volume 5

Interviews

ALLIED PUBLISHERS PRIVATE LIMITED
NEW DELHI MUMBAI KOLKATA CHENNAI NAGPUR
AHMEDABAD BANGALORE HYDERABAD LUCKNOW

ALLIED PUBLISHERS PRIVATE LIMITED
1/13-14 Asaf Ali Road, **New Delhi**–110002
Ph.: 011-23239001 • E-mail: delhi.books@alliedpublishers.com
Khasra No. 168, Plot No. 12-A, opp. Wisdom Academy School, Kamta,
Surendra Nagar, **Lucknow**–227105
Ph.: 09335202549 • E-mail: lko.books@alliedpublishers.com
17 Chittaranjan Avenue, **Kolkata**–700072
Ph.: 033-22129618 • E-mail: cal.books@alliedpublishers.com
15 J.N. Heredia Marg, Ballard Estate, **Mumbai**–400001
Ph.: 022-42126969 • E-mail: mumbai.books@alliedpublishers.com
60 Shiv Sunder Apartments (Ground Floor), Central Bazar Road,
Bajaj Nagar, **Nagpur**–440010
Ph.: 0712-2234210 • E-mail: ngp.books@alliedpublishers.com
F-1 Sun House (First Floor), C.G. Road, Navrangpura,
Ellisbridge P.O., **Ahmedabad**–380006
Ph.: 079-26465916 • E-mail: ahmbd.books@alliedpublishers.com
751 Anna Salai, **Chennai**–600002
Ph.: 044-28523938 • E-mail: chennai.books@alliedpublishers.com
5th Main Road, Gandhinagar, **Bangalore**–560009
Ph.: 080-22262081 • E-mail: bngl.books@alliedpublishers.com
3-2-844/6 & 7 Kachiguda Station Road, **Hyderabad**–500027
Ph.: 040-24619079 • E-mail: hyd.books@alliedpublishers.com

Website: www.alliedpublishers.com

First published, 2005
Reprinted, 2005, 2009, 2012, 2014

ISBN : 81-7764-713-X

Cover design : The Author

Artwork : S.M. Waugh

Published by Sunil Sachdev and printed by Ravi Sachdev at Allied Publishers Private Limited,Printing Division, A-104 Mayapuri Phase II, New Delhi - 110064

Invocatory Prayers

ॐ

Yogena cittasya padena vācāṁ
Malaṁ śarīrasyaca vaidyakena
Yopākarottaṁ pravaraṁ munīnāṁ
Patañjaliṁ prāñjalirānato'smi
Ābāhu puruṣākāraṁ
Śaṅkha cakrāsi dhāriṇaṁ
Sahasra śirasaṁ śvetaṁ
Praṇamāmi Patañjaliṁ

I bow before the noblest of sages Patañjali, who gave yoga for serenity and sanctity of mind, grammar for clarity and purity of speech and medicine for pure, perfect health.

I prostrate before Patañjali who is crowned with a thousand headed cobra, an incarnation of Ādiśeṣa (Anañta) whose upper body has a human form, holding the conch in one arm, disk in the second, a sword of wisdom to vanquish nescience in the third and blessing humanity from the fourth arm, while his lower body is like a coiled snake.

Yastyaktvā rūpamādyaṁ prabhavati jagato'nekadhānugrahāya
Prakṣīṇakleśarāśirviṣamaviṣadharo'nekavaktrāḥ subhogī
Sarvajñānaprasūtirbhujagaparikaraḥ prītaye yasya nityaṁ
Devohīṣaḥ savovyātsitavimalatanuryogado yogayuktaḥ

I prostrate before Lord Ādiśeṣa, who manifested himself on Earth as Patañjali to grace the human race in health and harmony,

I salute Lord Ādiśeṣa of the myriad serpent heads and mouths carrying noxious poisons, discarding which he came to Earth as a single headed Patañjali in order to eradicate ignorance and vanquish sorrow.

I pay my obeisance to him, repository of all knowledge, amidst his attendant retinue.

I pray to the Lord whose primordial form shines with peace and white effulgence, pristine in body, a master of yoga, who bestows on all his yogic light to enable mankind to rest in the house of the immortal Soul.

BY THE AUTHOR

This volume of *Aṣṭadaḷa Yogamālā* published by Allied Publishers, Delhi, is the fifth volume of the second part of the "Collected Works" of Yogācārya B.K.S. Iyengar. Each part comprises several volumes which are arranged according to the following scheme:

Articles
Interviews
Question and Answer Sessions
Techniques of *Āsanas, Prāṇāyāma, Dhyāna* and *Śavāsana*
Therapeutic Applications of Yoga
Garland of Aphorisms and Thoughts
General Index and Analytical Dictionary
Addendum

Also by the Same Author

Light on Yoga
Light on Prāṇāyāma
Concise Light on Yoga
Art of Yoga
Tree of Yoga
Light on the Yoga Sūtras of Patañjali
The Illustrated Light on Yoga
Yoga Ek Kalpataru (Marathi)
Ārogyayoga (Marathi)
Light on Aṣṭāṅga Yoga
Aṣṭadaḷa Yogamālā (Vols 1, 2, 3 & 4)
Yoga: The Path To Holistic Health
Yoga Sarvānasāṭhi (Marathi)
Basic Guidelines for Teachers of Yoga (co-authored with G.S. Iyengar)
Yogacandan (Marathi)

Also on Iyengar Yoga

Body the Shrine, Yoga Thy Light
70 Glorious Years
Iyengar His Life and Work
Yogapushpanjali
Yogadhārā

CONTENTS

PLATES

FOREWORD

Aṣṭadaḷa Yogamālā is coming forward again with the subtle intuitive essence of yoga through which the practitioner can become acquainted and practise keeping in mind these subtle qualities.

This volume covers the interviews I had with individuals and periodicals. I would keep in mind the background of the paper or magazine for whom the interviewer is interviewing. The answers have to be apt and short so that the readers are not bored, misguided or confused. But often the interviewer having only a background of bookish or theoretical knowledge, questions from the head rather than the heart. I have therefore answered the questions from that theoretical angle which may seem abstract. Answering in turn theoretically, I returned the interview back to earth with a concrete reply. Here, in this volume a reader will come across interviews which give the practical answers within a theoretical framework.

However, when pupils themselves approach me, their guru, out of inquisitiveness, doubt or sheer ignorance, then I have answered with a motherly touch to the issue.

Such interviews are like the diamond that shines through each of its many facets, bring illumination to the intelligence of the practitioner. The intelligence like a multi-faceted diamond guides the *sādhaka* with understanding to penetrate deeper and deeper with clarity and precision into the layers and coverings of the Self.

Just as a magnet magnetises and combs iron filings to move in unison, the magnet of yoga too combs the intelligence of the *sādhaka* to go deep within and cultivate a unifying awareness to the body, mind and Self.

BKS IYENGAR

THE INTERVIEWS

LONDON BROADCASTING COMMISSION
INTERVIEW WITH MR. IYENGAR*

Peter Murray: With me is the world's greatest authority on yoga, Mr. Iyengar.
Mr. Iyengar, I welcome you to the programme.

Mr. Iyengar: Thank you very much.

Peter Murray: Thank you very much indeed. You've literally only just arrived from the United States.

Mr. Iyengar: Yes, from New York. I just arrived this morning.

Peter Murray: Well I can say actually that I'm pretty sure of one thing, and that is that most people, when they arrive from America, suffer from what is known as 'jet lag'. Would I be right in saying that you don't suffer from jet lag?

Mr. Iyengar: Yes. I don't.

Peter Murray: Could you tell us exactly, when you fly, just as a matter of interest, what sort of position you take up just to get this sort of relaxation?

Mr. Iyengar: I have a great control over my nerves whereby I can slow down the speed of my breath, which creates complete passivity in my cells and I just relax on the seat itself. I neither feel disturbed nor excited. As the body is relaxed, it remains light and there is no rush in my mind either.

Peter Murray: What is the history of yoga, how many years does that go back?

---

* Edited transcription of Peter Murray's *Nightline* broadcast by the London Broadcasting Commission, 26th August 1987. This edited version was taken from *Dipika*, Winter 1987. № 16.

Mr. Iyengar: Yoga has existed from time immemorial. The subject of yoga is found in the *Veda*, the origin of all our literature including the philosophical and spiritual. However, *Maharṣī* Patañjali codified the science of yoga in the form of aphorisms.

Man was always inclined to know about the Ultimate Truth. For that, yoga came into existence. The urge to liberate himself from the bondage of ignorance led man to search out the paths, and yoga is one of them.

The *ṛṣī* yogis, who were treading on this path of yoga, found various body postures which generate energy in them, to peep within so that they could proceed towards serenity of mind and freedom. The common man began to realise that in order to live in this world, certain things to maintain health and happiness are necessary. An indisciplined way of living began disturbing his health and hence he worked out how to find methods whereby moving various joints, various parts of the muscles, supplying sufficient blood, he could keep himself healthy. That's how the science of yoga developed.

Peter Murray: And of course that was in India.

Mr. Iyengar: Yes! The origin of yoga is India alone.

Peter Murray: And how long did it take before yoga spread to the Western world?

Mr. Iyengar: Well, yoga was learnt by Westerners as they were ruling our country. Naturally there was a great deal of exchange between our arts, science and philosophy and their way of culture and art.

Peter Murray: So those that had been in India, the English people or the British people, studied yoga and brought it back.

Mr. Iyengar: Yes, many people wrote wonderful books on this subject. Even the High Court judge, Sir John Woodroffe, has written wonderful books on yoga.

Peter Murray: And was he a disciple of yours, by any chance?

Mr. Iyengar: No, I never met him personally. He is no more.

Peter Murray: Oh I see, we're going back many years now.

Mr. Iyengar: Yes, why years, centuries.

Peter Murray: Yes of course.

ꟷ

Peter Murray: Right, well we have a caller for you who would like to speak to you. Peter in Bayswater, good evening to you.

Peter: Good evening Peter Murray, I'm actually delighted to see somebody speaking about yoga on your programme and let me say one thing very clearly that I'm very much convinced regarding the yoga exercises which can help people tremendously. In my own divorce I was given a hell of a lot of tablets to calm my nerves and I realised that this is not the answer. As a child I remember my teacher taught all the students yogic exercises and at that desperate time of my life I remembered and went back to my childhood and practised certain yogic exercises with the result that within two days I threw all of my tablets in the dustbin. I hadn't been able to sleep for days and days before that, but with the help of yogic exercises I slept... So you see this is something very serious and wonderful.

Now my question to Mr. Iyengar is this, I have a very good knowledge of yoga. I do understand *buddhiyoga*, very little of course, *manoyoga*, very little of course, and *haṭhayoga*. I understand that *haṭhayoga* is to do with the physical side of the body but the problems which really affect people all over the world, especially in Europe, are the problems of mind itself, the difficulties which happen. Now *buddhiyoga*, *manoyoga* and *haṭhayoga*, there is one other form of yoga which I do not recollect or remember and could Mr. Iyengar elaborate about these various forms of yoga in the shortest possible way so that we can understand something other than *haṭhayoga*.

Mr. Iyengar: Yes, I will be very, very happy to inform you about yoga. First of all know well that yoga is one. Yoga means union. To unite ourselves to God is yoga.

People call yoga by different names to express their superiority compared to other types of yoga. The approach to yoga propounded by Patañjali cannot be termed as a kind of yoga. A human has a hierarchy starting from the body, senses, mind, intelligence, 'I'-ness, consciousness and conscience and the yogic line is applied to improve the human being from body to *buddhi* – intelligence – and the self. This being the essence of yoga, how can one categorise by naming yoga separately whereas methodology might be different due to the lapse of time and growth?

The word *ha* means sun, *ṭha* means moon; also these two syllables stand for Self and the consciousness. Similarly, according to the texts, *ha* stands for inhalation and *ṭha* stands for exhalation and it also covers different aspects such as physiological, psychological and mental levels. As far as *prāṇāyāma* is concerned, it means the harmony between the in-breath and the out-breath as well as the retentions following the in-breath and out-breath. The text says that *prāṇa* is to bring the consciousness to rest on the lap of the soul.

The intelligence and the mind are part and parcel of our mental body, including the cells. Yoga shows actual ways to quieten the cells so that the mind also becomes restful, the brain cells get rejuvenated and the intelligence sharpened. It does not mean that *haṭhayoga* is physical yoga. *Haṭhayoga Pradīpikā* speaks in the fourth chapter of what *samādhi* is, hence I advise you to read the fourth chapter which will give you a deep understanding of how to introduce the intelligence to each and every part of our body while performing the yogic *āsana* or while doing the *prāṇāyāma* or sitting in *mudrā*, *bandha* and *dhyāna*.

So, know very well that yoga is one. People have called it by different names for the sake of convenience. Patañjali author of *Yoga Sūtra* or Svātmārāma, the author of the *Haṭhayoga Pradīpikā*, do not differentiate yoga as the present yoga practitioners have differentiated. For these authors yoga is one and the same. Therefore do not get caught in the web of words.

As you mention that after your divorce you did *āsana* in order to calm down your nerves and your mind and found an improvement, did it not help you on a psychological as well as mental level? So, you find that all the other sheaths go on improving on different levels as you continue to practise.

Peter: Thank you very much, sir.

Peter Murray: Thank you very much, Peter.

Peter Murray: Now, Peter was saying just now how he went back to his youth and remembered his yoga and did certain yoga movements which helped him get over his nervous disability. What about the physical side, I mean how old have you to be to take up yoga? Is there an age limit?

Mr. Iyengar: For yoga, absolutely there is no age limit at all. One can begin from the age of six and practise until the last breath, and those who have not at all been introduced to the subject can begin at any age. For example, the late Queen Mother of Belgium began doing yoga, when she was eighty-four years old. She wanted to learn head balance, which I taught her.[1]

[1] See *Aṣṭadaḷa Yogamālā*, vol. 4, plate n. 31.

So age is not a problem at all, since the practitioners of yoga know how to utilise the energy of the body and mind according to the situation, that is the beauty of yoga.

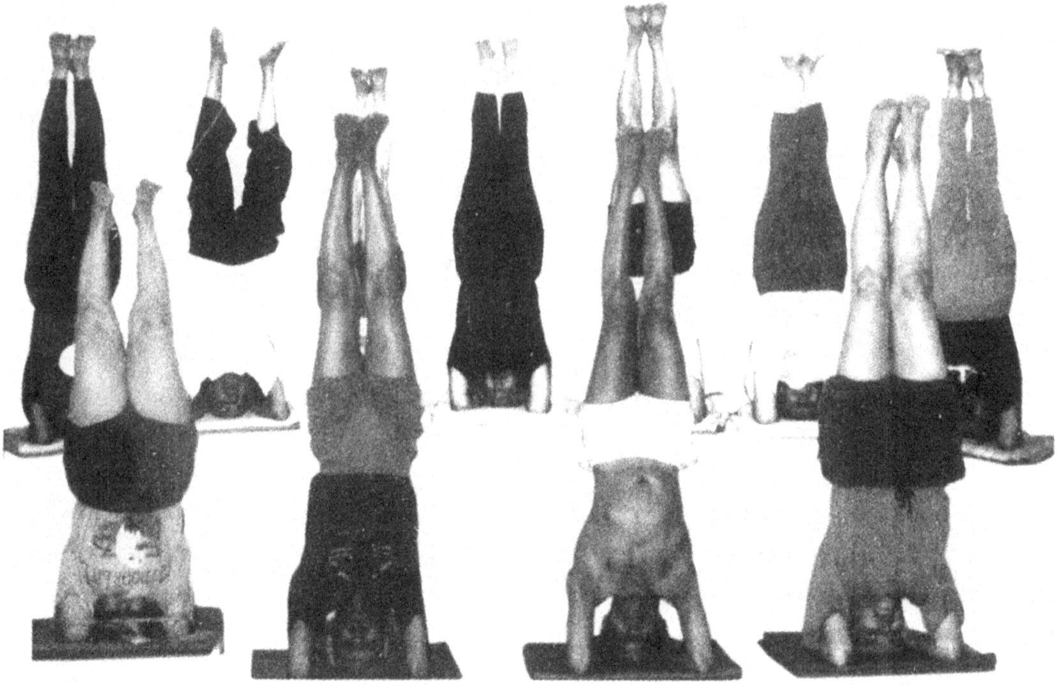

Plate n. 1 – Practitioners of yoga, 60years+ in *Śīrṣāsana*

Peter Murray: Right.

Steve in Bethnal Green would like to speak to you, Mr. Iyengar.

Good evening, Steve.

Steve: Good evening. I just phoned up, my wife is pregnant at the moment and I just wondered if it's all right for her to carry on doing any yoga positions in the predicament she's in at the moment?

Mr. Iyengar: May I know exactly in what month the pregnancy is now?

Steve: She's three months gone.

Mr. Iyengar: Three months? She can do comfortably for another two months without straining the abdominal organs. You have to create a vast space for the foetus to grow; hence she can do the *āsana* without compressing the abdominal organs but creating space and strengthening the spine.

Steve: OK, I see.

Peter Murray: Steve may I ask before you go, does your wife, or has she, ever done yoga before?

Steve: No, well, a person in the bank gave her a book.

Mr. Iyengar: No, no, I think if she has not undergone training with a teacher at this stage, and as there are two lives to be taken care of, she should not do anything by herself alone. Hence I advise you to consult a known yoga teacher who can help her exactly as to what *āsana* could be suitable so that even the labour pains could be reduced to a minimum.

Steve: OK, then I'll see.

Peter Murray: Yes, I see, so don't do anything until you've spoken to a yoga teacher, Steve. You got that, did you?

Steve: Yes.

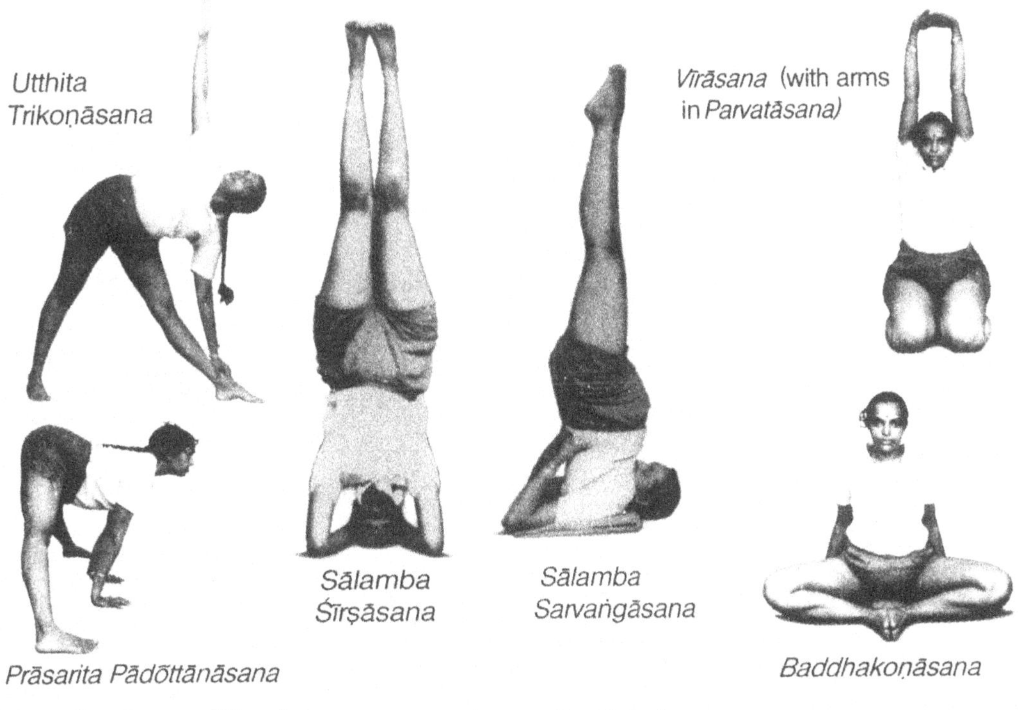

Plate n. 2 – Some of the *āsanas* commonly practised during pregnancy

Peter Murray: OK then. Fine. Thank you very much indeed for your call.

We go to Lyn who lives in Kenton.

Good evening, Lyn.

Lyn: Oh, good evening. I have a query regarding a hiatus hernia that I have. I don't suffer with it very much but I've been thinking about taking up yoga and I am not sure really whether I should be doing this, could you advise me please?

Mr. Iyengar: Well, you can certainly do some *āsana* for hiatus hernia. You can especially do the back arches with the help of props or on a chair so that the diaphragm develops strength and you will be able to create the space between the thorax and abdomen, which helps to recover. If you are particularly on the heavy side then you should not do the shoulder balance – *Sālamba Sarvāṅgāsana*, the forward bends, and the plough pose, *Halāsana* – but the rest of the *āsana*, such as standing *āsana*, concave extension of the spine in forward bends, can be done without any untoward incident.

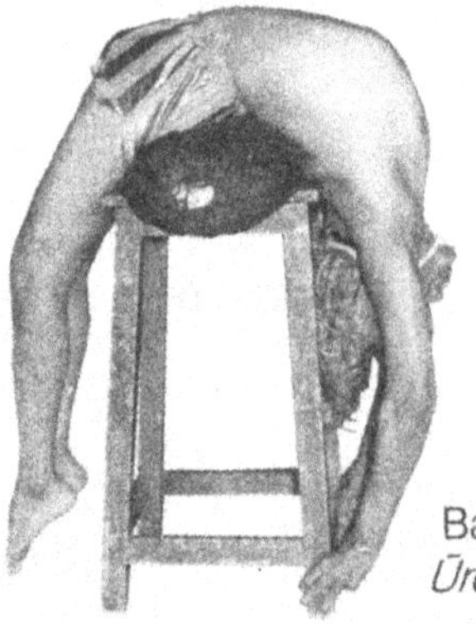
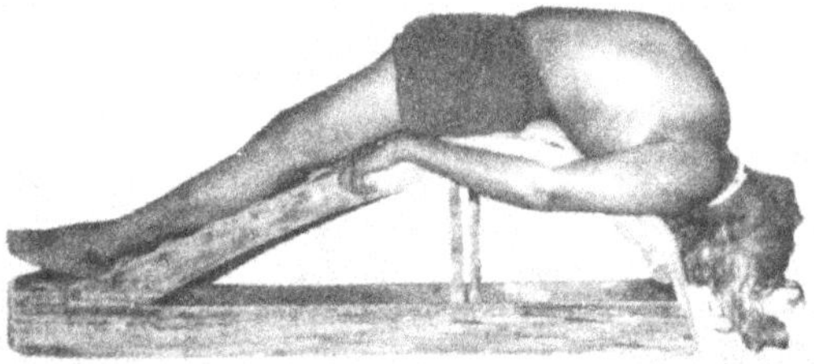

Back arches with help of a prop:
Ūrdhva Dhanurāsana and *Dwi Pāda Viparīta Daṇḍāsana*

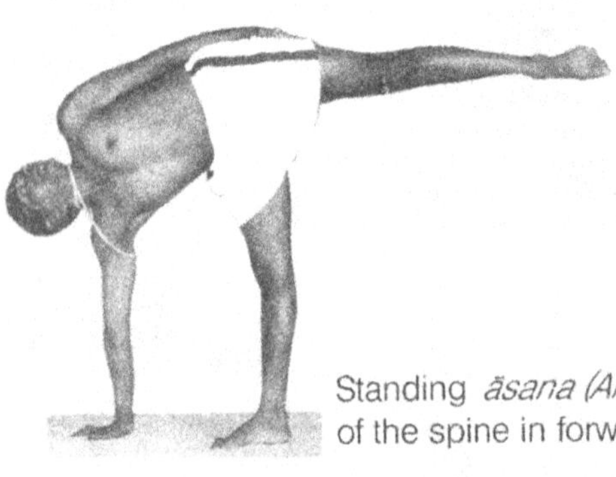
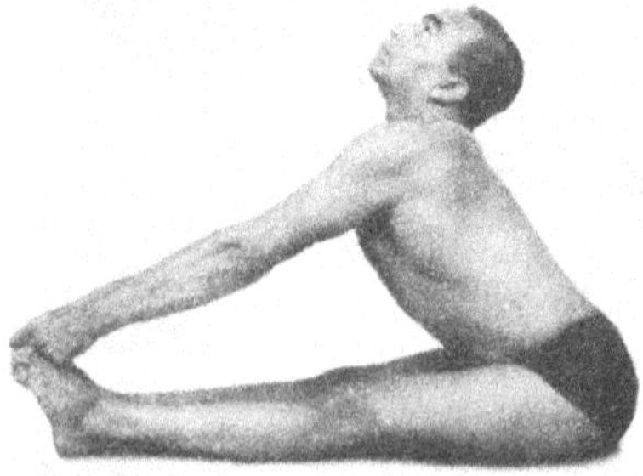

Standing *āsana (Ardha Chandrāsana)* and concave extension of the spine in forward bends *(Paśchimottānāsana)*

Plate n. 3 – Back-arches with props, and concave forward extension of the spine

Lyn: So if I go to yoga classes that I'm hoping to enrol in next month, then I shall be guided by the yoga teacher, shall I?

Mr. Iyengar: Yes, certainly, you should to any of my pupils who can easily guide you as I have given them ways and methods of handling such cases. You will be guided.

Lyn: Thank you very much for your help.

Peter Murray: Well, you live in Kenton don't you?

Lyn: Yes.

Peter Murray: Well, the Iyengar Yoga Institute is at 223a Randolph Avenue, London W9, and the telephone number 020 7624 3080.[1]

Lyn: Thank you very much for your help.

Peter Murray: That's a pleasure.

Peter Murray: One of the great problems with people here in Britain, I'm sure you know is the back problem, slipped discs and that sort of thing. Now once a disc has worn away and people have been using the wrong posture for a period of time, is there anything that yoga can do for a bad back?

Mr. Iyengar: *Yogāsana* is not merely just an exercise. They are postures; the alignment in the posture of the body is very important while practising the *yogāsana*. Due to the perfect alignment, even the worn-out discs develop a certain strength to bear future pressure on those areas. Secondly, we have got thirty three spinal vertebrae. If one vertebra is damaged that does not mean we have to neglect the other thirty-two vertebrae, hence I say that it is better to protect the other areas so that the disease may not increase and make the person a cripple.

Peter Murray: Obviously the person who starts yoga at about eight years of age, his chances of getting a bad back are practically negligible, aren't they?

---

[1] Contact the Iyengar Yoga Association IYA(UK) who can direct you to a teacher near you.

Mr. Iyengar: Children never get backaches.

Peter Murray: No, but I mean they won't get it in later life if they.....

Mr. Iyengar: No, not at all, not at all. Since they know the alignment, they can adjust both sides of the spinal column accurately in all the movements, creating space between each vertebra. But they need to practise regularly. If they neglect then it cannot be guaranteed.

Peter Murray: It's interesting too that just before we came on the air we were talking about how most people think in terms of yoga of people standing on their heads, just one of the movements. Could you tell us exactly what that does for you?

Mr. Iyengar: Yoga is actually to associate oneself with the body cells, associate oneself with the mind so that they conquer the impediments of the body and the fluctuations of the mind to live in peace and happiness. That's the aim of yoga. But only standing on the head does not mean yoga, it's part of yoga but...

Peter Murray: Yes, of course, but that's what most people think of it as.

Mr. Iyengar: Maybe, but before doing the head balance – *Sālamba Śīrṣāsana* – there are so many other things which have to be done and standing on the head cannot be equated to the whole of yogic science. We have got *āsana*, we have got *prāṇāyāma* – the breathing techniques, we have got to know how to control the senses, how to sit for meditation, how to concentrate, all these things put together are yoga.

As far as the head balance, *Sālamba Śīrṣāsana* is concerned, it is called the king of the *āsana*. The brain is the seat of intelligence, determination, knowledge, wisdom, will power, memory and discrimination. To keep these functions of the brain healthy and efficient, the practice of *Sālamba Śīrṣāsana*[1] is essential. It increases its capacity.

Peter Murray: A lot of people suffer not only from bad backs but varicose veins. Is there anything that can be done?

Mr. Iyengar: Yes, all inverted poses are good. Inversions like standing on the head, standing on the shoulders, forward bends and flexing the knees and sitting on the legs in certain positions, reduce

---

[1] See *Aṣṭadaḷa Yogamālā*, vol. 3, plate n. 28.

the load on the varicose veins and make the blood flow back to the heart, so that the quality of the blood as well as the venous circulation improves.

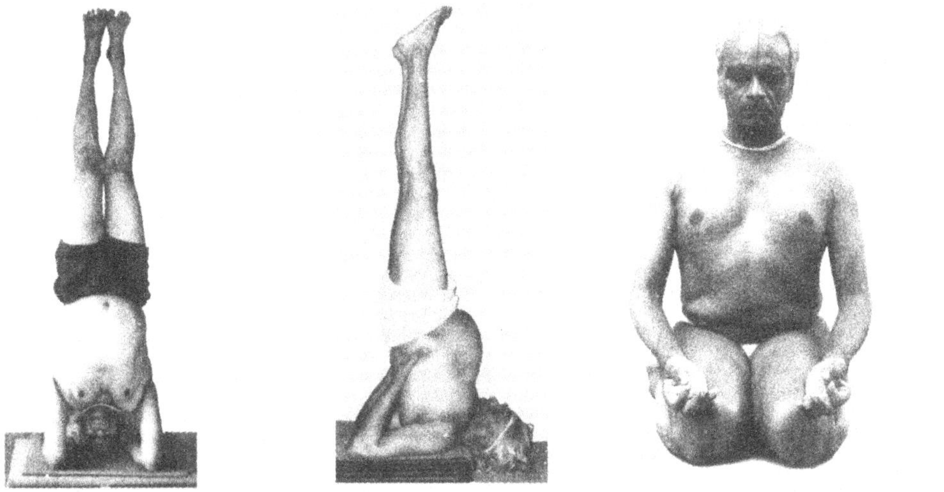

Plate n. 4 - *Sālamba Śīrṣāsana, Sālamba Sarvaṅgāsana* and *Vīrasana*

For bad backs one needs to do standing *āsana* as well as the lateral twists to eradicate the deformities of the back.

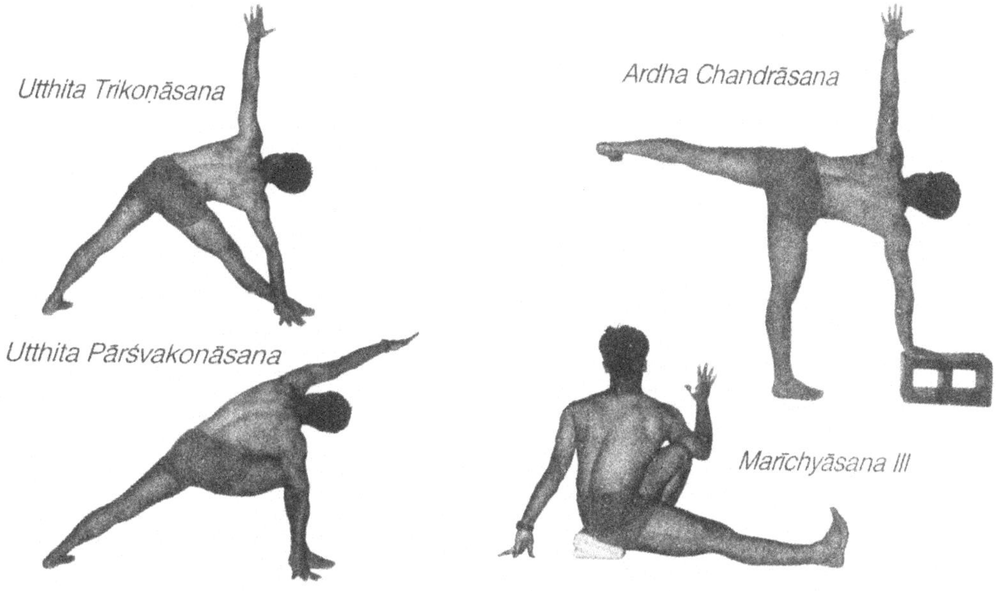
Utthita Trikoṇāsana
Ardha Chandrāsana
Utthita Pārśvakonāsana
Marīchyāsana III

Plate n. 5 – Standing *āsanas* and lateral twists for deformities of the back

Peter Murray: Right, we go to Bob now, in Southall.
Good evening, Bob.

Bob: Good evening, Peter, and good evening to Mr. Iyengar. It is very nice to speak to him. I think actually he might slightly have stolen my thunder because I was ringing in regarding a bad back and I have had diagnosed a slightly deformed spine and I wonder if there is any form of yoga which would be helpful or on the other hand would be harmful to me.

Mr. Iyengar: See, the standing *āsana* are known as educative *āsana* to improve the deformed spine. We need to correct our posture. In order to do that we have to educate and culture our muscles by understanding where they have been affected or disabled.

The standing *āsana* strengthen the weak muscles. The *āsana* are taught as if you are in traction. Many yogic *āsana* work as natural tractions and create space in those compressed or painful parts so that the relief comes immediately. That is the way one has to consciously know exactly what has to be done with full awareness.

Bob: I see, so it could be quite beneficial to me then.

Mr. Iyengar: It is definitely beneficial because ninety-nine per cent of the people have these backaches not only in England, but the world over. For several years I have conducted classes on lower backaches and they have tremendously improved. Even people who had to go for an operation were completely rid of it without an operation.

Bob: Right, fine, thank you very much.

Peter Murray: OK Bob, thank you very much indeed.

Now we'll go to Ian in Ilford. Good evening, Ian.

Ian: Good evening. I've got a question for Mr. Iyengar. Could he please explain the *Samavṛtti prāṇāyāma* – that's from his book *Light on Yoga*.

Mr. Iyengar: Yes, *prāṇa* means energy, and *āyāma* is to make the energy move with extension and expansion to store the energy in the storehouse of the lungs. *Prāṇāyāma* teaches how to use that drawn-in energy so that it is properly distributed into the system. You know, we are made up of five elements: earth, water, air, fire and ether. Out of these five elements, water and fire are 'anti-elements', or antagonistic to each other. The normal breath, which we draw in, fuses the element of fire and the element of water in our systems and produces a new energy, known as 'bio-energy'. This bio-energy is produced by elongating the inhalation and exhalation and creating pauses in between these two breaths. *Prāṇāyāma* creates energy and allows the energy to reach the remote parts of the lungs where the alveolar cells get feedback from the long breath we take and the breath we release without any tension so that the residual energy that was drawn in, is retained in the process of exhalation. That is why it is called *prāṇāyāma*.

Āyāma has got three movements: extension, expansion and circumduction. While doing *prāṇāyāma* the muscles of the chest and lungs get all these movements. All the three actions of *prāṇāyāma* put together make the lungs function at their optimum level.

In *Samavṛtti prāṇāyāma*, the duration of all the four aspects of *prāṇāyāma*, namely inhalation, inhalation retention, exhalation and exhalation retention are kept in an equal ratio. *Sama* means equal or identical. *Vṛtti* means the movement or a course of conduct. Since there are varieties of *prāṇāyāma*, when all the four aspects of breath as just now mentioned are kept in equal ratio and with identical flow, it is termed as *Samavṛtti prāṇāyāma*.

Ian: Thank you, I see, that is very helpful.

Mr. Iyengar: However, as a practitioner, read *Light on Prāṇāyāma* several times before you attempt *Samavṛtti prāṇāyāma*. First you need to watch your own capacity and the movements.

Ian: Thank you.

Peter Murray: Thank you very much for your call. Welcome back to Peter Murray's *Nightline*. With me is the world's greatest authority on yoga, Mr. Iyengar, and we go straight to a caller. It's Richard in Hackney. Good evening, Richard.

Richard: Good evening, Peter, good evening, Mr. Iyengar. I want to ask a question on behalf of my girl friend, because she's a bit shy to ask, to phone up, but she does yoga every night and she wants to know how long before she does the exercise should she stop eating food.

Mr. Iyengar: Well, after yoga practice she can take light food after half-an-hour or forty-five minutes, and three hours after food, she can practise.

Richard: Forty-five minutes after, it would be all right?

Mr. Iyengar: A minimum of forty-five minutes is enough.

Richard: And half-an-hour before?

Mr. Iyengar: No, not half-an-hour before. If you have a good lunch, then there should be about three or four hours' interval between food and yoga. She should stop eating food three or four hours before the practice of yoga and eat forty-five minutes later after practice. I hope it is clear.

Richard: Right, I think that's all she wants to know really.

Peter Murray: All right, Richard, thank you very much indeed. In fact would I be right in saying that you cannot be a perfect yogi until such times as you stop eating meat? Is it essential to be a vegetarian?

Mr. Iyengar: Well, as you progress in your yogic practice, the system does not accept any other food than what it really wants. The system rejects meat, heavy and spicy food, so one becomes a perfect dietician by oneself through the practice of yoga. That is why, in the beginning, I do not restrict food for my pupils. As the practice improves, the body dictates what food it needs, not through the taste of the tongue or choice.

Peter Murray: I see... We now go to Nora in Redbridge.
Good evening, Nora.

Nora: Good evening, Peter. May I speak to Mr. Iyengar?

Peter Murray: Yes.

Nora: Thank you very much, Mr. Iyengar.

I wanted to know whether there are different types of yoga and the reason I ask this is because I went to yoga to relax, I am the type of person who finds it very difficult to relax and I found it so depressing and I got so depressed I had to give it up. Why?

Mr. Iyengar: First of all, yoga is one, which I answered in the beginning of the programme. God is one, but people give different names. Yoga is also one but people call it by different names, according to the method they have chosen.

As far as the second part of the question is concerned, in order to get *Śavāsana* or relaxation, first of all one should know how to diffuse the mind throughout the body like the rays of the sun that shine evenly when the clouds are not there. Similarly the rays of the mind should spread in the body, diffusing evenly over each and every cell of our body. Then *Śavāsana* comes automatically, there is no fear at all, and there cannot be any depression in yoga.

Nora: Well, why did I get so depressed then with yoga? I found it so dreadfully depressing that I just could not go on with it.

Mr. Iyengar: Probably you must have jumped to meditation immediately without knowing the capacity of your nervous system. First you have to strengthen your nervous system and get the stability of the body, then you can go towards meditation, which definitely brings calmness but without any depression.

When you say that you find it very difficult to relax yourself it means that you are a restless person with unsteady thoughts. So you need to do some other *āsana* to strengthen the nervous system and gain steadiness.

If the centre of your chest sinks inward or is empty from within, in *Śavāsana*, you get depressed. So with the support of pillows elevate your chest in *Śavāsana*. You feel comfortable and relaxed.

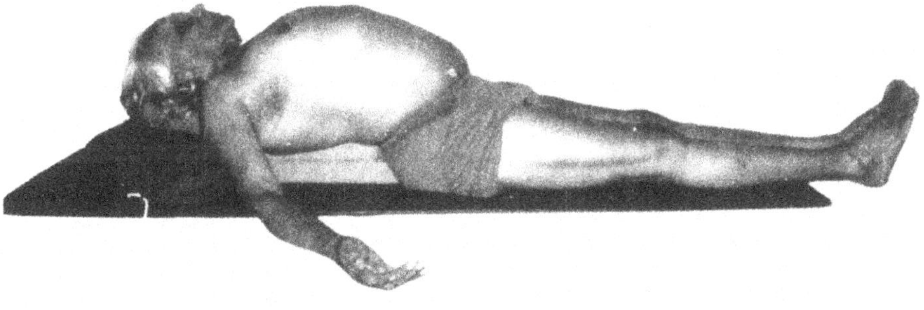

Plate n. 6 – *Śavāsana* with chest elevated

Nora: Thank you. Now what type of yoga... I mean, are there different types of yoga?

Mr. Iyengar: No, there are no different types of yoga at all.

Nora: There is just yoga?

Mr. Iyengar: Yes, yoga is one.

Nora: Oh, well perhaps I had the wrong teacher.

Mr. Iyengar: Patañjali is the authority on yoga. He asks us to seek ethical discipline, the physical discipline, the sensorial discipline, mental discipline and intellectual discipline. People say, "I am doing *buddhi yoga* and controlling the intelligence". Some say, "I am stilling the mind", they call it *mano yoga*. They use just words, but yoga engulfs the entire system of man, from skin to the self, from the self to the skin.

Nora: Would you think that perhaps I had the wrong teacher?

Mr. Iyengar: I do not like to comment on such matters. But I can only say that if I had seen your condition I would have told you what to do with ease.

If you cannot do *Śavāsana* – relaxation – easily, then I would have certainly taught you certain *āsana* where relaxation sets in unconsciously before you go for *Śavāsana*. There are various *āsana* namely, *Supta Vīrāsana, half Halāsana, Setubandha Sarvāṅgāsana, Viparīta Karaṇi*, and if you do them then your body, the organs of action, nerves, the senses of perception and mind begin to relax and then when you do *Śavāsana*, there comes an automatic conscious relaxation.

Nora: I see. Well, thank you very much indeed, I am most grateful to you. Perhaps I will try again and perhaps I will try some different teacher.

Mr. Iyengar: If you contact some of my pupils, they will certainly show you how to prepare the body to go into the relaxation position.

Nora: Thank you.

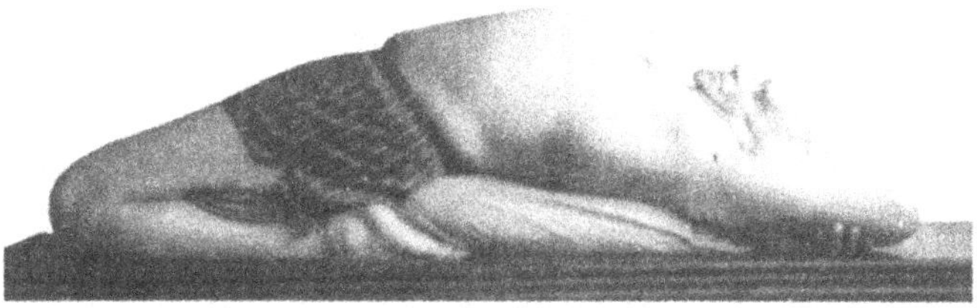

Supta Vīrāsana

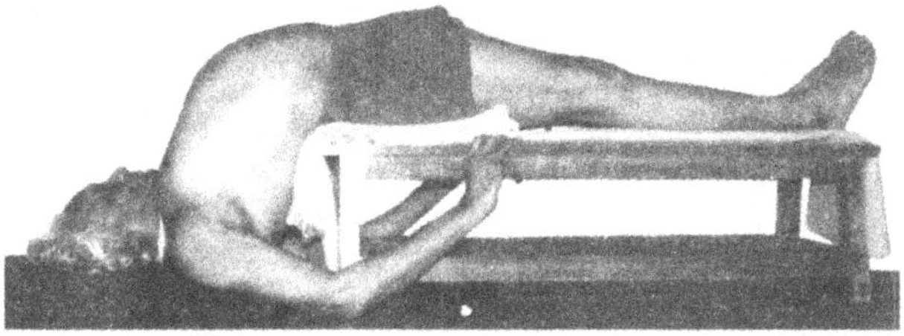

Setubandha Sarvāṅgāsana

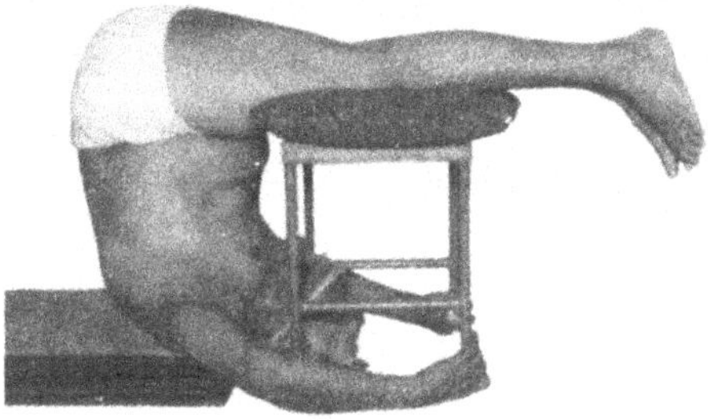

half Halāsana

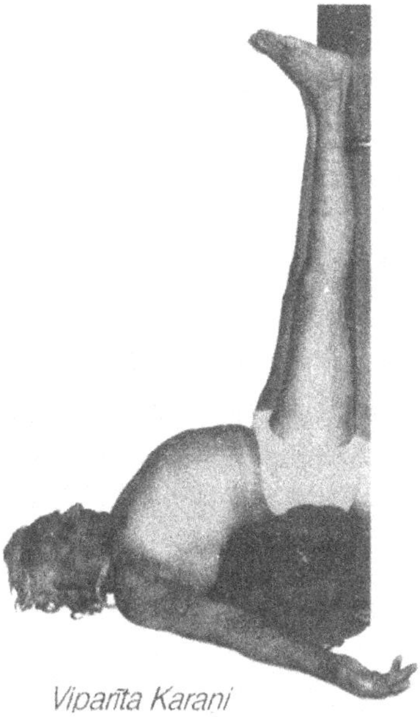

Viparīta Karaṇi

Plate n 7 – *Āsanas* for relaxation to set in

Peter Murray: Now we go to Lucy in Lingfield, in West Sussex. Good evening Lucy.

Lucy: Hello Peter, hello Mr. Iyengar.

I have been doing yoga now for about two years and I try to do some every day and when I get into the postures I feel much better mentally and physically if I do it every day, but my body does creak and crack terribly. Could you tell me why this is so? The more I seem to do yoga, the more I creak and crack. It doesn't hurt me.

Mr. Iyengar: Yes, the creaking and cracking sound in joints does not hurt at all. In the beginning you get this sound because you do quickly and with speed. Start gradually by moving the joints and muscles, so that you don't get these creaks and cracks.

Lucy: Ah, so it is all right.

Mr. Iyengar: Yes, yes. It is all right as long as it does not pain.

Lucy: Well, I do feel a lot better but every time, as I do a lot of them, the spine creaks and cracks.

Mr. Iyengar: You need not become nervous. It stops automatically. Only see that you do not do the *āsana* very fast one after the other and over-exert. Slow down the speed.

Lucy: Oh, I see. How long will that take, because I have been doing it for two years.

Mr. Iyengar: Well, maybe another six months or so.

Lucy: Another six months or so?

Mr. Iyengar: Yes, you should continue. I know, it sounds terrible to the ears, it sounds offensive. It is an indication of the dryness of the joints. The blood circulation has to improve around the joints and muscles, so continue to practise and see that you do not over exert yourself. The moment you get the natural movements while going into the postures, then it will stop.

Lucy: Ah, superb, thank you very much.

Peter Murray: All right, Lucy, thank you very much indeed for your call.

Peter Murray: We will now take one from Damian, in North Paddington. Good evening, Damian.

Damian: Good evening. Good evening, Mr. Iyengar.

My problem is I have been suffering from tuberculosis and I allowed the tuberculosis to progress very far, while doing yoga exercises, not wishing to take medicines. In the end I was directed to take medicines with the result that the tuberculosis is gone but my lungs are pretty badly damaged.

In your book *Light on Yoga*, you state, for recovery from tuberculosis, to seek guidance of a qualified instructor, and since you are probably the most highly qualified instructor, I wonder could you mention some of the *āsana* which would help me the most?

Mr. Iyengar: Yes, my friend, happily! I was a tuberculosis patient in the year 1931-32. Now I am sixty-nine years old. So when the doctors said I was suffering from tuberculosis when I was a boy of thirteen years they thought that I might not survive at all. However, I survived due to yoga and not only have I got my health back but I have served humanity with love for good health and made use of my life fruitfully.

However, *Light on Yoga* will not help you at this stage, because I haven't introduced any prop in that book, but only gave the *āsana* which help to rejuvenate the lungs, in the section about the lungs. Do with props or support. You will find a sea of change in you.

Damian: That is the one I try and do.

Mr. Iyengar: No, no, that is not what I am saying. If you visit the Iyengar Yoga Institute, they have got props, where the same *āsana* is performed without any strain. You can rejuvenate your lungs without strain. So if you look into the props, you can do all those *āsana* including the head balance, which is in the book, with the help of the rope, how to hang oneself in an upside-down position.

Damian: Well, the headstand I do naturally without any problem and the shoulder stand.

Mr. Iyengar: When you do shoulder stand there is compression of the lungs and the ribs cave in. So do first *Setubandha Sarvāṅgāsana* and then *Sālamba Sarvāṅgāsana* with the help of a chair, then you definitely derive better benefit than what you are deriving now.

Damian: OK

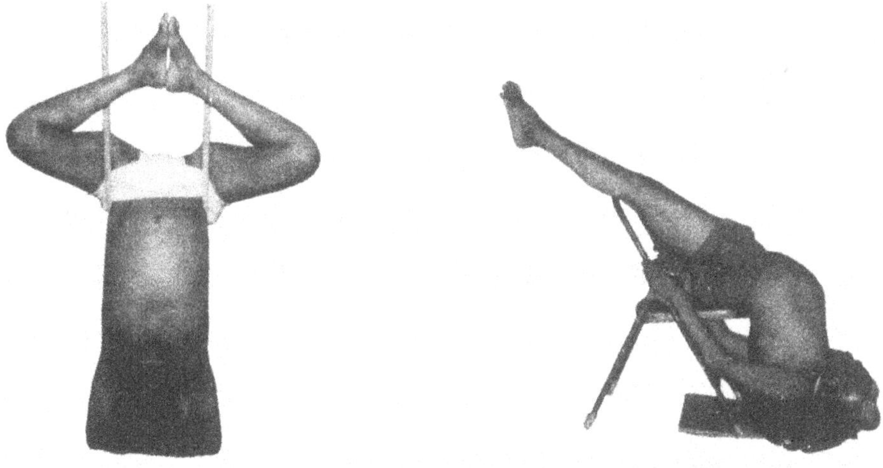

Plate n. 8 – *Śīrṣāsana* with the help of a rope and *Sarvaṅgāsana* on a chair

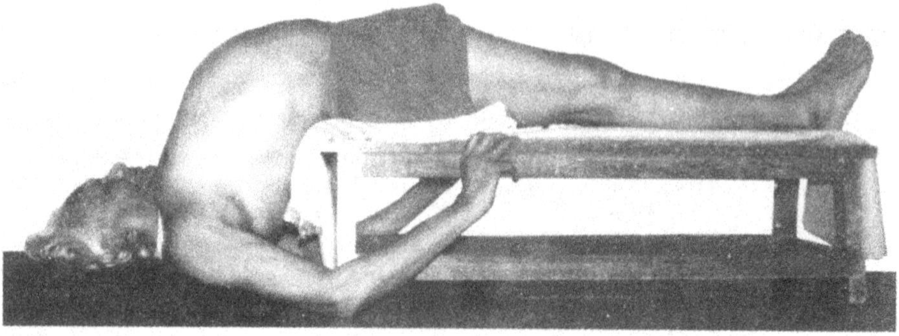

Plate n 8 cont. - *Setu Bandha Sarvaṅgāsana,*

Peter Murray: OK, Damian? Thank you very much for your call.
We now go to Jane, in Welling. Good evening, Jane.

Jane: Good evening, Peter. Good evening, Mr. Iyengar. I have been doing yoga for quite a number of years as I find it is the most gentle form of exercise for me, but there is just one thing that worries me. I have got three slipped discs that are fused together in my neck and I wondered if it is safe for me to do the shoulder stand?

Mr. Iyengar: No. I will not advise you to do the shoulder balance. But if I am teaching you directly, then I can show you exactly how to keep the cervical spine in a concave position without injuring that area in the shoulder stand. However, I advise you to do the standing *āsana; Utthita Trikoṇāsana, Utthita Pārśvakoṇāsana, Vīrabhadrāsana* I&II, *Ardha Chandrāsana,* curving the neck backwards, *Bharadvājāsana* on a chair, which are introduced in my book *Light on Yoga* and some rope work which is known as *yoga-kuruṇṭa* where the discs move to their positions. Thereafter you will be able to do some shoulder balance without any injury at all.

Jane: Only one teacher said that it was all right to do it.

Mr. Iyengar: No. First you have to treat yourself for the slipped discs of the neck. After getting all right, you use four or five blankets or mats, and keep the shoulders on them and the back of the head on the floor, then there is no strain or injury on the neck at all.

Jane: Oh! I know, thank you very much.

Peter Murray: All right, Jane, thank you very much indeed.

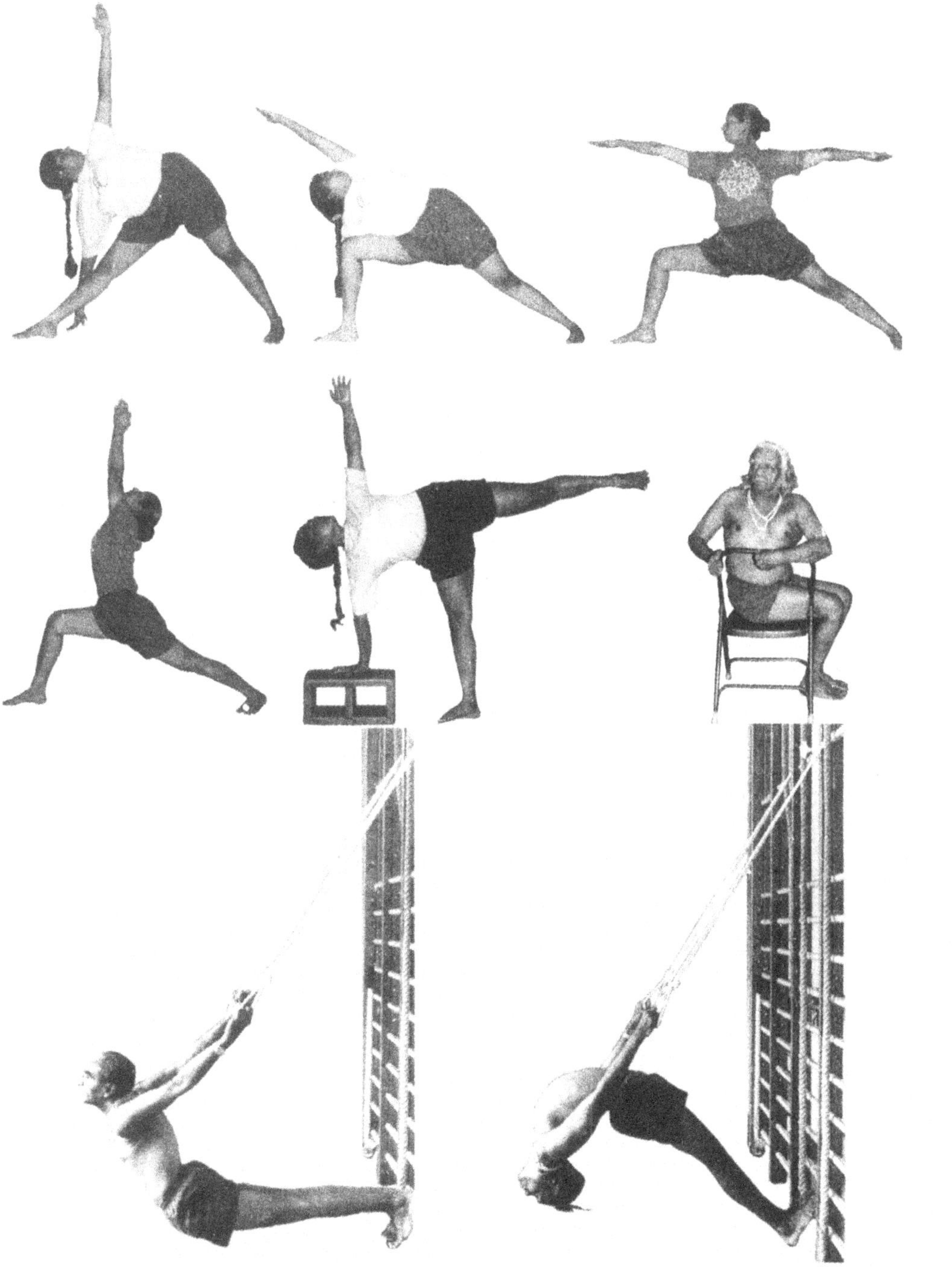

Plate n. 9 – Standing *āsanas* curving the neck, *Bharadvājāsana* on a chair, *yoga-kuruṇṭa* (*āsanas* using a rope)

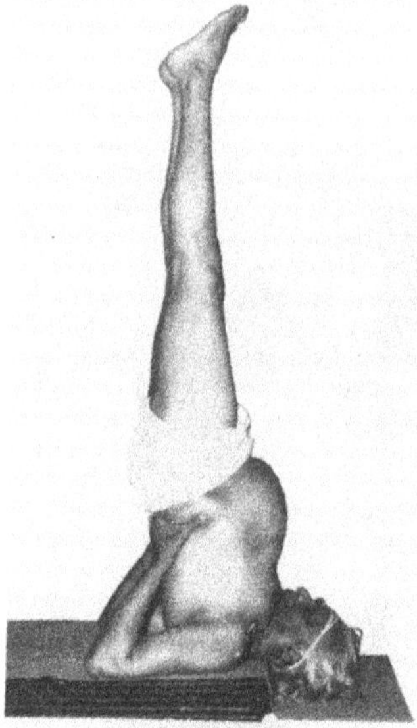

Plate n. 10 - *Sālamba Sarvaṅgāsana* on mats

Peter Murray: Mr. Iyengar, did you want to come back to the subject of breathing?

Mr. Iyengar: Yes, my friend, because there was a person who asked me a question about breath. We normally do fifteen breaths per minute. The respiratory system is a semi-voluntary system. It can be voluntary at times and at times it can be involuntary too. Knowing this fact the yogis found out how to pump air to the extremities of the lungs and so they learnt this art of doing slow, soft, rhythmic inhalation and slow, soft, rhythmic exhalation. *Prāṇāyāma* is not at all dangerous if people do not hold their breath too long beyond their capacity. There is a danger if they hold the breath beyond their capacity. If anything untoward happens, then it is better to stick to normal and deep inhalation and exhalation, feeling the flavour of the breath through the intelligence, then I say *prāṇāyāma* will never do any damage to anyone.

Peter Murray: Right, thank you very much indeed.

Peter Murray: We will now go to Mike, in Southgate. Good evening, Mike.

Mike: Good evening, gentlemen. I have been doing yoga now for about five months and find it extremely beneficial and I am going to a very good teacher and physically I find it absolutely wonderful. I have got rid of backache, I have got rid of cramp. What I wanted to ask Mr. Iyengar was, when does relaxation of the mind come? I am a very, very tense, highly-strung person and does that come naturally with the *āsana* or does one have to do special exercises to relax the mind?

Mr. Iyengar: It comes by regular practice of *āsana* because you develop inter-penetration while performing the *āsana*. Because of that inter-penetration the rays of your intelligence from the brain diffuse throughout the body. The moment it starts diffusing more and more, the brain becomes quiet and silent and this is the gateway for total relaxation.

Mike: Oh, I see, so by practising the *āsana*.

Mr. Iyengar: Yes, yes, you are going to get it.

Mike: It comes automatically to you.

Mr. Iyengar: Yes, it comes automatically, provided you do the *āsana* correctly. You should not remain tensed while doing the *āsana*. You need to do a couple of *āsana* which make your brain to get quietened and the nerves pacified. There are some *āsana* for the inert body and dull mind to make them active and there are other *āsana* that make the nerves quiet and stop the mind from rushing. You need to choose those passive *āsana* such as *Supta Vīrāsana*, *Setubandha Sarvāṅgāsana*, *Viparīta Karaṇi*[1] so as to calm yourself down.

Mike: I would just like to add, yoga is the most wonderful thing.

Mr. Iyengar: Undoubtedly.

Peter Murray: OK. Thank you very much indeed. Thank you, Mike.

Peter Murray: We now go to Pam, in Waltham Cross. Good evening, Pam.

---

[1] See plate n. 7.

Pam: Good evening, both of you. Mr. Iyengar has almost answered a question that I was going to ask and that was about breathing exercises. There was one point that I would like to ask, if I may, about blockages that could be caused maybe in the body through practising breathing exercises at home without a teacher. And I was interested to know what these blockages could be and should you not practise breathing exercises at home such as *Bhastrikā*.

Mr. Iyengar: Always it is better to see a good teacher. And if you do not find one, a good book is better than a bad teacher. Do you understand? So, have you got my book *Light on Prāṇāyāma?*

Pam: Yes.

Mr. Iyengar: You can follow that very statement where I have taught how to observe normal breath. The moment you observe the normal breath with your intelligence, you will see that I have shown how it becomes deep automatically. In the beginning of the book itself I have shown the safest method. It is enough to develop the quality of improving the art of breathing and of filtering the breath so that it can enter the lungs without any dust or pollution. All this I have explained in the book for the good of all.

Peter Murray: Do you understand that, Pam?

Pam: Yes I do, thank you. I found the breathing exercises beneficial but does Mr. Iyengar think it is better to practise with a teacher rather than on your own?

Mr. Iyengar: Yes, yes, many of my senior teachers may be conducting classes on *prāṇāyāma* in your area. If it is possible for you to attend these once or twice a week, you will get a good background of the art of inhalation, the art of exhalation and also you can learn how to keep the cells in a receptive state while practising *prāṇāyāma*. One should learn that *prāṇāyāma* is not a muscular breathing process, but a cellular breathing. It works on the cells. Without disturbing the cells, without disturbing the fibres, you have to learn the art of inhalation and exhalation. This is *prāṇāyāma*.

However, as far as *Bhastrikā* is concerned, read in *Light on Prāṇāyāma* the notes and cautions given for *Bhastrikā* and *Kapālabhātī*. These two should not be done too long with strain. The sound of exhalation should not vary or diminish. Or, if irritation is felt, one should stop. When there is blockage, in order to remove it you can do alternate nostrils *Bhastrikā* and this only for a few cycles.

Pam: I see then. Thank you very much indeed.

Peter Murray: Thank you very much, Pam.

ઉ૪ ૪૦ ૪ઈ

Peter Murray: Let's go to John, in Soho. Good evening, John.

John: Good evening and thank you very much, gentlemen. I have two questions. One of them has to do with aerobics. I would like to know if you consider aerobics to be a safe and helpful form of exercise or if it is dangerous for people generally.

Mr. Iyengar: See, if you ask me about yoga I will certainly give you my guidance for the simple reason you can do yoga without disturbing any system or function of the body. It does not disturb your harmony, it does not strain the muscles, and it does not strain the nerves.

Peter Murray: I think that more or less answers your question, John, doesn't it?

John: Yes, it does and also in doing *prāṇāyāma* there are times when the breathing ceases for periods of time, after doing a series. Is this beneficial and should that be encouraged?

Mr. Iyengar: If it ceases by itself, take it for granted that it is very good. But if you force it deliberately more and more, then it will have a pressure on the nerves which may affect your nervous system. So I advise you very much to accept as it is coming.

John: Thank you very much.

Peter Murray: Thank you, John.

Peter Murray: We go to Anita, in Clapham. Good evening, Anita.

Anita: Hello, good evening, Peter, good evening, Mr. Iyengar. Well, I have got a question. I have been doing yoga a little bit, for a couple of months, and I have been reading your books as well. I get a lot of pain in my knees. Should I continue or...

Mr. Iyengar: If the pain persists too long, then you should know that you are doing the *āsana* a little bit wrong. You should choose the *āsana* which give a soothing feeling. First of all you should know that when there is knee pain you need to stretch the legs. If you cannot manage to stretch, then use

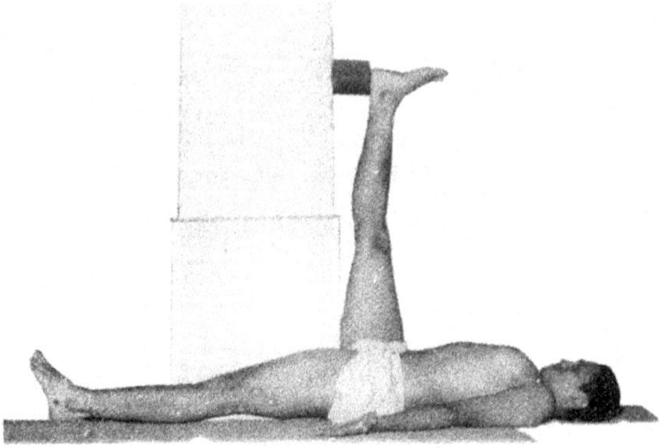

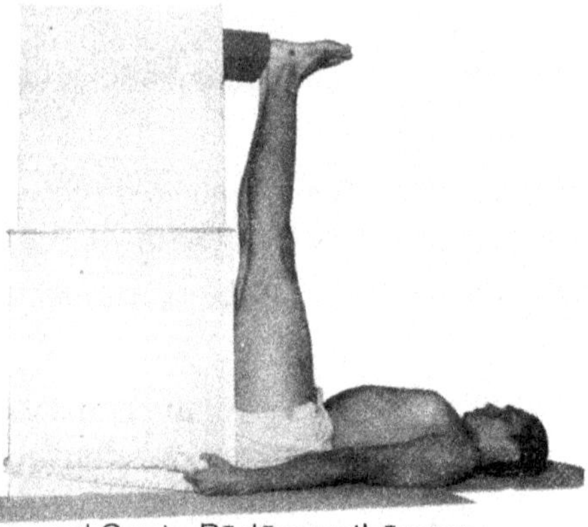

Ūrdhva Prasārita Pādāsana and Supta Pādāṅguṣṭhāsana against a corner wall

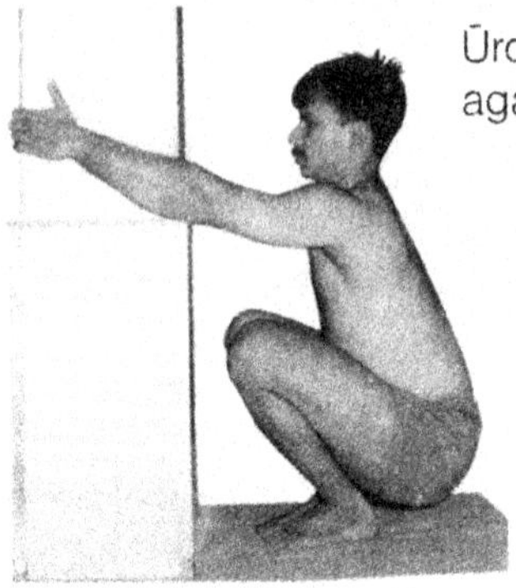

Mālāsana with support with folded napkins behind the knees.

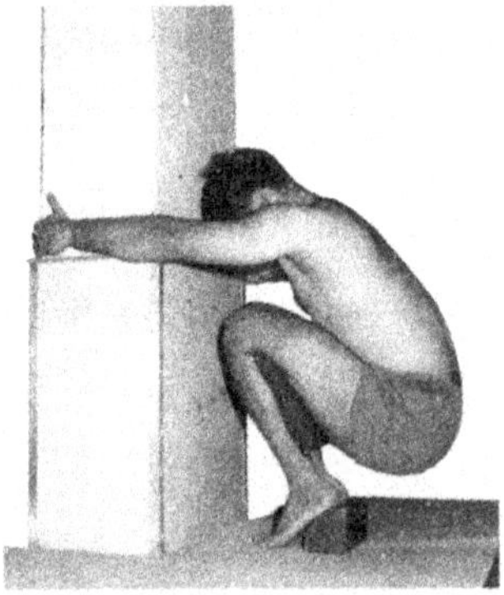

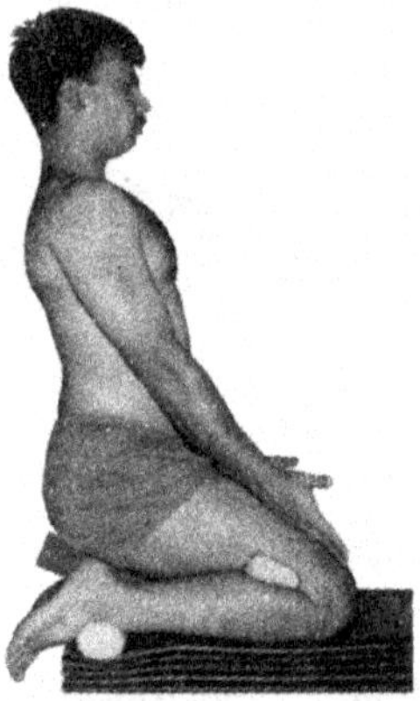

Vīrāsana, sitting on an edge feet hanging over and padding in between the thighs and calves.

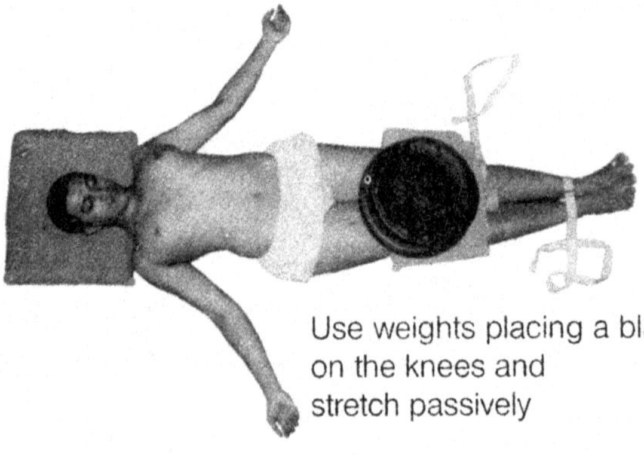

Use weights placing a blanket on the knees and stretch passively

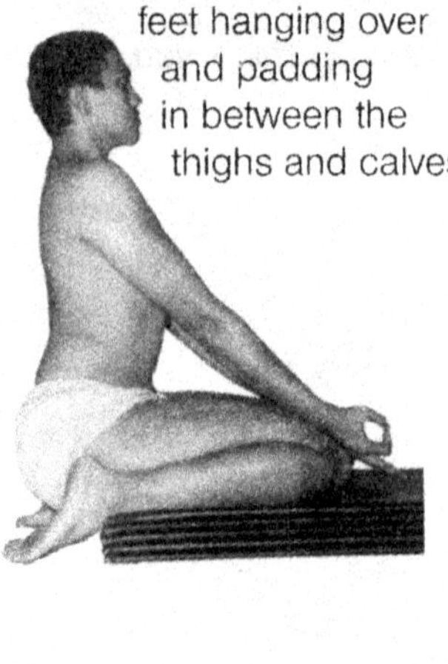

Plate n. 11 – Some *āsanas* for knee pain

weight placing a blanket on the knees and stretch passively, or put your legs up against the wall. This is called *Ūrdhva Prasārita Pādāsana.* Similarly do *Supta Pādānguṣṭhāsana* against a corner wall. When the legs are kept anti-gravitationally like this, the knee pain reduces. Next go for flexion of the knees. Do *Vīrāsana*, sitting at the edge of a table, feet hanging over the edge and pillows or bolsters in between the thighs and calves. This sitting posture gives great relief.

When the above practice is done with comfort, then I advise you to fold two napkins and place them underneath the knees where the two ligaments are resting. If you insert the cloth between the two ligaments at the back of the knee and then flex, you don't get pain. Later do the *āsana* gradually bringing the dangling feet to the surface on the floor. When this is achieved, then you do not get the knee pain at all. Similarly, you can do *Mālāsana* with support, having the folded napkins behind the knees.

Anita: I see, so in between the ligaments.

Mr. Iyengar: Yes, in between the ligaments.

Anita: I see, thank you very much indeed.

Peter Murray: Thank you very much indeed, Anita. It certainly has been a very interesting hour. I hope you have enjoyed being with us.

Mr. Iyengar, I would like to thank you very much indeed for the privilege of us having you here tonight. Thank you.

Mr. Iyengar: Thank you.

THE LATEST NEWS OF THE MOST ANCIENT SCIENCE – YOGA*

Q.- What are the mechanics that working through the *yogāsana* stop the progress of illness and stimulate the beginning of recovery?

It is not easy to answer this question in a few words, especially because the healing mechanisms of yoga vary broadly in each *āsana,* as well as in each illness, from diabetes to asthma and from hypertension to depression. Mind is the root cause of many diseases. The continuous increasing mechanisation of our modern ways of living have an unavoidable undertone of stress. It is impossible to abolish it, but it is possible to learn to use our own instruments, the body, mind and intelligence, in a correct manner and endure it. Today one learns to use machines to increase production, and it seems that man is gradually becoming a part of this machinery, instead of being a rightful beneficiary.

Yet, I would like to inform you that I have helped people suffering from skeleto-muscular disorders, organic defects, and neurological imbalances to psychosis cases. Similarly, I have helped many people through yoga and those who had no children got children, those with disturbed family life got back solace and good relationships, and the growth of hereditary diseases has been checked.

Q.- Coming to the first part of your answer, what is the relation between the external stress-producing mechanisation and the illness producing internal stress of the human body?

I think that the human body is, in a sense, a machine, but the mind enormously brings on the body the sensitivity to the action either in stress or relaxation. Let's take the problems of heart and coronary arteries. Western physiology agrees that the coronary's blockage may be due to a reduction of the space disposable for the continuous pumping action of the heart. This space in the cardiac region

---

* Exclusive interview with Iyengar, living legend of yoga, "Doctor Guru", by Giuliano Ferrieri. Published by the magazine *L'Europeo,* 64th year, no. 8, 19th February 1988.

is sometimes reduced by the incorrect position of the shoulders and the chest or the hardened diaphragm that limits the amplitude of the breath and contracts the arteries.

In today's way of living external mechanisation might have lessened our physical burden, but in that place competition for power and pelf has taken place too. Therefore, as a human being, the stress has become inevitable both ways whether one exerts physically or doesn't. With all the physical and material comforts, the stress gets built up, if there is no mental peace. As the laziness and slowness burden the intellect with stress, mental perverseness like anger and desire build up the emotional stress.

Q.- And what is the yoga action on the therapeutic plane?

Yoga uses specific *āsana* that correct the structural defects and the muscular faults that cause the imbalance of the positions taken by the body. Sometimes I see that in some *āsana*, the patient's left small toe does not touch the ground. This is a signal that his left chest is compressed – this makes him a candidate for future heart attack. Take *Ūrdhva Dhanurāsana*. Here the body is arched like an upward bent bow. It helps the energy to flow inside as well as outside of the banks of the heart. This *āsana* elongates the heart muscles longitudinally and helps the heart to pump blood and clears out that which blocks the free flow. The inner coatings encircling the vessels that make the passage narrow are made to move out and clear the passage. This way yoga helps to fight heart attacks and coronary diseases.

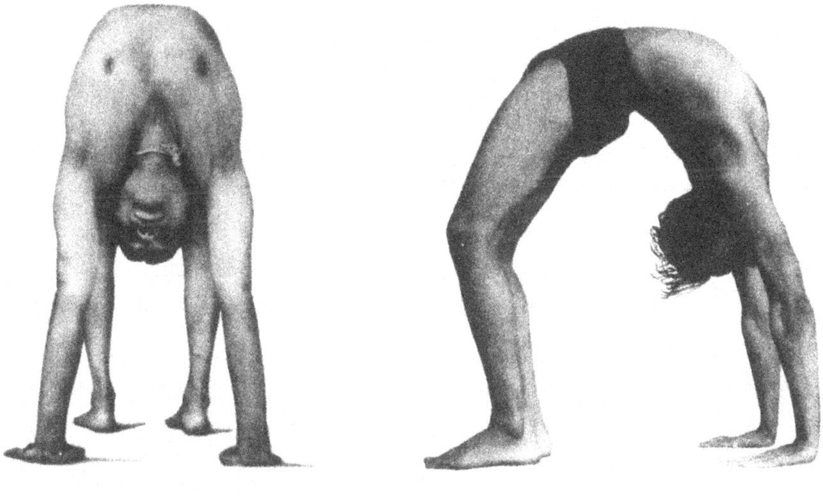

Plate n. 12 – *Ūrdhva Dhanurāsana*

Yoga has a lot to contribute in the field of therapeutic and healing science.[1] It corrects the body as well as the mind. As the body gets caught in the web of diseases, the mind gets caught in the tug of war of dualities such as pleasure and pain, success and failure. The whole yogic treatment is for the body and mind. The *āsana* improve the respiration and circulation of the body. They bring the chemical changes within and charge the body with bio-energy. The *prāṇāyāma* generates vital energy. *Āsana* and *prāṇāyāma,* when accompanied by the *yama* and *niyama,* play wonders on one's body and mind by bringing the required changes.

Please know that yoga being a subjective therapy, one has to do it personally, individually in order to bring the change in oneself or to eradicate the defects, if any, in oneself. It is not something like swallowing tablets. Rather one has to personally practise to experience and derive benefits from it.

Q.- Western gymnastics tend to contract the muscles; is it in this sense opposite to the yoga muscle exercises?

Right, this is one of the differences. We aim to lengthen the fibres of muscles in every *āsana,* instead of putting pressure on the various muscles or organs.

The western callisthenic exercises stimulate the sympathetic nervous system, resulting in the increase of the rate of the metabolism and accelerating the heart's function. This is one of the reasons why after a long gymnastics session one is physically tired. The yogic *āsana,* by lengthening the nerves and the fibres of the muscles, act directly on the parasympathetic nervous system, stimulating one mentally. After a session of *yogāsana* one finds oneself with a lower metabolic rate and in a more relaxed state, a lower heart beat and a positive diffused feeling of relaxation.

Q.- Is the contrast existing between western gymnastics and yoga showing that biological and cultural tradition divides the East from West? Is yoga exportable to us, then?

The question is not about the difference between East and West. The culture and tradition may be different but the gymnastics, callisthenics or any other such type of exercises are adopted by one and all, irrespective of differences in culture. Biologically, all human beings are alike.

Now, as far as the cultural difference is concerned, yogic culture is such that it is applicable to one and all.[2] We, human beings, ultimately want to be free from pains and sorrows. Our problems

[1] Refer to *Aṣṭadaḷa Yogamālā,* vol. 3, section II – "Yoga, Health and Therapeutics", and section III – *Āyurveda.*

[2] See *Aṣṭadaḷa Yogamālā,* vol. I, section II – "Yoga explained".

are basically the same. We all need to improve the human relationship. The principles of yoga, in this sense, are applicable to all problems of the human race. Yoga is universal. It is not a matter to be exported or imported. It has to be adopted.

On the organic plane, I do not see any difference between East and West as both, having increased in the margin of comfort in life style, tend to use their limbs less and less. This lack of movement in joints causes the shortening of muscles and nerves which restricts the arterial passages, leaving the door open to many illnesses. Therefore whether it is East or West, both need yogic culture, yogic therapy and its techniques for sound health and contentment.

Q.- But after all, yoga is India.

Yoga is not India. Yoga is not Indian. It was discovered and built up in India. So its origin may be found in India. Is there an American electricity, a Russian cancer or an Italian tuberculosis? Electricity is for all, it is universal energy. The diseases too are universal ill currents. Hence, yoga might have had its origins in India, but it belongs to everybody. Yet is it not surprising to see that today yoga is practised more in the West than in India? Knowing this, how can you ask whether yoga is exportable to you, when it is already accepted and adopted?

In India, yoga was practised by a few in the thirties and forties. When I was teaching, there were hardly a dozen yoga teachers in those years. Now yoga has not only become popular but a household word, and one can find yoga teachers in every lane.

You say "cultural differences". If so, are the feelings of joys, emotions like lust, anger, greed and physical pains the same or different in humans? To think that a country's borders are barriers to yoga is equivalent to refusing to admit that there is a universal consciousness in every man.

Q.- And in this sense, both India and Iyengar must be proud of the increasing interest in yoga which has attracted even Italy.

This may be right and wrong. But I do not know. Perhaps the West has a more marked attitude expecting miracles from yoga. This mental stance has to be kept aside when better health or complete healing occurs in yoga. The credit for healing must go to the science as well as the person who had to work with determination not only in the technique, but above all, with faith in himself. Very little is gained by a mind that is full of doubts. Conversely, it is the duty of the person who takes care of the patient to create confidence so that the patient heals himself through the method taught. Hence, learning is as much an art as teaching, and every teacher knows that he can learn from his pupils too.

It is true that when yoga was not at all respected at that time, I made up my mind to work on the subject and made presentations to attract people towards it and this is how you see yoga is bracketed with my name.

Yes, like other European countries, Italy too got fascinated in yoga and took it well.

Q.- This in theory. In reality the patient depends upon his doctor, and the student of yoga on his *guru*. Your students depend on you, then.

It is not true. Please read my answer again. Creating confidence builds 'self-help' in one. He who credits me with his newly found well being, is giving a sign of gratitude and not of dependence. I am nothing more than an instrument. I reached a certain standard not because I am a genius, which I am not, but because I struggled and cultivated this art and attained a certain level to help those suffering people to recover faster. From this essence which I got, I went out to give to my students within a limited frame of time. I aim at that while teaching, that everybody reach the standard I reached, using reasonable effort and labour and which is possible for many who work to help the needy.

Q.- But Iyengar's yoga is reputed to be painful, violent, "cruel".

(The yogi shakes his head smiling, and the movement goes to the white hair framing his face).

The father educating his child may make a show of supremacy on many occasions, though he may not like it. Those who come to me as pupils and patients are like a child to me. Sometimes I may behave as if I were their father: using a toughness, showing a father's love, sometimes even compassion. Here, compassion does not mean showing pity. A surgeon does a surgical operation on patients, which is painful for the patient. Only he does not feel it since he is under the influence of anaesthesia. As a yoga teacher I have to do this operation when the patient is conscious. Obviously, it is painful. Only in this way we learn to act, to live, to grow. Do you mean to say that it is not painful to me when I physically help the patients to guide them into the *āsana*, where I need to extend their muscles, lubricate their joints, bend their bodies? So in a way, there is sharing in suffering together.[1]

[1] The author has a special, innovative way of teaching. He does not stand away and aloof from pupils while imparting the knowledge of yoga, but when the pupil or the patient does not get the required position, he runs and skillfully adjusts those parts with his own hands, with the required accurate pressure. While helping, many a time, he invites certain physical pains. With all these inflictions on his students, the results appear to be fantastic.

"Perhaps this question regarding the difficulties with Iyengar's yoga should have been directed to the teachers that grew from the School of Pune," says Grazia Melloni who directs in Rome the B.K.S. Iyengar Association of Yoga.

"This is the most unfounded and dislikeable accusation. Of course Iyengar is a 'tough' teacher, meaning he demands a lot of effort from his pupils. At the same time he too works very hard with more effort than what he asks from his pupils, to keep them getting what they need. This effort is so, because yoga itself makes demands at every step, whether therapeutic or in those higher aspects such as dhyāna *and* samādhi. *Without sacrifices one cannot easily gain the control on the body and the mind.*

"Once I heard Iyengar say to a patient: 'I am sixty-nine and you forty-five, and you say you cannot get into this āsana. *Therefore <u>you</u> are the older man. Now let's start again: when you reach your objective that is to do like me, then you will know that age is more a mental concept than a physical reality.'*

"Iyengar and the yoga he teaches never hurt anyone, and thousands have practised āsana *with him. To fool Iyengar during his classes is impossible but when he is out of the class, he can easily be taken for a ride. The spontaneous laughter he often abandons himself to, is the true reflection of his great heart and his innocence."*

Yoga is in some aspects an 'impossible' science, often much criticised. Today the western scientific culture, using its own technology, is testing this compound of philosophy, religion, art of yoga which is five thousand years old on machines, and it finds itself staring at results confirming this ancient Indian art. Quoting Mr. Romolo Rossini, director of Milan's clinic for mental nervous illness, and his past studies, "The E.C.G. signals the visible macroscopic modifications induced into the brain by yoga practice."

Dr. R. P. Kaushik who works in India says: "Practising yoga results in a volumetric increase of the brain." Yogi Swami Rama who agreed to a series of controlled experiments done by Dr. Elmer Greeb, of the Menninger Foundation, in America, showed he could raise the temperature of one of his hands by 10º C more than the other, could reduce voluntarily his heart beat from 74 to 56 beats per minute and showed to the E.C.G. a number of alpha waves that normally occur only in the phase preceding sleep and represent and confirm a psychophysical state of maximum relaxation.

Q.- What are yoga's limits, as a preventive and curative treatment?

In my personal philosophy I do not see limits to the power of man; the horizon is the limit. After saying that, I cannot honestly consider yoga as the panacea for all the ills. I know that yoga could cause damage if practised the wrong way. I corrected many mistakes done by people who came finally to me. I know that inverted *āsana* are risky for heart sufferers and for hypertension patients.

Certainly I never said that yoga could cure leukaemia and cancer. But even in these cases, why not try? I do not say this because of my pride, because I want to find out how yoga works on such cases, but with humility; we know so little of this scientific field and even less of that regarding human powers; who are we – scientists or yogis – to judge?

The miracle is really in man, in each and every one of his cells, and even if we firmly say that yoga cannot cure cancer, there might be some people who could have a new cellular reaction that might reverse the process of one of those illnesses superficially defined as "incurable" by medicine. I have treated people having cancer, who could arrest the disease, prolong their life and died peacefully when they did yoga until their last breath.

Every illness is in reality a part of ourselves; it is a part of our manifestation. According to yogic philosophy, the diseases are the fruits of our past *karma*, results of our own action done not only in this life but the previous lives too. Though the soul or self does not get affected with disease, we as a compound of body, mind and soul, or the soul, which is called empirical soul, feel the affliction. The practice of yoga brings the new awareness of tolerance and endurance. These qualities indicate the degree of development we have reached.

Why not take pain and disease positively so that we can face life positively through practice of yoga? Is not pain both the alarm signal and the indicator for the remedy? Then why should we be surprised to see that the maturing of the mind, a healthier attitude towards life, a more serene frame of mind can bring an ill body back to health?

Q.- Following yoga therapy, a better oxygenation caused by better breathing could re-activate a malfunctioning cell. Is this the way?

This is one of the ways: Here, *prāṇāyāma* helps to a great extent: *Prāṇa*, meaning the breath, energy, life, or even soul, and *āyāma*, meaning disciplining of the breath voluntarily.

Yes, the breathing techniques specified by yogic science rejuvenate, energise and cure many diseases. When we want to make some coffee, we normally use a filter to obtain an optimal brew. Let's say that we must filter our breath to extract the essence from each particle. The air is the content, *prāṇa* is the final filtered product of that content. And this filtered essence is circulated everywhere. As the lymphatic system goes parallel with the circulatory system, I can say that with *prāṇāyāma* the *prāṇic* energy is circulated along with these two systems, though anatomically you don't find a special tubular body to circulate the energy. According to yogic science these are called *nāḍī* through which the vital energy is circulated.

Q.- In Christian culture, man is dust, and to dust shall go. Is it right to say that in your culture man is air?

No, we too say that the body is dust which merges into dust after death.

We are made up of five elements of nature, namely: earth, water, fire, air and ether. After death, these five principles of nature go and reunite with those respective elements. The *Haṭhayoga Pradīpikā* says, regarding the effect of *prāṇāyāma*, that as long as there is breath in the body, there is life. When breath departs, the life goes (*H.Y.P.*, II.3). This is the end of the mortal body. When breath leaves this body, we call it *pārthiva śarīra*, or the body belonging to the element of earth. You call the body dust, we call it the earth matter. Both are the same.

But let me explain to you that before life, *prāṇa* is with cosmic air and after death it mingles with the cosmic air, so to some extent man is air. You see we have five *prāṇa* or energies[1] in us namely: *prāṇa*, *apāna*, *vyāna*, *udāna* and *samāna*, each contributing itself to the whole functional mechanism of the body. These are accompanied by other five *upavāyu* – supporting *vāyu*, namely *nāga*, *kūrma*, *kṛkāra*, *devdatta* and *dhanamjaya*. The last, *dhanamj-aya*, is the one which helps the body to degenerate to the dust. So the *vāyu* helps there too.[2]

I further say that by practising *prāṇāyāma*, if a *yogi* conquers *prāṇa*, he is a *prāṇajayin*. After death, such a *yogī*, though he leaves his elemental body to the dust, his subtle body or *sūkṣma śarīra* accompanies him to proceed towards further evolution. Death makes him either to be in an incorporeal state called *videhin* or makes him to merge in nature, which is known as *prakṛtilaya*. However, life after death for him is upgraded since he will be merging his individual energy into the cosmic energy.

---

1 For further details please see the author's *Light on Prāṇāyāma* and *Light on the Yoga Sūtras of Patañjali*, published by Harper Collins, London, and *Aṣṭadaḷa Yogamālā*, vol. 2, pp. 99-100.

2 For further details, see the author's *Light on Prāṇāyāma*, chapter 3, sections 1-7, and *Aṣṭadaḷa Yogamālā*, vol. 2, pp. 99-100. See also *Light on the Yoga Sūtras of Patañjali*, under I.19.

GLIMPSES OF YOUNG *GURUJĪ**

PROLOGUE

The morning of Sunday, August 14th dawned with a bright sunny sky, probably reflecting the chirpy moods and anticipation of a group of youngsters who had a big day ahead. We had planned to have an informal chat with our Gurujī, *B.K.S. Iyengar, the focus being his youth.*

We all assembled at the Ramāmaṇi Iyengar Memorial Yoga Institute wearing our best clothes, trying to wear expressions appropriate to the occasion though our hearts fluttered at the very thought of being with Gurujī *in this setting. The youngsters present for the event were Sharmila, Priti, Namrata, Varsha, Sandhya, Ashok, Parth, Aboli, Bhavnesh, Devki, Arti, Kirti, Roshan, Jasmina and Urmila. To make sure that the program would go on without a hitch we prepared ourselves thoroughly, even going to the length of having a practice session with Shri Prashant Iyengar. This not only released our nervousness but also gave us a very good insight into what we consider a mysterious personality.*

A few mats were arranged near the marble platform with a mike and tape-recorder making the hall look totally different from usual. The atmosphere was charged with mixed emotions, a palpable excitement, a bit of apprehension and a great sense of awe.

Gurujī *arrived, sporting a white yoga T-shirt and* dhoti *much to our delight; the long red vermilion mark on the forehead, and a beaming, benign smile that lit up the place. He was in a pleasant, carefree mood that did wonders for our increasing heartbeats.*

After paying our respects we requested him to sit on a seat that had bolsters on each side, a royal arrangement for the Royal King of Yoga. *We sat around him and crossed our fingers before we could launch our barrage. Our energies geared up, we inhaled deeply and started off.*

What happened afterwards is history. There was a marathon session of almost three hours where we sat with bated breaths; hunger and thirst all forgotten. One could say we were

---

* This interview was conducted in August 1988, by students of the Ramāmaṇi Iyengar Memorial Yoga Institute. First published in *70 Glorious Years of Yogacharya B.K.S. Iyengar – Commemoration Volume*, by the *Light on Yoga Research Trust*, Mumbai, 1990. Reprinted in *Newsletter*, the BKS Iyengar Yoga Association of Australasia, January-February 1994.

floored by Gurujī's *replies, wit and repartee, and of course his utter frankness. We are sure that the length of the interview is warranted in the situation and hope that our readers derive from it the same pleasure that we did.*

Bhavnesh: *Gurujī*, we have been wanting to talk to you for quite some time now.

You are examining or frightening me?

Bhavnesh: Not really; it is more like an informal chat. Your autobiography *Body thy Shrine – Yoga the Light*[1] and film *Gurujī* have given us glimpses of your youth, your hardships and trials. We are eager to know what you were like in your younger days. Would you define youth as being a period of exuberance and ambition, strength and vitality?

Youngsters should have tremendous ambitions to make life worth living. I was merely fifteen years old when I took to yoga. I had no other education or training, hence I decided to master what I already knew rather than work under others. I faced challenges from all directions – no funds, no friends or relatives, rejected by society – I decided to fight and succeed. Utopian ideals are hard to achieve when faced with practical difficulties. I made up my mind to fight the situation and came to a drastic decision that I would either mar my life or make my life worthful on this earth.

Sharmila: Were the youngsters at that time like you?

Absolutely not. The affluent are able to acquire knowledge easily – they lose fervour or zeal. I have realised that poverty is a garland for knowledge. My appearance in those days, coupled with my illness – tuberculosis and malaria – strengthened my determination to fight destiny; either to sink with this art or convince people that I had something they needed. I possessed the guts to do or die.

Arti: How do you view today's youth?

---

[1] Published by B. K. S. Iyengar 60th Birthday Celebration Committee, Mumbai, in 1978.

With your enthusiasm and having a will power like me, you could become the gems of the coming century.

– Thank you Gurujī. –

(Gurujī is always optimistic. He does not blame the youth of today like many do. Often, he opines that it is the fault of the parents more than of the children. Similarly he finds today's children's lack of contact and selfish approach drifts them away from their parents. Also today's social problems, poverty, joblessness, bad habits like smoking, drinking, addiction to drugs, depression, add to further complexes.

For him, the youth have a great physical and intellectual potency. It needs to be channelled with right guidance and thinks yoga would certainly play a major role in building them up as worthy children through good health and a balanced state of mind.)

Namrata: Which was the greatest blessing of your youth?

My friend, it is obvious, eh! A person who was unsteady at the age of fifteen, considered a good for nothing, ignored and ostracised, is now being dubbed a very proud man. The greatest blessing was the determination to prove the worthiness of my life.

Perhaps, my ill health, poverty, lack of education, strictness and discipline of my *guru* acted as blessings at a later stage to make me continue with yoga *sādhanā*. Also, now I consider the deprivation and underprivileged state were the great blessings to reach the state of what I am today. Do not think that youth and yoga go together. But it did on me and my early self-training helped me to attract the youth of today towards this ancient but dry art.

Priti: Tell us something about your impulsiveness.

Impulsiveness in youth is universal. It can be positive or negative. I carefully watched this element of impulsiveness in me and nurtured it for good use in developing my practice in the art of yoga, no matter how long it took, and I eventually succeeded in making people respect the art that I was practising.

I was timid in my early days. Being such, I had no guts to lose my temper on others, but I used to lose it on myself whenever I failed to make progress in yoga. Perhaps my will power turned itself into anger. Even now, it is for the sake of students that I become imaginatively impulsive so that they learn to pick up soon. I do not like the art of yoga being taken casually.

(Gurujī seems to be impulsive from his student days in the Yogaśālā *of Mysore. Whenever he failed, he says he used to lose his temper on himself. His strong will power and commitment to his* sādhanā *was making him restless whenever he failed to reach what he wanted.*

Being sincere and devoted to his art, even today he cannot tolerate if his students take to the practice lightly. His insistence to respect the art that one practises is to be valued.)

Sandhya: We would like to hear about an unforgettable adventure/experience in your younger days.

(Gurujī was always a courageous person. In fact he stayed in a so-called haunted house, since the rent was low and nobody dared to enter that house. In his youth he had the courage to run after those who came to rob the dynamo of his cycle, or his clothes, and used to catch them.)

In my younger days, I was humiliated and insulted by friends in general and close relatives in particular. I think no youth can bear it. My wife was the only person who knew my life inside out. When I first came to Pune in 1937 I was eighteen years old; nature threw responsibilities upon me and taught me the art of teaching. I was teaching college students who were not only elders in age but intelligent with better-built bodies than me.

I had a *śendi* (*śikhā* in Sanskrit) – tuft of hair – in those days. I was the only person having the tuft of hair, while the rest of the college students were polished and westernised. My family members were tradition bound and very orthodox too. Hence, it was difficult for me to enter the homes of my relatives without a *śendi*. However, this tuft of hair became a laughing and teasing factor for the college students. They used to make fun of me. The humiliation at the hands of those students made me realise that I had to prove to them that I was at least superior in the presentation of *yogāsana*. I put them to shame by performing *āsana* with them and made them pant, in spite of my seemingly weak physique, *śendi*, and the fact that I could not speak even one correct sentence in English when I first came to Pune.

(He says that the members of his family were very orthodox. All his elders had a tuft. In those days, if a family member had a haircut, he was not allowed to dine with others, neither was he allowed to go into the kitchen. So the fear of family members, who may debar him by seeing his hair cut, made him keep it. Slowly he began lessening his tuft and one day made up his mind to remove the tuft as people of Pune were highly westernised then. So he thought he should live according to the change of time and changed his hairstyle.

He gives also an example of what orthodoxy prevailed in his home. When in 1954, he went to Europe and returned, he went to Bangalore to pay his respects to the eldest of his family – his maternal uncle. The uncle was so wild on him that he never allowed Gurujī to enter his house or prostrate to him as Gurujī had crossed the ocean. Crossing the ocean was forbidden even to Lord Rama who had to build a bridge to cross over the ocean to rescue his consort Sita.

This continued even in his time that he could not go inside the house of his relations for having crossed the ocean.

Gurujī continued to have the tuft of hair (śikhā) *until 1951. He had very long, thick and black hair.)*

Varsha: How did you learn English?

I could not use effective words like *Swāmi* Vivekānanda or Shri Radhakrishnan did. In spite of the fear complex I managed to master enough courage to stand on the platform when people asked me to give lecture demonstrations. I used to write and prepare the lectures by heart, learn those sentences that are needed to start the demonstrations, and end up with thanks. I was addressing the same to my wife as an audience, much to her amusement. I used to say that I am not a man of expression and people could judge for themselves what I present.

We were taught English in schools but that was not enough. I picked it up gradually, while talking to people. I could never imagine that one day I would become an author to write books on the subject of yoga in English.

Kirti: You started teaching ladies in the beginning, were you not self-conscious?

I was the youngest man among my colleagues. Being young the ladies agreed with my *Gurujī* that they would learn yoga only from me.

In those days, in the thirties and forties, women were shy to come in front of men. However, looking at me, who was like a village boy with a tuft of hair, they were happy to learn from me. I did not feel self-conscious at that time as I had no feelings at all. My mind was tuned to stand on my own legs when I accepted to teach. My main worry was that I should not injure anyone. Therefore, my mind would not go on any other thoughts. I was very cautious about pains experienced by them, which helped me teach some *āsana* without causing pain. This attitude of mine helped me to concentrate on my work rather than on what the youths have in their minds today. Therefore, I was not self-conscious. When the college students teased me for my tuft, perhaps I became a little self-conscious which helped me to improve my performance of *āsana*, whereas, while teaching ladies, I did not become self-conscious, I could become a good teacher. With perseverance I succeeded and won them over.

However, a serious repercussion of my teaching women in Pune, spread by my relatives in my hometown, was that it began to earn me a bad name. Especially since I was unwilling to get married, all kinds of aspersions were cast on my character. Teaching in a girls' school also posed difficulties from parents and society in general. But the principals of schools, teachers or girl students as well as the people who were in direct contact with me could not point a finger at my character. My nature was totally different. I was neither allured by girls or women, nor did they allure me. Hence, my mind only gravitated towards yoga.

Another problem I faced at that time was the jealousy of my competitors. I used to be the youngest teacher then, just eighteen years old and these people created a lot of furore over my being given a chance to teach in Pune.

(Dr. V.B. Gokhale had invited Gurujī to Pune being impressed with the extent to which he could move and bend his body, which seemed to be impossible anatomically.)

Roshan: Do you remember your first student?

Oh, yes! One Prof. Deolalkar of Dharwar Karnataka College, Mr. Mudaliar and Sakhalkar of Pune, both dead now. Almost all my students then were elderly, in their forties to seventies. Mr. Bal Gadgil, Principal of Fergusson College, did not believe it when I told him that I had taught the Principal of the same college, the Late Sri Rajwade, who was 87 years in 1937, who was unable to stand, and performed *Supta Trikoṇāsana, Supta Vīrabhadrāsana*,[1] under my guidance.

Roshan: Who was your first lady pupil? How old was she then? How old were you?

My first lady pupil was one Mrs. Gulati – wife of Dr. Gulati – who must have been twenty or twenty-one then, while I was teaching in Dharwar in 1936.

Urmila: What were your views about the general public then?

In those days, one who practised yoga was a laughing stock and ridiculed as if no constructive work was possible from such people, but today I see that yoga has gained a tremendous respect in society. Yoga practitioners were considered as subhuman, even less than animals. I was called a madcap whenever I passed by.

[1] See *Aṣṭadaḷa Yogamālā*, vol. 1, plates n. 7 to 10.

Certainly I say that this subject then was really not known to the public in general. A very few who were aware of the subject thought that it was meant for those who renounce the world like *swamis* and *sannyāsīs*.

Urmila: How has the transition come about?

People felt that yoga could only be taught individually or practised by a person who had been thrown out by the family or was half mad or had lost interest in life or had nothing else to do in life. People ridiculed me, they used to laugh at me. This negative attitude of people made me arrogant and rough. I had the will to show what self-respect is. I knew what I was doing. I had faith in what I was practising. If you were in my place you would have left off the practice or developed this arrogance. Thank God, I brought respect to the subject. Now people appreciate you when you say that you are doing yoga.

My hard work of introducing the subject of yoga to a mass in schools and colleges in 1937 for three years changed the mentality of the people. Then I passed on the subject to the army. All these were the period of transition. Of course, in order to bring the transition I had to introduce the subject to the masses in such a way that they could appreciate and develop interest. They never wanted to know the philosophy. They wanted the direct, visible, cognisable results. So I had to introduce it in the beginning as a physical exercise. When they started finding better results than physical exercises, I started introducing *āsana* as organic exercises on the organs and spine, then on stabilisation of mind to reach one day the ultimate aim, *mokṣa* or emancipation and freedom.

Devki: What was your guiding force during your severe financial and other hardships?

Determination and courage were the keys for me to face the problems. Also as we all know that every cloud has a silver lining, I was sure that one day I would see the silver lining of my life.

Secondly, my family members had branded me as a perverse but intelligent boy. No doubt I was haughty in my younger days, which kept me away from any favours from family members or relations. I had no encouragement from anyone. As I had said many times that if I get ill or die no one is there to cry for me and no one to praise my life, that gave me the spirit of "do or die" in yoga. Perhaps their hatred for me was the driving force for me to prove that I am something in the world.

Fortunately, after years of trial, God blessed me and today not only my family members but also all relatives are proud to use my name in arranging marriages or for seeking a job.

Jasmina: We youngsters are usually very obstinate about what we do. Were you also like us during your youth?

I was very obstinate. It was very positive. I had no selfish motives. With only one determination and that is to master the *āsana.* I was not worried about negative remarks on my practices.

You, youngsters of today, no doubt are obstinate but this quality, if focussed in the right direction, may make you all become the gems of my country.

Jasmina: Did you make any changes or compromises?

As far as my practice was concerned there was no question of compromise. As I had nobody to guide me, I had to work with the pros and the cons if I found I went wrong, as I had nobody to guide me.

As far as teachings are concerned, I had to find alternative ways. So a certain kind of compromise in the art of teaching was needed for my survival. I had to guide the students for them to benefit as well as create interest to pursue the subject. Hence, I changed my techniques, with subtle and finer points so that they continued without fear. Yet, I did not enforce my discipline, determination or obstinacy on them as these were for me to improve myself.

When I look back now, I don't think that it was any kind of compromise. On the contrary, it shows how clear I was in my approach. Undoubtedly I forced the discipline on my body and mind but while teaching I learnt where I have to give leniency, where I have to be mild, where I have to divide the techniques into smaller units so that they learn with ease what I learnt quickly.

Namrata: So, in order to give it to others you made it a sugarcoated pill?

Yes, you can say a sugarcoated pill, as I wanted them to continue the practice of yoga. Now I give non-sugarcoated pills, because it is popular. Sugarcoated ones are useless, as the essence of reality disappears. Now I have to fight to make people do yoga with integrity and honesty. Earlier, I had to create integrity in them, build honesty in them, because it was an unknown subject. I took each disease or disability in a patient as a challenge and worked on the ways to give relief.

Sharmilla: Can you tell us about your youthful dreams?

What kind of dreams could I have when I had to struggle to earn my bread? Often hunger at nights put me into a sleepless state. For me, day-to-day a square meal was important. Now, when I look back, I myself remain surprised about my success and achievements.

Let me put it this way. I did not cherish youthful dreams as such. Even when I was forced to marry, I did not dream of getting a wonderful wife. But fortunately, I got a wonderful partner in my life. However, when I was in Mysore, *Swāmi* Yogananda, the author of the famous book *The Autobiography of a Yogi*, had come to Mysore. I had to give a yoga performance. When he saw my demonstration, he tried to tempt me to accompany him to America, which I refused. But this episode left its imprint on me that one day there could be a possibility to go to the West. And when Sir Yehudi Menuhin approached me, I did not take it as a surprise.

But let me tell you about dreams. Rarely I get dreams. But some dreams were very significant. I had dreamt I was in Anantapadmanabhapuram – now Tiruvanantrapuram. I was looking at Lord Padmanabha in his sanctum sanctorum. As my gaze moved from the face to the foot it seemed that a great fire arose from the foot and was approaching me as if to burn me. I thought I should prostrate before my *guru* before it consumes me; as I did so, the entire scene vanished.

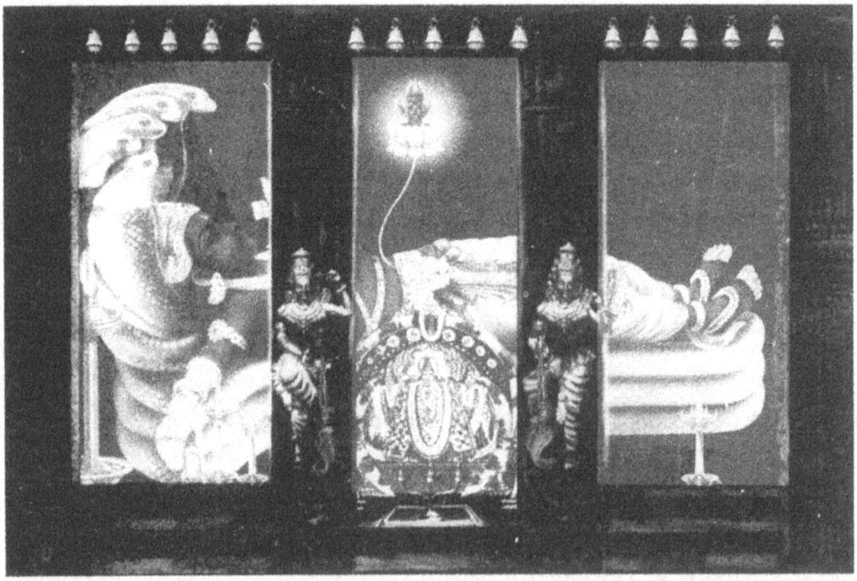

Plate n 13 – Lord Padmanabha in His sanctum sanctorum

The second one was near Mandya (Karnataka) – a temple in Tirunarayanapuram. I entered the innermost quarter where no one is allowed. The priest was annoyed and asked me to go back. I was also firm – the Lord had called me and I would remain rooted on that very spot. The Lord, then pacified me by stating that He was always with me, so I should not mind the angry priest and leave the place in peace.

Aboli: *Gurujī*, if you had the opportunity to be young again, what would you add or subtract from your personality?

If I were blessed with this maturity and freshness, I think I would be a revolutionary in this world, I would change the mental calibre of the entire generation.

I don't think that I have to subtract anything from my personality. My firmness, anger against ridicule and insults, intolerance towards injustice, all such things may remain the same. Good education devoid of undue responsibility at a young age may add to my responsibility.

Basically, I am bold, courageous, a hard worker so it won't make much difference. Who knows, if my family was well to do I would not have gone to my brother-in-law, T. Krishnamacharya, and yoga would have remained far from me. The adverse circumstances sometimes too, help for further achievements. For me it proved a blessing.

Parth: Youth is generally faced with all kinds of temptations. How did you keep them at bay?

Temptations were there, but it was up to me to make or mar my life. I think my firm determination helped me throughout. When I taught at Bhave Girls' School in Pune, I was faced with embarrassing situations. I would keep aloof from them mentally and tide over such situations.

Priti: Do you feel the Lord was protecting you then?

It may be the fear that saved my life or it may be the destiny in the form of God that protected me – I don't deny it. So I withstood the temptations for the simple reason that if I became a victim of temptations, my ability to teach yoga would disappear. So yoga has protected me from being a victim of external appearances. I decided to marry when my *guru* told my mother, brothers and sisters that I had gone astray with my female students. I lost my temper at my *guru* and said that if I went to a prostitute, I would make her my wife.

Devki: You had a strong character.

You may say now seeing me that I had a strong character. It is more of ambition than of character to survive in life and make yoga popular. This attachment to life with respect and to make yoga popular overruled all other temptations. Because I did not fall into the trap, you may now attribute this to my strong character. I decided to marry in order to put an end to the stories and rumours.

Varsha: About your married life.

Initially, I was against marriage because of my economic situation. I was prepared to bear God's punishment, but did not want another person to suffer on my account. I made the decision after carefully considering my situation, especially vis-à-vis my lady pupils who left no stone unturned in luring me. Often I used to drive away the prospective brides by not shaving for 10-12 days at a stretch, or apply oil on my head, which was considered a bad omen in those days. Once I went to Malur for a demonstration. My *Guru* had surreptitiously arranged for a party to be at my home. We reached about 9.00 p.m., and found that the girl had been there since 9.00 a.m. The fact that she waited so patiently made me think that God had kept this girl there, so I said that I would marry without a word.

Varsha: Had you seen her before?

Never, I just saw her on that day. She was tall, of medium build and I just agreed to marry. By chance the next day, as I was going to see my maternal uncle, I saw her in a shop bargaining; there and then alone, I thought she is the right person for me.

Sandhya: You mentioned that you did not have friends to confide in during your difficult time. Was there anybody besides your wife?

No, nobody. I had only my wife to talk to; she was my wife, my friend, my guidance, my solace.

Namrata: After marriage, when you practised yoga, did your wife know anything about it?

No. Only it seems, her brother explained to her *Paśchimottānāsana* and said that that was yoga.

Namrata: Did she find it funny when you did yoga?

Well, that did happen. But I had already told her that my profession was yoga and it was the only way to earn a living and she accepted it. When I left my *guru* in 1937, I was a raw student and my body was stiff – I could not do *āsana*. When I got married, I would ask my wife to help me in order to get a better *āsana*. So I trained her to help me master the *āsana*. So in one aspect she acted as my *guru* also, though I had to guide her how to assist me.

Sharmila: She must have been a great inspiration.

She was, no doubt, a great inspiration. Did I not tell you that yoga was a ridiculed subject in those days? A wife who never said a word or interfered in my daily practices, was that not a gift of God for me? She never asked me to stop my practice in order to go for a walk. She would tell me to practise first and then take her out. I used to be out most of the time to take private classes by cycle covering twenty to thirty miles a day. What little time remained at my disposal was consumed by my own practices. So my wife bore the major burden of looking after the family.

Jasmina: When and how did philosophy enter your life and influence you?

Gradually and chiefly with the suffering I underwent. As I taught yoga to scores of invalids, I realised that yoga could be a boon to suffering humanity. I was at the same time compassionate and merciless to all who came to me. I did feel for the sufferer and so in order to relieve him quickly from his pains, I had to be merciless when dealing with him. If a person can improve in two or three days, why should it take him two-three months to come back to normal? That was my line of thinking. I used to be attached and detached at the same time. Compassion led me to be attached to a person for his improvement, and detachment led to mercilessness so as not to spare any effort in the healing process.

As days and years rolled on, I got interested in philosophy and the simplest philosophy I could learn was the *Mahābhārata*, *Rāmāyaṇa* and the *Bhagavad Gītā*.

Bhavnesh: Can you share your spiritual experience with us?

Can spiritual experience be explained? How can you precisely demarcate a human being on a physical, intellectual or spiritual level? Can we express compassion or friendliness though we experience it?

– *Well, not really.* –

Similarly, spiritual life has to be experienced though explanations may guide you to get a dip in the ocean of knowledge. Reading gives a view on spiritual life but when you put what you have read into practice then the glimpses of experiences set in.

Spiritual life exists when there is no difference between the thoughts and the path one follows. If there exists a difference between the two, I am playing with the intelligence or exhibiting an image that is not actually what I am. It is far more important to live in it rather than express it.

The present generation is perhaps exposed to exhibitionism. If one wears a saffron cloth, *mālā* around his neck, you take it for granted that such a man is leading a spiritual life. It is a subjective experience to be experienced and not through expressions. It is an intrinsic matter and it has nothing to do with public appearances.

Kirti: Have you experienced what we have read about?

By the grace of God, yes, I can see that your inner being is not different from mine. It is the age and intelligence which makes the difference and forms your attitudes and way of thinking. But I have to show the difference outwardly to enable me to impart the knowledge I have.

If asked to give a demonstration in front of thousands of people, the element of egotism is bound to be present. I can practise with humility because no one is watching. If one can prevent the inevitable egotism from becoming a part and parcel of one's life, it means one is a spiritual man.

Ashok: What are your records of *Sālamba Śīrṣāsana* and *Viparīta Chakrāsana*?

My friend, I have done *Sālamba Śīrṣāsana*[1] for one hour to observe its ill effects. I did it one day twice with an interval of ten minutes. The brain became a log of wood and I felt as if I haven't slept for months, and dehydration continued for days and days. Skin was dry and it had lost the sense of touch. I have to practise this way to experience the good and bad effects of *āsana*. Over the years, God used to punish and injure me first in order to learn on myself before I could teach people with such problems. All pains and injuries have come to me before a patient approaches me with problems akin to my sufferings. *Viparīta Chakrāsana*[2] record is 218 times non-stop, in 1976.

---

[1] See *Aṣṭadaḷa Yogamālā*, vol. 3, plate n. 28.
[2] See *Aṣṭadaḷa Yogamālā*, vol. 4, plate n. 29.

Ashok: At what age?

It was in 1977 to be precise. I used to finish *Ūrdhva Dhanurāsana* (up and down) 200/250 times in five minutes. I used to do *Viparīta Chakrāsana* 108 times in four minutes. Today I do the same in twenty minutes (at the age of seventy).

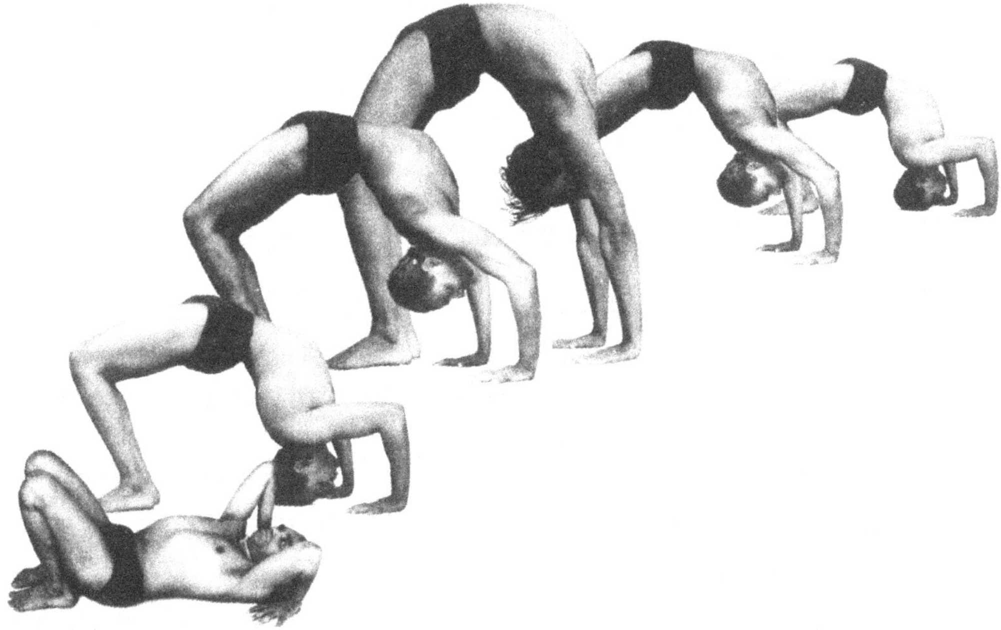

Plate n. 14 – *Ūrdhva Dhanurāsana* (up and down)

Sandhya: Can you narrate your experiences related to *prāṇāyāma*?

I was not taught *prāṇāyāma*. I would do it for two-three minutes and start gasping. I also realised the utility of back bends and forward bends in *prāṇāyāma*. Being a patient from infant stage, I had a difficult time with my weak lungs. I used to feel that I was too young to do *prāṇāyāma*. I began to do it as late as 1944-45.[1] I would wake up around four o'clock in the morning, when my wife would prepare coffee for us. Often I would go right back to sleep, but I somehow persevered with whatever will power I had. And I kept building up fro m there.

[1] See *Aṣṭadala Yogamālā*, vol. 1, section I, pp. 62-65, "How I learnt *prāṇāyāma*".

Urmila: Was it your weak body that could not respond to *prāṇāyāma* or your stubborn. demanding nature and high expectation that did not make *prāṇāyāma* possible? When you explain in *Light on Prāṇāyāma, Ujjāyī* in *Śavāsana*, how did this idea occur to you when *prāṇāyāma* was impossible? Can you tell us?

Due to the overdoing of backbends, as they are very attractive for demonstrations, my back used to become sore in five minutes of sitting. Due to this over-mobility of the spine I could not take deep inhalations or exhalations. When I thought of doing *Śavāsana*, in a few minutes time I used to go to sleep. So I could do *prāṇāyāma* neither in *Śavāsana* nor in *Padmāsana*. This gave me the will to strengthen my spine by practising forward extensions and lateral twists.[1] When the spine became strong and stable I began practising *prāṇāyāma* for a few minutes. The moment the spine started to become sore I used to stop it.

Urmila: Did you not ask your *guru* for guidance?

I did ask, but he told me categorically that I was unfit to do *prāṇāyāma*. In the olden days and even today, scholarly people have generally been reluctant to impart the knowledge they have. They are quite abrupt in their manner, and do not consider pupils deserving enough. It would be difficult indeed to have a free, frank discussion as we are just having. For, example even Ramana Maharshi's philosophical approach was for the wise pupils who helped him to understand his philosophy, as many were highly qualified scholars. This was the way of life in the early days.

Roshan: Can you tell us something about your first trip abroad?

I went abroad for the first time in 1954. I underwent mixed reactions. The culture was totally different. Being invited by a celebrity also made me learn how to deal with famous people. I have found that they have their own prestigious interests and can exploit you to their own ends. I was a total stranger without friends but with a determination to succeed. My aim was to establish yoga throughout the world. Being a member of an orthodox family did make me uneasy at late-night parties thrown by celebrities, which included drinks. Being a pure vegetarian, I used to live on boiled potatoes, fried peas and carrots. I did lose weight but I had to control the fried food to protect my liver. I would take a few fruits, though they did not taste better than Indian fruits. Eating at the same table where fish

---

[1] *Āsana* from *Paśchima pratana* and *Parivṛtta sthiti*. See *Aṣṭadaḷa Yogamālā*, vol. 4, "Yoga in Educational Institutions".

and meat were served was unbearable. I would concentrate only on my plate, not daring to look beyond it. There is a dramatic transformation when I go there today. No one smokes or drinks in my presence. They serve vegetarian food at parties when I am invited. This about-turn is without uttering a single word of criticism.

Priti: Who was the first celebrity you met?

In India or abroad?

- Of course abroad. -

Yehudi Menuhin, the famous classical violinist. He came to India in 1952. At that time he was suffering from a nervous breakdown and couldn't even hold a violin. Many concert artistes need to take tranquillisers. It takes them days to relax and return to normalcy. When he came to India he wanted to meet yoga teachers as he had heard of the efficacy of yoga. At the recommendations of the then President of India, Dr. Rajendra Prasad, and Prime Minister, Jawaharlal Nehru, he met several *gurus* of Delhi, Calcutta, Mumbai and Madras.

In Mumbai, a prominent cardiologist, Dr. Vakil and his wife, who were my students, recommended me to him. I got a telephone message saying that Menuhin would see me for five minutes of a certain day. I refused as the distance and expense of the journey were too much for a five minute's meeting. Eventually they agreed to pay for the expenses and I took my wife and children to Mumbai for the first time to show them Mumbai.

I arrived on time at Raj Bhavan where Menuhin was an honoured guest of the government. He got up late from bed saying that he got exhausted each morning due to pressures of work and social occasions every night. I said that I would make him relax him before we spoke. I made him to lie down in *Śavāsana*, asked him to close his eyes to relax him. Then I placed my index and middle fingers on the eyes to relax and quieten the eyeballs, ring fingers on the nostrils for slow rhythmic breathing, little fingers on the upper lip and thumbs to arrest sounds entering his ears. (This is *Ṣaṇmukhī Mudrā* in yogic terminology.) Within a few minutes, he began snoring. I realised that he has gone to deep sleep. I maintained this *mudrā* for 45 minutes. When my fingers felt the movement of his eyeballs , I took off my fingers. He woke up and said that he never experienced in his life this type of rest. When refreshed, He told his hosts to cancel all appointments for the day, as he wished to spend his time with me. He then asked me to show him what I could do. I demonstrated from the start to finish in one hour. He was awe-struck and wished that his wife, a ballet dancer, had seen the demonstration. He felt that I was like a ballet dancer presenting the *āsana*.

He wanted me to come again. So we met again the next day and that was the beginning of a long-standing relationship. Whenever I used to touch him while he performed *āsana,* he felt exhilaration in his system.

In India, I taught Shri J. Krishnamurti, Achyut Patwardhan, Jayaprakash Narayan, Virendra Patil (Chief Minister Karnataka), G.S. Pathak (Vice President of India), Major Gen. Habibulah, Gen. Sri Nagesh and many more.

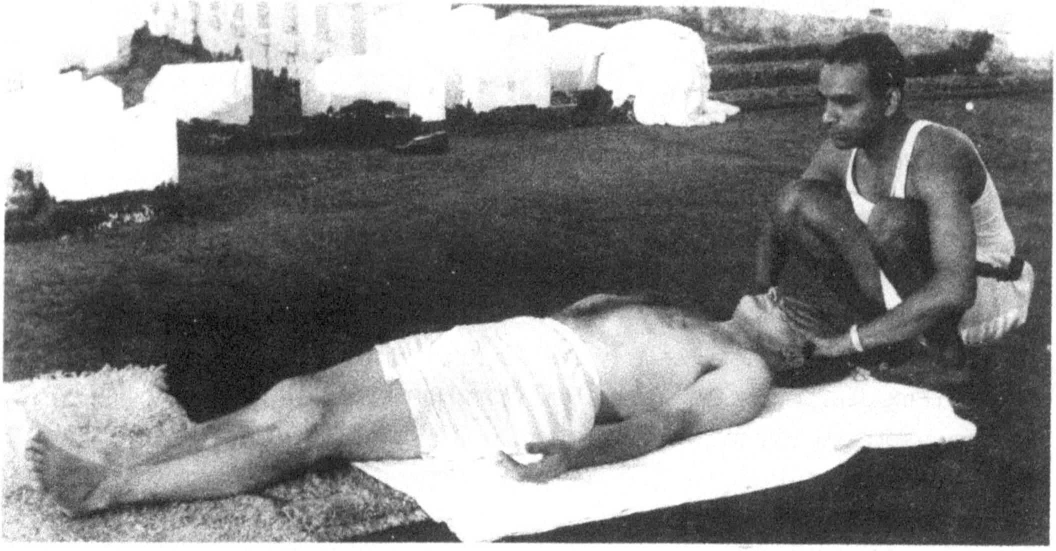

Plate n. 15 – *Ṣaṇmukhī Mudrā* for Yehudi Menuhin

Kirti: How did you inculcate values among the youth then when you were young or in Western countries?

I have always stressed that the youngsters should always be guided by their conscience. While teaching the students in the Inner London Education Authority (I.L.E.A.) and other areas of the western world, I was asked not to teach religion or use Hindu terminology. So I had to devise roundabout ways of building the youth without philosophising, and I did manage to bring them to higher levels. Formerly yoga was associated only with older people. Geeta and Prashant are fortunate that they have a lot of youngsters coming to learn. I was tired of teaching old people.

And when I was young, teaching youngsters, I always kept in mind that I was teaching youngsters. In those days I could not convey the moral values with conversation or talk. Nobody would have listened to me as I was young. But one thing was a fact. While teaching *āsana* to the youngsters I was very strong and strict, though I was not so with the elderly and diseased as I explained to you that I offered yoga as a sugarcoated pill to them. However, when *āsana* are done precisely and meticulously, the attention is drawn in. Therefore youngsters cannot let their minds wander.

I used to make the youngsters do the *āsana* varying the movements from one *āsana* to another *āsana* with rhythm and grace constantly changing the sequential order (the *vinyāsa* way)[1] which was not only a great fun but alertness in body and mind. This way helped them towards concentration and exhilaration.

In this manner, I applied a practical method and attracted them towards yogic discipline.

Bhavnesh: How did you feel about your teaching vis-à-vis that of your *Gurujī*?

My teaching has undergone a tremendous transformation over the years. By keen observation of my own practice of *āsana*, as well as the performances of my students, I built up a comprehensive style of teaching. For the last thirty years, I am constantly penetrating deeper inside, as such my techniques express with a deep understanding as I absorb more and more. My performance tomorrow may be different from that of today as I am building up from the feedback though the foundation does not change. You may find my performance of *āsana* an improvement over my *guru*'s since I came to Pune in 1937, because I have not stagnated at all.

However I have not changed the base that he gave. I brought further refinement and depth to it.

Sharmila: Did you develop any *āsana* on your own?

I have developed most of them through innovations. I was always curious to see how the *āsana* would be if I did them another way. This experiment enlightened me further. There are many *āsana* and *prāṇāyāma*, which I worked out in such a way, how it could be further simplified or how it could be further developed knowing the intricacies. This way of thinking and approaching brought new *āsana* into the picture.

The use of ropes, boxes and other props has been entirely devised by me. I used my memory, attention and observation to build from previous knowledge.

---

[1] See the article *Vinyāsa Yoga*, in *Aṣṭadala Yogamālā*, vol. 2.

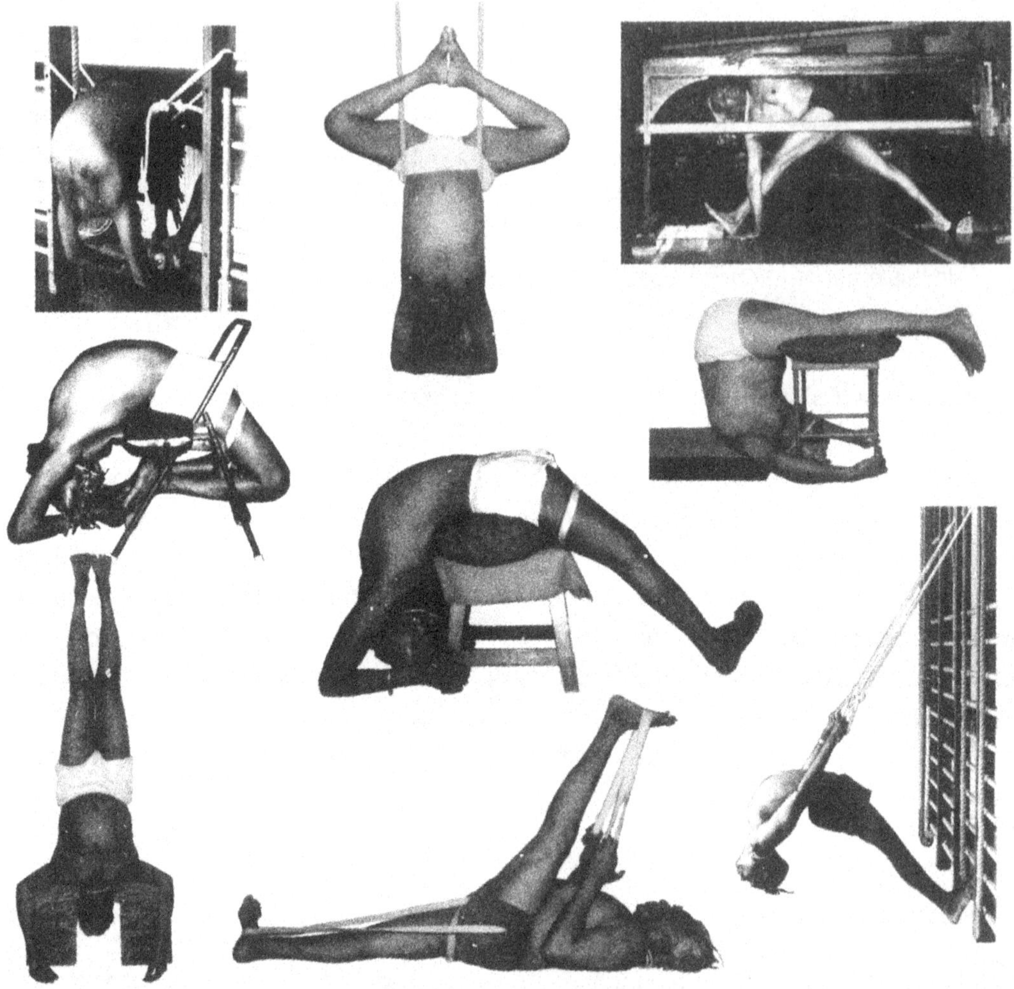

Plate n. 16 – Memory, attention and observation based on previous knowledge developed the props.

Sandhya: What about disappointments in life? Can you identify a turning point?

Disappointment was the key to raise me up. There was no specific turning point, as disappointment continued. I did not have much choice – I had to sink or swim. Even though failures continued in different forms, I did not fail in yoga. With constant practice and perseverance I would go on. Condemnation by society was more painful than personal disappointments. Many people took advantage of me in the early days in Pune. Wealthy industrialists would neglect paying my fees. Sometimes the imprint of those difficult times comes up and I tend to get wild, especially when attacked.

Sandhya: How did you get over them?

The credit goes to yoga. It generated energy in me to face disappointments. It protected me from complexity of the mind and from a fall. It destroyed the evils such as vanity and false prestige. I grew stronger and stronger to face all the opposition, failures and condemnation. The subject of yoga, which Patañjali describes in his *Yoga Sūtra,* became clearer and clearer. Now you find yoga or any spiritual subject is offered on a golden plate. This was not the situation then. The people from Mumbai were broadminded; the Mumbai press knew about me much before the Pune reporters. I did not settle there as the weather is not congenial to me. I worked hard in Pune but Mumbai recognised me.

Kirti: What advice would you give us, the youth of today?

Once you have decided on a course of action that is good for you, you should not oscillate. A strong determination and discipline are necessary to succeed. If you waver, you will lose the track and disappointments are bound to rise. The onset of temptations is very powerful when one is young. You must be watchful and not surrender to the lower pulls. Do not heed what your friends say right away. Measure them, find out the motive behind their statements. You should be careful so as not to be misguided by your so-called friends and well wishers.

Parth: We have heard that the practice of Iyengar Yoga is problem killing?

Yes, the impossible becomes possible. A girl with ear trouble was referred to me. Her doctors advised an operation, but agreed to let her do yoga for two months before that. In that period, her ear problem had gone. A boy who couldn't stand came to me. By the third lesson he could stand on his own.

You learn to face the world boldly and courageously. The clarity of intelligence gives a solution to each problem.

Aboli: What inspires you to make the impossible possible?

It is experience along with intuition. Experienced knowledge is something like the river flowing from the source reaching the sea, it ought to inspire me from the inner voice to make things possible.

Namrata: Can you narrate your best experiences?

I have risen from sub-human to a human level; that is enough for me. I was a nobody, shunned and condemned by society, damned at every step. Today I am full of joy and happiness, with all my pupils eager to do my bidding lovingly. Is it not my best experience?

Sharmila: Your message?

I have always been and shall remain an ethical man. Spiritual life is in the grace of God, but to stick to ethics is our duty. We are all children of God, but when we follow certain principles in life, He does look after us at all times, making the path much smoother. So trust in your undertakings and aspire to reach the goal accepting all drawbacks coming in your way.

Jasmina: We had an immensely enjoyable session, and if we could draw some inspiration from you it would make our lives worthwhile.

Thank you, God bless you! Let yoga guide you throughout.

NEVER GIVE UP HOPE*

Q.- Why is not yoga taught in schools? We all take it up late and wish we had started earlier, because we find we have to work harder.

My friend, that shows we become wise only after the event. But why should not we as parents create an interest in yoga in our children, so that they get used to yogic movements as *yoga-kriyā?* It should and must be done. But without understanding the need for children's growth the politicians and administrators interfere, thinking they know what is best for children's education. They do not come in contact with those educationists who know what children need. Armchair bureaucracy is the cause of not allowing children to develop discipline as well as physical and mental health. Regarding your other question, it is a good question. Your friends who are parents should demand that yoga be taught in schools, so that body and mind grow together in unison, and when they are advanced and ready they may receive the light of the spiritual knowledge that is taught later on.

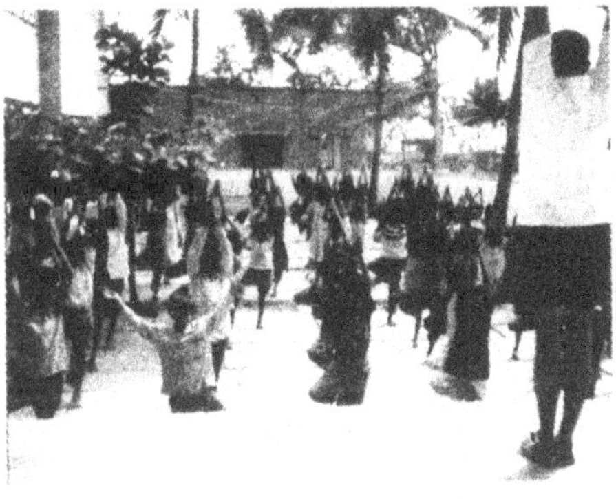

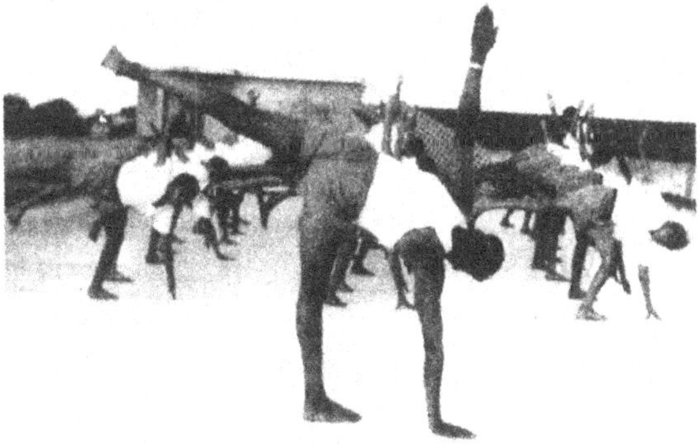

Plate n 17 – Teaching children

* Interview at Bharatiya Vidya Bhavan, 1st September 1988. Published in *Dipika*, n. 20, Winter 1990, London.

If the armchair bureaucracy is one of the reasons, the other reason is the lack of knowledge on the subject of yoga. This subject is often considered as an "old-age-programme". Many think that yoga has to be done when there is nothing else to do in life and when the body is diseased, deformed and aging.

If yoga has to be introduced in schools one has to have a thorough knowledge of what has to be taught to make them worthy citizens of the country. Often, people think on a theoretical level and not on a practical level.

Q.- What should we do to promote the fact that it is never too late to start yoga?

You should be happy even though you begin later in life. Only, when aged you may not be able to perfect yourself in this subject easily. You have implanted this seed of yoga in yourself, which may flow in your children. At least you will create the right environment if you are blessed to be born again. It is never too late. You consider yourself lucky to start at this age knowing the world, and you may begin to work in a reverse way, to make the return journey towards non-attachment and renunciation, to experience the pleasures of the kingdom of the soul.

Q.- Mr. Iyengar, I have never come to terms with pain. How do you cope with it?

Life and pain, life and pleasures go together. There is no pain without pleasure, there is no pleasure without pain. Only a person who has reached bliss is free of pain. We are caught between the joys of the world and the beauty of spiritual realisation. But the art of yoga makes each individual bear pain with contentment. I have not conquered pain, it is there in my body, but I have accepted it as a natural process in my evolution.

You all call me a stern teacher, but do you know how stern I am on myself. Compared to my sternness as a teacher, I am definitely more compassionate towards you. Healthwise I suffered a lot when I was a child. My *guru* said, "Do some yoga, you will improve". Eventually he said, "Tomorrow you will do *Vṛśchikāsana* – the scorpion pose."

– "*Sir, I do not know how to do it.*"

– *"Bend the elbows, do elbow balance, bend the knees and place your feet on your head – that is the Vṛśchikāsana."–*

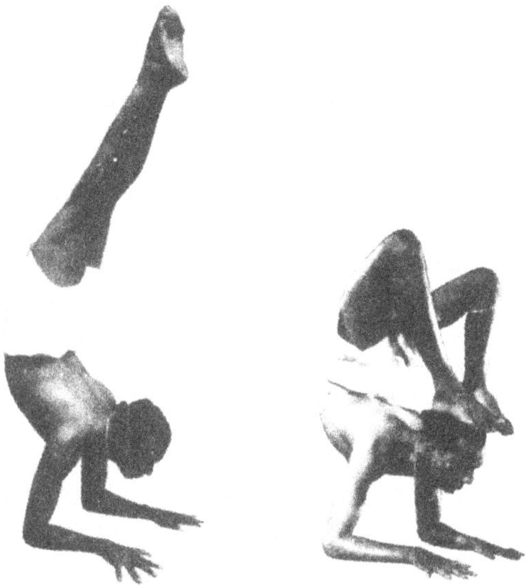

Plate n. 18 – *Pīnchā Mayūrāsana* and *Vṛśchikāsana*

– "*Sir, I have never seen it done.*" –

– "*You have to do it tomorrow because we have visitors.*" –

Similarly, one day some dignitaries were expected. My *guru* told me to do *Hanumānāsana*. I said, "What is it, sir?" I had not heard of *Hanumānāsana*.

He said, "Go straight with one leg stretched forward, and the other leg backward and sit on the floor."

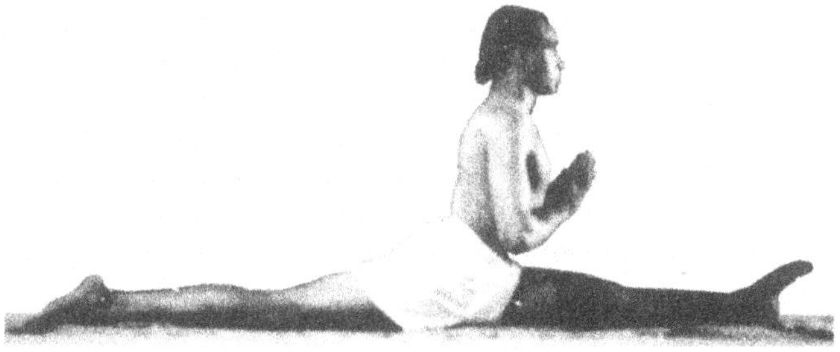

Plate n. 19 – *Hanumanāsana*

– *"I have never done it, sir."* –

He said, "Do it".

In those days we wore very tight, stitched underwear (*langot*) and I told my *guru*, "Sir, it's too tight, I do not think I can spread my legs".

He said to one of his senior students, "Go to the office and fetch some scissors." And he cut the underwear on both sides and forced me to do it. Well you can understand what excruciating pain I felt to get into this *āsana*. He said, "If you had not done it, you would have spoiled my reputation."

He often behaved like this, with all the complicated *āsana* – like instant coffee. That did not make me forget the pain. It took years to remove these excruciating pains, as I had to find out means to lessen them. Sitting was a pain; standing was a pain; walking, a pain; sleeping, a pain. On account of this, if someone makes a mistake I cannot bear it, and say, "Why do you want to suffer? So I am quick to correct with appeasement or a stern warning. Because of this going out to help to free one suffering from pain, I am branded as a stern teacher. Now, I have worked out simple ways to certain actions in the complicated *āsana* without going through excruciating pain. The roughness in the movements is misused. With this process I have minimised the pain, even though I can't eradicate it totally, and my pupils should be grateful for this research.

Unfortunately we have become pleasure-seeking or comfort-seeking people. *Tapas* is the base (foundation) for yoga-*sādhanā*. Comforts and *tapas* cannot go together. So a practitioner has to remember that towards pain, even if it is just a body ache, we need to develop forbearance and tolerance. Our ancestors have already said that knowledge does not come to one unless one takes pain to earn it.

Please bear with it: do not think it cannot be reduced. If your pain is one hundred percent, perhaps I can reduce it to half or even less, which itself should be a great joy to continue the *sādhanā*. When you prepare your mind, your pain becomes a friend. If you do any of the *āsana* without any reaction from the body or the mind, that posture has a bad effect. Like two stones that produce a spark, each *āsana* produces a response in the muscles, the nerves, the mind, and the intelligence. If it comes easily, something is wrong. If it produces resistance equal to your challenge, then the pain is soothing, not irritating. If you get a splinter in your finger, you prick your finger again to get it out. The first prick hurts, but the second one does not; it is soothing because you know you are removing the first pain.

Similarly in yoga, if you have a pain like a needle, you have to find which type of needle you need to remove it. Any pain that comes while you are doing *āsana* and disappears afterwards is not a real pain. If it continues for days, then you know that you have done something wrong. You need to use your discrimination to correct the wrong to become a better yoga *sādhaka*.

Know well that the body, which is our instrument, needs to be used properly, judiciously and systematically. If we show comforts to the body, it gets attached to the comforts. Obviously, it does not want to suffer with pain. When the body, the muscles, the bones and the joints are not used or misused, it becomes a habit to the body. When the body gets habituated to a wrong *āsana* it does not want to get corrected. The muscles are more adamant than we are. Instead of serving us they boss us about. When in pain the mind and body do not co-operate with your will, which you need to put it in a right perspective. To break the wrong habits and pick up the good habits is a painful process. And that is the pain, which you suffer from.

Again, the beauty of *āsana* lies in the fact that they bring the hidden diseases to the surface. The body expresses a pain if the disease is hidden.

So, in short, the pain is because of wrong musculo-skeletal structure, misuse or disuse of muscles; lack of blood circulation, faulty practice of *āsana* such as over or under-doing, or body afflictions, which have yet to be seen or diagnosed.

Q.- How soon after beginning *āsana* can you start learning *prāṇāyāma*?

Nowadays, pupils like to jump and they corrupt the teachers to teach them as they want. Pupils come and ask, "Sir, can you teach me *prāṇāyāma*, can you teach me meditation?" They think that a teacher has to teach according to the demand of the pupils. But as far as yoga is concerned it cannot be taught or learnt in an instant. People think that I practise and teach only *āsana* and not *prāṇāyāma* and *dhyāna*. Though I touch all aspects of yoga, they have a wrong notion that I teach *āsana* and hence I am a physical yogi and one who teaches *dhyāna* is a spiritual yogi. If I dance according to the wishes of the pupils, they may call me a spiritual teacher. Yoga is inclusive of ethical discipline, physical discipline, *prāṇic* discipline, mental discipline, intellectual discipline and ego discipline.

Similarly, *prāṇāyāma* too cannot be taught by asking. One begins *prāṇāyāma* only when *āsana* has been perfected, the body is under control, and the practice has been maintained over a long period.

For example, *bandha* are essential in the practice of *prāṇāyāma*. If you cannot do *Sālamba Sarvāṅgāsana* and *Halāsana*, well, you cannot do *Jālandhara Bandha*. In *Sālamba Sarvāṅgāsana* there is a natural *Jālandhara Bandha* (a chinlock). If you cannot do *Sālamba Śīrṣāsana* you cannot do *Uḍḍīyāna Bandha*, because the moment you do *Sālamba Śīrṣāsana*, there is a natural *Uḍḍīyāna Bandha*. These *bandha* are essential factors in *prāṇāyāma*. In order to save stress on the brain and acceleration of heartbeats as in jogging, you need to do *Jālandhara Bandha* by bringing the head down to rest on the notch of the chest. Strain should not be felt in *prāṇāyāma* and the heartbeats should be very rhythmic and slow. *Uḍḍīyāna Bandha* is the gripping of the lower abdomen. So too with *Mūla Bandha*, in *āsana* like *Ūrdhva Dhanurāsana*, *Dwi Pāda Viparīta Daṇḍāsana*, *Kapotāsana*, *Vṛścikāsana*, *Chakrabandhāsana* and *Mūlabandhāsana*, one learns *Mūla Bandha* wherein the anus is contracted and gripped up to the anal sphincter muscles. It needs to be done in *prāṇāyāma*, so that the energy does not dissipate in an untrained body. These are examples of why *āsana* is said to be so important before *prāṇāyāma* is started.

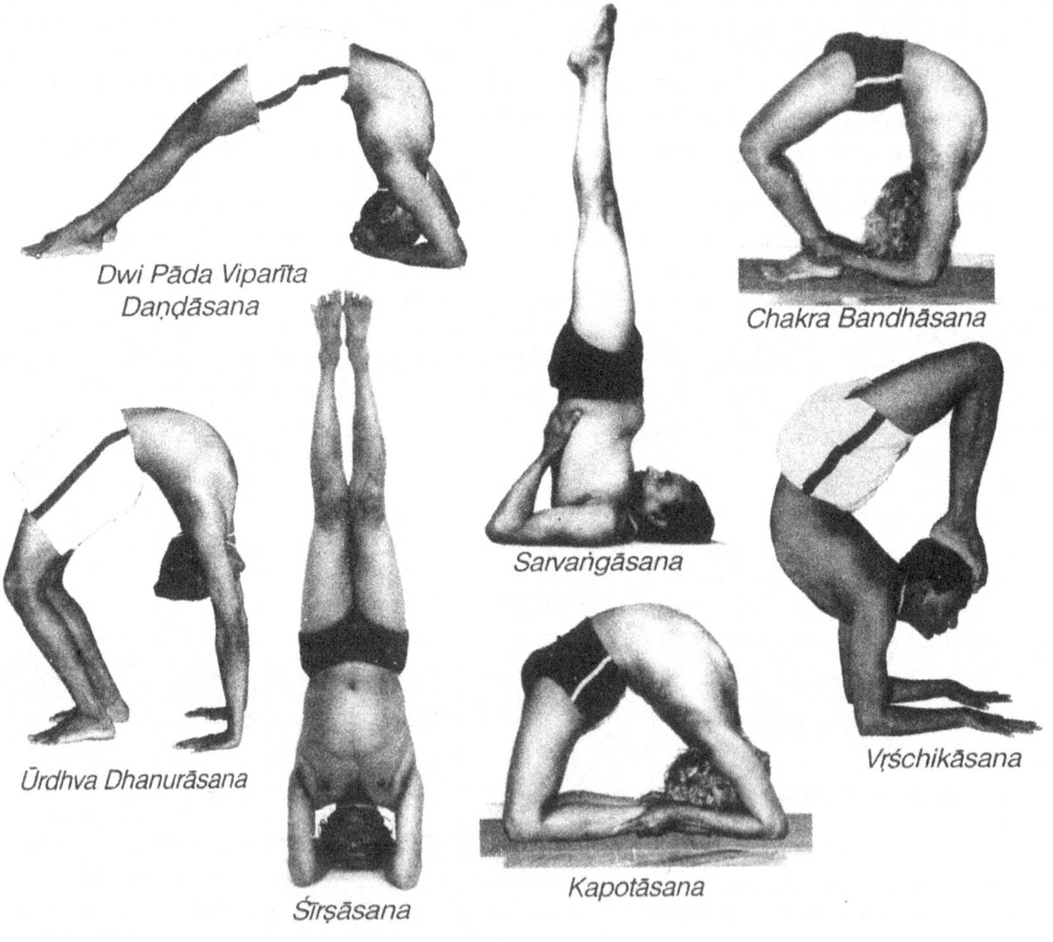
Dwi Pāda Viparīta Daṇḍāsana
Chakra Bandhāsana
Sarvangāsana
Ūrdhva Dhanurāsana
Vṛśchikāsana
Kapotāsana
Śīrṣāsana

Plate n. 20 – *Āsana* to learn the *bandhas*

You have read Patañjali's definition, *sthira sukham āsanam* (*Y.S.*, II.46), interpreted as, "Any steady comfortable *āsana* is enough". Please know that *sthiratā* is nothing but *dhāraṇā* and *sukhatā* is *dhyāna*. In my experience, all comfortable *āsana* eventually become uncomfortable. You may sit comfortably for two minutes or five minutes, but then you shake your foot or move your toes.

Patañjali has defined what mastery of an *āsana* means: firmness in the body and a pleasant feeling in the brain; in other words, when the effort becomes effortless and you feel you are pumping fresh blood to reach the cells. If the blood does not reach the cells, it means the cells are not working towards health, so the *āsana* is of no more use as a treatment for a disease.

Prāṇāyāma should only be started when the lungs have been developed through the practice of *āsana*, and the intercostal muscles have gained elasticity both internally and externally. Then one can measure the slow, soft depth of inhalation and exhalation, and that is the time to begin *prāṇāyāma* in order to master it.

The practice of *āsana* makes one fit to do *prāṇāyāma*. People think that *prāṇāyāma* is only a breathing technique. It is not so. In order to do *prāṇāyāma* one needs stability, steadiness, vitality, energy and liveliness, which come through the practice of *āsana*.

Q.- Mr. Iyengar, I think many western businessmen like myself suffer from stress, which I regard as a mental illness. Do you think the *āsana* can provide relief from stress, or do we have to go into meditation?

Meditation is not going to remove stress, my friend. Meditation is only possible when one is in a stress-less state. To be stress-less the culture of the cells, the build-up of calmness and coolness in the brain is a must. By learning how to relax the brain one can remove stress. How to keep the brain cells in a receptive state is the art which yoga teaches. And remember that *dhyāna* – meditation – is part and parcel of yoga, it is not separate. *Yama, niyama, āsana, prāṇāyāma, pratyāhāra, dhāraṇā, dhyāna* and *samādhi*, all these are the petals of yoga. There is *dhyāna* in everything; in all these aspects one needs a reflective or a meditative mood.

Learning postures certainly helps. If I say, "Relax your brain", you cannot do it. If I put you in a certain *āsana*, your brain relaxes and you become quiet. This is the beauty of yoga. If you do *Halāsana*[1] your brain becomes completely quiet. If you are dejected mentally, do *Setu Bandha Sarvāṅgāsana*[2] for ten minutes; your depression disappears, though you do not know how.

It has been beautifully said in the *Haṭhayoga Pradīpikā*, "Mind is the king of the senses; breath is the king of the mind; and the nerves are king of the breath". If you know how to stretch and how to keep the nervous system elastic and lively, it can take any load and therefore the word stress does not strike at all.

People go to the cinema if they want to be free from stress. But even watching the movie is stressful. Even *Śavāsana* is a stress, but it minimises the stress factor. In sleep there is also stress:

---

[1] See *Aṣṭadaḷa Yogamāḷā*, vol. 4, plate n. 27.
[2] See *Aṣṭadaḷa Yogamāḷā*, vol. 4, plate n. 5.

you move from one position to another because of stress. You sit in meditation and there is stress. If you drop your spine while meditating you go to sleep, so you have to keep your spine erect and that is stressful. Walking, eating, reading – everything is stress. There is nothing in this world free from stress until death. Even death is stressful. After death we are not there to tell how stressful it was. So the degree of stress is important. Rather than asking "Can I be completely free from stress?" how stress affects your nervous system – that is what matters. When the stress is constructive it is a positive stress, which does not harm the nerves. But when it is destructive it is negative stress, which is harmful.

When you say that western businessmen suffer from stress, it is not so. All suffer from stress. The main cause behind stress is anger, fear, speed, greed, unhealthy ambition and competition, which show a negative effect on the body and mind. When one does good work without selfish motives, the mind is open though there is the stress of work, but it is a positive stress. The practice of *āsana* and *prāṇāyāma* not only make you stress-less but also energise and invigorate the nerves and the mind for positive stress.

If it rains heavily, the water does not necessarily penetrate the earth. The rainwater flushes and floods. If it drizzles for many days continuously, then the water seeps deep into the earth, which is very good for cultivation. Similarly in ourselves, when we use our brain, the peripheral nerves act, but they do not penetrate inwards. If the peripheral nerves are made to interpenetrate the autonomous nervous system and the central nervous system, you will find that the nerves appear so deep that their depth seems immeasurable. This is due to the extension and expansion given by the various *āsana*, and stretching the various parts of the body diffuses stress. The stress that saturates the brain is also diffused, so the brain is rested and there is a release from strain. Similarly, while doing the various types of *prāṇāyāma* the whole body is irrigated with energy. *Prāṇāyāma* requires physical and nervous strength, intellectual and conscious application, persistency, determination and enduring power. These are all learned through the practice of *āsana*. The nerves are soothed, the brain is calmed, and the hardness and rigidity of the lungs are loosened. The nerves are made to remain healthy. There is a certain vibration, whether it is rhythmic or not, which you can make rhythmic and subtler in your *āsana* and *prāṇāyāma* practice without force or stress. You are at once one with yourself and that is meditation.

Dhyāna does not achieve this. You need to achieve all these for *dhyāna*. *Dhyāna* cannot be done by those with the stress factor, weak body, weak lungs, hard muscles, collapsed spine, fluctuating mind, timidity and mental agitation. Often people think that sitting quietly is meditation. This mistaken notion is the cause of misunderstanding. *Dhyāna* has to lead necessarily towards *jñāna*. *Jñāna* and *dhyāna* go together. For that one needs all these preparations. Stress is related to nerves and cells. *Dhyāna* is related to higher mental faculty.

Q.- Mr. Iyengar, what do you think about the western obsession with jogging?

Yoga is known as a *sarvāṅga sādhanā*, a complete discipline. Jogging is not considered as a whole exercise. When I speak of *āsana*, they do not work only on your body; they work on your vital organs, your body, your mind, your intelligence, your consciousness, on your very self. Does jogging do this? It is *aṅga bhāga sādhanā* – only a certain part of the body is involved. Your heartbeat gets accelerated. Do you call this stimulation of heart or strain in the heart? Is it education? Inside your body is an indescribable geographical map. It needs a lot of study. You have to educate yourself and judge what is congenial and healthy. When a child runs, it does not gasp for breath, but when elderly people run at the same speed as a child, they do gasp for breath. Is this not a sign to know whether jogging stimulates or irritates the heart? Practice of *āsana* does not irritate but stimulates the heart. So this question should have been put to those who jog and not to me.

Q.- Why is it that different yogis prescribe different *āsana*, and sometimes even the basic posture is different? Does Patañjali in his *Yoga Sūtra* describe the *āsana* themselves, or are they an interpretation?

If Patañjali had described everything, his work would not have been in *sūtra* form. The *Hathayoga Pradīpikā* is not in *sūtra* form; it is a technical book, whereas Patañjali's is a philosophy of self-culture. If you do not keep the *Haṭha Yoga* text before you, you will never understand Patañjali's *Yoga Sūtra*. They complement each other.

Now, why do different people give different basic *āsana*? Speaking for myself, I have disciplined myself and explored this field for fifty-two years. When I wrote *Light on Yoga*, I gave a six-year course having in mind that all would attempt practising like me. Hence, I forgot to think of those who are mild and average in intelligence, who may not muster the strength to complete their stipulated course and I failed to mention that it was intended for intensive students to master in six years. But today I could add many basic stages for those that cannot master in six years and can make the course last eighteen years for them.

Over the years I have studied not only the anatomy of human beings, but the anatomy of the *āsana* also. I studied by observing the anatomy of each and every movement of the body watching the mobility and the rigidity of the joints, such as foot, knee, hips, arms, elbows and fingers. I looked into the movements of extension and function of each and every muscle, such as the spinal muscles, neck muscles and the degree of movement in the *āsana*. I codified the *āsana* and accordingly showed the stages to learn with ease. If I had not studied the structure of each *āsana* I should probably have given whatever method was easy for me.

If I find *Utthita Trikoṇāsana* easy and *Utthita Pārśvakoṇāsana* difficult, naturally I introduce *Utthita Trikoṇāsana* first. But if I find that some people cannot do *Utthita Trikoṇāsana* and can do *Utthita Pārśvakoṇāsana* easily; then I ask them to do that first and then the *Utthita Trikoṇāsana*. This helps them to learn the later one with attention and care. The reason behind this variation is that in *Utthita Trikoṇāsana* when the trunk moves and bends to the right side, the right root of the thigh and groin fail to bear the weight of the trunk, causing the knee to bend. In *Utthita Pārśvakoṇāsana*[1] the knee in any case has to bend. Obviously the groin becomes soft. That causes one to go to the *āsana* with ease. This is how the teacher has to see and guide the pupils to understand their own body, its movement, placement and so forth. This is a process of study in developing, understanding and evolving the quality of intelligence. If people teach the *āsana* according to their mobility, they are not good teachers. You have to see hundreds of people, find out their reaction and listen to what they say when you are teaching them and then work on one's own to understand which points co-operate and which do not. That is how I studied and learnt to build flexibility of my mind. Teachers need to see what one is doing and what one needs to do.

If you go to two different doctors, they may give you two different medicines for the same ailment according to their understanding. It is similar in yoga, but we could meet and iron out some of these differences and agree on a new programme. Unfortunately, many of today's yoga masters are not practitioners at all, but have become masters because they may be having an urge to get on in life or have a commercial frame of mind. Today yoga has become such a popular subject that people want to cash in on its name and fame.

In my country, the people know me, but I am not sure whether the government officials know me. If I say children cannot be taught meditation, they say, "Oh, this man does not know anything. Don't invite him". I once told them, "Children know only two things. Either they remain active or go to sleep. They do not have emotional disturbances and hence they do not need to meditate. Even if at all they have emotional disturbance due to family problems, or for being a single child with no companions or due to the demand of studies, meditation is not the answer or solution. Why make children intellectually impotent at that age by making them remain in a state of void? Let them be active, teach them to focus their intelligence on studies, so that they develop properly." But my advice was not liked. This is where the differences arise between an experienced person in the field and armchair thinkers. One has to strike a balance in building up children in a constructive way. Yoga teachers ought to be broad-minded. They should not be adamant in their known system and with the idea of growing popular. Let yoga become popular, not me, you or the teacher. Art is immortal; but we are mortals.

---

[1] See *Aṣṭadaḷa Yogamālā*, vol.3, plate n. 25 & 26.

So my suggestion is that we sit together, chalk out a system, and present a syllabus that is beneficial for everyone – and I have done this for other countries.

Q.- Mr. Iyengar, could you comment on how our indulgence in the pleasures of the senses affects our energy levels and our ability to pursue the domain of the spirit?

Patañjali made an authoritative statement, like a *Veda*. He said, "The contact of nature with *puruṣa* is the cause of all unhappiness in the world."[1] So with a sweeping statement he says, learn to be completely detached from the world and you are liberated. Realising this to be a sweeping statement, he reflected a little on it and later said that nature has certain virtues or qualities – *sattva, rajas* and *tamas*. In order to learn and understand about the world without being part of it, one has to understand the interplay of the qualities of *tamas, rajas* and *sattva*.

In the second chapter he clearly mentions that the senses are there for the evolution of the soul. Understand their purpose: "As soon as they have fulfilled their purpose, they withdraw and you realise your position the moment they withdraw."[2] So use them as instruments for your progress, but do not become part and parcel of them. If you are caught in the web of nature, your energy levels get diverted in pleasures and pains and lose the ability to pursue the domain of spiritual knowledge. The organs of action, senses of perception, mind and consciousness are only there to serve the self and not to rule over the self. So yoga is the method that teaches you to draw the senses towards the soul. When you are doing *Paśchimottānāsana*, when your head is down and your legs are straight, you cannot look at the world: you have to look within yourself. When you do *Adho Mukha Svānāsana*, the moment you stretch the spine and feel by looking backwards, you see inwards as your attention is drawn inwards at once. Draw the senses of perception and organs of action towards the seer, so that the seer benefits from these vehicles or garments of the soul.

Similarly, you have to know about the nervous system. The peripheral nervous system triggers the external part. See how far this triggering sensation reaches inwards. Is it feeding the intelligence, or is it only asking for repetition of pleasures? The mind and the memory fight with each other. The memory tells the mind, "Do not listen to the intelligence but listen to me, because I know things from past experience." So the mind is drawn by the memory, but neglects to listen to the wisdom of the intelligence. It is only when the mind or the senses lose their potency, they say, "I should not have listened to my memory. I should have consulted the intelligence." Only through the contact of intelligence does judgement come. This is *pratyāhāra*, where the memory is superseded

[1] *Draṣṭradṛśyayoḥ saṁyogaḥ heyahetuḥ* (*Y.S.*, II.17).
[2] *Sva svāmi śaktyoḥ svarūpopalabdhi hetuḥ saṁyogaḥ* (*Y.S.*, II.23).

by and subjugated to the intelligence. This is the way the yogic discipline guides us to use our senses for understanding and evolving towards the soul.

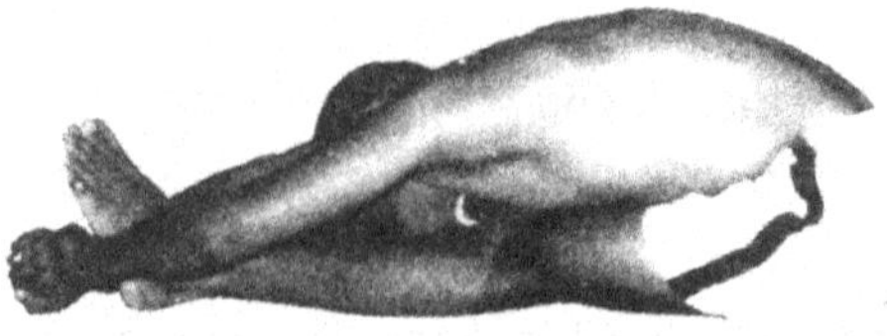

Paśchimottānāsana

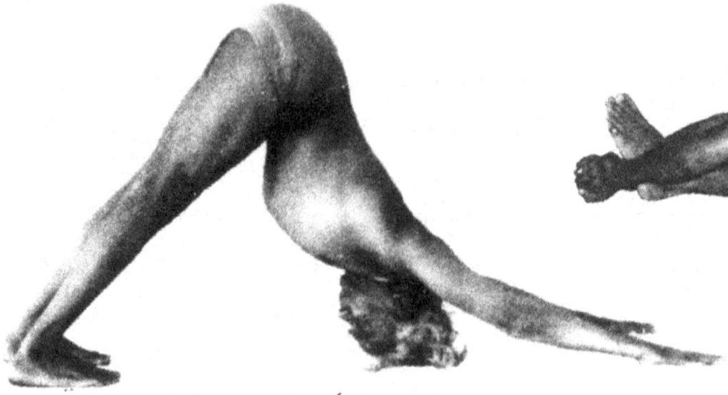

Adho Mukha Śvānāsana

Plate n. 21 – Attention is drawn inwards in *Adho Mukha Svānāsana* and *Paśchimottānāsana*

Unfortunately, we misuse our senses, our memories and our intelligence. We make the potential energies of all these to flow outwards to get scattered. We may say that we want to reach the domain of the soul but there remains a great tug-of-war. We neither go in to pursue the domain of the self *(apavargārtha)* nor out in the pleasures of the world *(bhogārtha)* and that saps the energy.

Q.- When doing *Śīrṣāsana*, should you be balanced only on your head, or should you use strength?

When you do *Sālamba Śīrṣāsana* you have to think. When I do *Sālamba Śīrṣāsana*, I watch where my head is, where my shoulders are, I question the position of my neck. For example, first I stand in *Tāḍāsana* and study the space between the ears and neck, as well as the neck and shoulders. When I do *Sālamba Śīrṣāsana* do I watch my shoulders collapse and go nearer my ears or do I retain space between my ears and neck as in *Tāḍāsana?* You should study like this, using your intelligence and lifting the muscles of the neck and shoulders that collapse. If you raise the inner deltoids higher, see whether they are in level with the outer deltoids. By this adjustment, see if there is a load on your neck or not. Your awareness and intelligence in head balance should produce a straight line on your body from your head to your heels. The inner intelligence should be parallel to the back body, the front body and the side body. It is hard to learn this *āsana*, yet I hope you understand and learn to do comfortably by extending and elevating the sides of the trunk. Then to hold on to the *āsana* is easy. If the head goes back, the legs come forward. If you take your shin back, the foot comes forward and everything goes wrong. There should be right extension without strain.

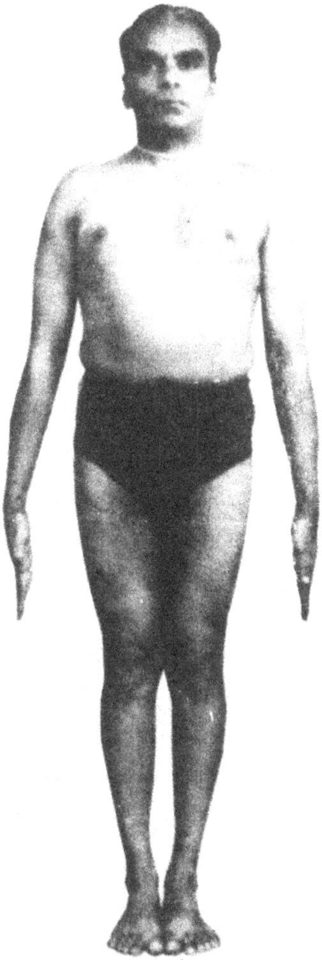

Tāḍāsana

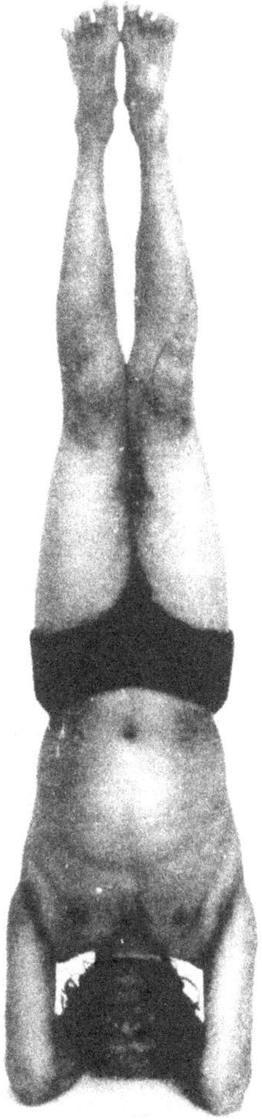

Śīrṣāsana

Plate n. 22 – *Śīrṣāsana* and *Tāḍāsana*

When you do *Sālamba Śīrṣāsana*, the upper arm should not rest on the lower arm. If it does, that is not *Sālamba Śīrṣāsana*. It puts the load on the spine, and shrinks the neck muscles bringing neck pain, head pain and so on. If the hands are not protective, your shoulders collapse and the neck feels the weight. If you use the arms like the legs of a tripod, you do not feel the weight of the body on your head or neck any more. Do you feel the weight of your legs when you are walking? Similarly when *Sālamba Śīrṣāsana* is done regularly, the doer feels no weight on the head.

So, the secret of head balance is that you should not feel your body weight on your head and that is perfect *Sālamba Śīrṣāsana*.

Q.- If certain *āsana* are difficult and make you dizzy and sick, should you continue or give up?

If an *āsana* makes you dizzy, you should ask whoever is teaching you what are the *āsana* that remove the dizziness. Suppose your eyes are tense when you are doing standing *āsana*, or you held your breath getting dizzy after three or four *āsana* and feel as if you will black out: at once we say, do *Adho Mukha Śvānāsana* or *Uttānāsana*. With your head down the dizziness goes. Any pose that makes you dizzy means that it is not coming easily; Dizziness means over exertion which sends you a message of discomfort. When you sense that message, don't continue. Do *Uttānāsana* or *Adho Mukha Śvānāsana* in between, then a standing *āsana*, again a head resting *āsana*, then another standing *āsana* and so on.[1] This kind of sequencing is called *viloma vinyāsa*.[2] This way you will not get dizzy.

This applies particularly to people with stomach upset or low blood pressure, or if they hold the breath while staying in the *āsana*, or if they have liver or ear problems. We do not let them do *āsana* which increase dizziness. With these adjustments we teach them forward bending *āsana*, so that their problems are brought under control. Then we advise them to do standing *āsana* with the introduction of forward bends in between. We do not stop their practice. Rather adjust the faulty action and faulty posture.

Basically, you need to find out the reason behind the problem. You need to know why you feel dizzy. It could be from a simple cause such as sleeplessness, mental fatigue, heavy meals, indigestion, the liver problem or tumour in the brain. So, one needs to find out the cause. By giving up the *āsana*, you do not find the remedy. You need to experiment to find out which *āsana* help. You have to consult your teachers. If they do not know, you have to write to me, and I will answer you. It depends totally upon the cause of the problem.

Q.- What do you think of yoga for the mentally handicapped?

]It is not a question of thinking, my friend, but of acting and applying. I look at a handicapped or mentally retarded or challenged person's eyes, behaviour, and power in the legs, I see such defects and I teach accordingly, stabilising their eyes and legs. Yoga, as you know, works one hundred per cent on the respiratory and circulatory systems, the windows and gates of the soul. If they are trained properly, then the four lobes of the brain get sufficient energy for right function. Otherwise they may remain imbalanced. We have to learn to see the mentally challenged child from their eyes. The eyes are nearest to the brain and in all mentally retarded children their eyes are unsteady.

---

[1] See *Aṣṭadaḷa Yogamālā*, vol. 4, plate n. 19.

[2] See the article *Vinyāsa Yoga*, in *Aṣṭadaḷa Yogamālā*, vol. 2, section III.

The moment the eyes are steady, the brain becomes stable. Then we say, look here, look there, stand this way, and pay attention here or there. You have to look at their eyes that need to be stabilised in each position. You need to teach them to focus. They need to be given the direction to focus their eyes while doing the *āsana.*

Then they improve. The eyes are the index of the brain and the ears are the index of the mind and consciousness. The eyes belong to the element of fire; ears belong to the element of ether or space. If there is harmony between the eyes and the ears, the process of focussing the attention becomes easy.

So if you are teaching the handicapped children, always teach them to stabilise their eyeballs. Make them follow your finger, and increase their gaze.

Ask them if they can bring their eyes to look at a particular point. Stability will come and the fluid in the brain will float evenly. The same with each limb. If the feet are turning out, bring them in. Teach them each action separately, one foot at a time. You should not confuse them by introducing several motor actions at a time. The confusion develops reluctance in them. Then they hate you and the subject as well. You should not expect skilled and complicated movements or actions. You should make them extroverted. You have to cheer them up. You have to learn to act quickly so that the child does not lose attention. You, as a teacher not only need the patience but more effort from your side in order to bring a small improvement in them.

Q.- Mr. Iyengar, do you have some words of encouragement for us to remember when we are struggling with laziness and lack of discipline in our *āsana* practice?

About ten years ago I had two severe accidents. But for yoga, you probably would not see me now. I lost control even in *Utthita Trikoṇāsana.*[1] I could not lift my shoulders or move them back. Even bending my knee was painful because the accident was so bad. But I did not go to a doctor – remember that – otherwise where was my faith in my own art? I said to myself, I have practised yoga for fifty-two years, let me try again. So this is the encouragement I would give you, that I began again from scratch in 1979 and I am eighty-five percent recovered: fifteen percent still eludes me. I do not give up hope and stop the practice, which would be pointless. Better practice to fail rather than not try at all. This resolution of mine is my encouragement for you to persist in the *sādhanā.*

I do *Vṛśchikāsana*[2] today, which was impossible for me five or six years ago. Even when I gave the demonstration at the Barbican I could not move properly at all. A friend asked me how I put up with the pain. You all know I am stern with myself. I said, let me finish with the demonstration, I will

1 See *Aṣṭadala Yogamālā,* vol. 3, plate n. 25.
2 See plates. n. 52 and 25

take care of the pain later. So even in the Barbican video,[1] which you have all seen, if you observe carefully, I was not in a very good shape because of injury – though it is a good guide for you all!

Today I do better *Vṛścikāsana* after ten years of suffering. You know, it is all about the mental frame. When you are doing *āsana*, every single line of the body has to be observed carefully. Is it straight from the source to the periphery or is it crooked? That is what I have learned from my injury, and it makes me a better teacher and a better performer. So I hope this is sufficient encouragement for you, that I have not lost heart. I say, I will do my best under any difficult condition or adverse circumstances. Do not be dissatisfied, but do not be contented either. Otherwise, you become dull. Whatever I have done today, can I progress one hair's breadth tomorrow? If you have that attitude I am sure you will all enjoy yoga.

When you are not physically or mentally challenged, why not thank God and put in a little more effort to kill laziness and to progress?

Q.- With head balance, how important is it to learn to fall safely? How can we learn that – can we ask our teachers to help?

All teachers are supposed to help, so they must. You cannot come down slowly since you are a beginner, you have to flex the knees and aim to bring the back of the crown of the big toe down to touch the ground, then you will not hurt yourself. Sometimes you feel you are going to lose balance. Do not fight to keep it because you won't succeed. Let yourself come down. Even if you bring one leg down, you will be all right. You should not bring your knees on the floor or fall on the face.

You cannot be taught to come down slowly till you can balance well in *Sālamba Śīrṣāsana*. Until you know how to come down you cannot learn how to go up! Coming down follows the current of gravitational force whereas going up is against the current of gravity. You jump up quickly against the wall because it gives you confidence and stops you from the fall. But on the way down, the floor is so far away that you are afraid. That is why the teacher is there to help you lift up and bring you down so that you develop the confidence to balance *Sālamba Śīrṣāsana*.

In *Sālamba Śīrṣāsana* the spine becomes rigid, so it is important to know how to move it again to come down. In coming down, the secret is to take off the tension in the spinal muscles and flex the legs. Coming down is an art; it has to be learned, because you are going with gravity. Going up is not an art, as you are moving against gravity. You have to ask your teacher to guide you to come down in three or four steps: bending the knees, knees touching the stomach, rolling the spine slightly to touch the toes to the ground. Rolling the spine and dropping the toes to the floor should synchronise, that is the art.

---

[1] This video is still available and is known as *Yogamālā*.

Q.- What is *kuṇḍalinī?*

Why do you bother about *kuṇḍalinī?* We do not know our bodies at all, we do not even know how to keep our tailbone erect and yet you think of *kuṇḍalinī*, which is a divine energy or *divya śakti*. Patañjali speaks of the abundant flow of energy in a yogi. Previously it was known as *agni*, fire. Later it came to be called *kuṇḍalinī* as the central nerve is in *kuṇḍalākāra*, coiled three and a half times. The awakening of *kuṇḍalinī* comes with the divine union of body and soul; it can be awakened, but not simply with hard effort, as people would have you believe nowadays. Reading the texts, people often misinterpret and do *prāṇāyāma* forcefully which is wrong. It damages the brain cells, the nerves and the central nervous system. Often people get deranged. Recently one of my friends died. I told him he was doing it all wrong but he laughed at me. In fact, he criticised my practice of *āsana* and *prāṇāyāma* and thought his was a spiritual practice. Finally, he became vegetative and died.

One needs to watch one's practice very carefully. Suppose I am standing in *Tāḍāsana*, I watch what the lobes of my brain are doing in *Tāḍāsana*, or does the pressure in my brain change from the front to the back? Even to float the brain on the fluid of the spine requires attention and intelligence. If we know how to balance the fluid, the lobes of the brain do not shake. Often people do a lot of *Bhastrikā*, or prolonged *kumbhaka* or even chronologically controlled breath by force like *viṣama vṛtti prāṇāyāma*.[1] Such forced breath does damage the electrical nerves of the brain.

In the *Bhagavad Gītā*, Lord Krishna said to Arjuna, "Now I am going to show you my real form called *viśvarūpa darśana*. But you can't see my form with these eyes, so I bless you with divine eyes", which Lord Krishna did. There is no pupil like Arjuna nowadays. You will have to read it for yourself, because I cannot recount the life of Arjuna. What an intense pupil he was – that is why Krishna could grace him with that divine eye, which is *kuṇḍalinī*. You and I cannot achieve that. We are still looking for the pleasures of the world, even though we are not satisfied with them, and we cannot have it both ways. So unless and until you discipline your entire inner system to such an extent that it becomes divine, you will not experience *kuṇḍalinī*. It means the divinity of the body united with the divinity of the soul. We have a huge gulf between body and mind, mind and soul. Let us work to bring them closer. Then I think I shall not have to explain *kuṇḍalinī*, because you will experience it for yourself.

Q.- I have a question about yoga and vegetarianism. I know a number of people who are actively involved in promoting vegetarianism, the principles of non-violence and so on, but I notice that in all your writings you have never stated them as

[1] See the author's *Light on Prāṇāyāma*, Harper Collins, London

prerequisites for a yoga practitioner. In my opinion violence and eating meat are in conflict with *yama* and *niyama*. What is your view on the promotion of vegetarianism?

The reason I have not dealt with it is this. Many of you have not read about my life at all. When I was young I was very sick. Poverty kept me undernourished. I practised yoga to gain health. When I grew up, there was a time when I couldn't get a meal for three or four days. I used to live on water, so who am I to talk about nutrition? Today God has given me everything, but I have not forgotten my early life. Is yoga meant only for the well off, or is it for the under-nourished also? I was under-nourished, but I have done a great deal in the field of yoga. So I say, if the salivary glands do not act, do not eat. When hungry, you see dry bread and it stimulates saliva, then that is the nourishing thing for you, as it has been for me very often.

Coming to vegetarianism, "As you sow, so shall you reap". The growth of the mind depends on the food you eat. If you eat animal food, this is what goes into your system. At the time of slaughtering they are in great fear. This instinctive fear changes the chemistry of its body at the time of its death. That instinctive fear that has spread in its body is what one eats. Eating that flesh of the animal which is disturbed at the time of slaughtering goes into the system and affects the minds. The psychological or mental thread of fear or feelings continue to flow in the system. The animal may not communicate its feelings but the fear psychosis flows in our blood. If you do not use vegetables they go rotten; although there is life in them, you do the minimum of harm by eating them. They are soothing to the system. Today, of course, vegetarian food is also commercialised and there is tremendous rapaciousness in growing vegetables for money – so there is also violence involved.

All I would say is that if there is no saliva when you eat, then that food is injurious, whatever it may be. I will not talk about diet because I cannot forget my early life. I have lived on water continuously for days. So you have to choose food that refines your mind that keeps you lighter and makes you happier. If you do not feel heavy in your alimentary system one hour after eating, then that is good food. You must judge for yourself, even with vegetarian food, what is soothing to your practice.

The beauty of yogic practice is that when you get involved in it, your system does not accept the non-vegetarian food or meat. *Sādhanā* brings the natural transformation, which I feel is more genuine and effective.

Q.- What is your special diet?

To be honest, I do not like to be special. I am one like you. I take the same food as you consume. Only I choose what is light to digest in the given circumstances. I am a vegetarian and I have not even touched eggs.

As a man who has come from dire poverty, how can I take affluent food when millions of my brothers and sisters do not get one square meal? In my early days, I have lived on tea and coffee. When I wanted to eat, God did not give me. When everything is there, my mind goes back to the early days and it does not allow me to indulge in food. One thing is certain, that I never over-eat or choose foods. If one chooses food, one is not a yogi.

However, I love sweets; yet people call me bitter or violent! But one thing is that I never try to sugarcoat any talk or behaviour.

Q.- Would you say that yoga is international?

We are all human beings, but we have been taught to think of ourselves as Westerners or Easterners. If we were left to ourselves we would simply be individual human beings, no Africans, no Indians. People tell me I come from India so I develop certain characteristics to appear Indian. But when you and I meet together, we forget ourselves. There are no divisions and we talk mind to mind, soul to soul.

Yoga is not an international culture but a universal culture as it universalises each individual from the body up to the seat of consciousness. There is no difference in the seer. The difference comes only between the "garments" of the seer – the consciousness, the mind, the senses of perception and the intelligence. Break them; do not feed them with divisive ideas. That is what yoga teaches.

Patañjali used the expression *sārvabhauma* – universal – some 2,500 years ago. So yoga is a universal cult. When it is universal where is the question of internationality? We have divided the nation according to the political ideas and differences. The veda says *vasudhaiva kutuṁbakam*. *Vasudhā* means Earth – our planet and *kutuṁba* means family. The earth is one family. The veda did not divide the earth into parts. So the question is not of internationality. It is a universal art for every human being that is wanting in his emotions, his instincts, his intelligence, to improve. So if yoga can build up right knowledge, stabilise the emotions, transform instinct into intuition, take it from me that you and I lose all differences and we all become one. That is the universality of yoga.

Despite my limited knowledge, I have tried to give clarity and not confusion. If there is any confusion, please do not ask my pupils but write to me directly and I will clear it up. God bless you.

MOULDING LIFE*

Q.- Is there a humorous side to B.K.S. Iyengar?

I do not know whether I have a humorous side. Yoga is serious devotional work. But I give them enough to laugh at. I joke in class not only with my pupils but also with myself. My students immensely enjoy my imitation of their defects. Life cannot be always serious. Without humour, teaching cannot be fresh and it cannot easily be absorbed.

Q.- More than half the participants at your birthday celebrations were Westerners. Why is it that they are so drawn towards you?

We, in India, over-notice foreigners. There were only ten to fifteen percent of foreigners. They come to me possibly because they have nowhere else to go to learn and understand the true aspects of yoga!!

Q.- You and Rajneesh share the same zodiac sign. Who is the real *Bhagwān*?

There is only one *Bhagwān*, Krishna, Narayana, Śiva, by whatever name you call. We are all *Bhāgvata*[1] of the Lord, i.e. particles of God and not *Bhagvāns*.

Q.- Rajneesh has so many physical ailments. Can you fix him?

Yoga is a therapeutic as well as a spiritual science. From the therapeutic point of view, it is the duty of a doctor or healer to help if the patient approaches him. But ultimately the cure is not in my

---

* Interview for *Poona Digest*, December 1988.

[1] *Bhāgvata* – The devotee of the Lord. The one who follows the path laid by God.

hands. I am an instrument of God. Only through His blessings can cure come as sleep comes. Whether it is Shri Rajneesh[1] or any one on the street, if approached, I may attend immediately or a little later according to the time that is at my disposal. The yogic path is not denied to anyone.

Q.- A slightly personal question. Despite your incredible capacity for body flexibility, why do you have a paunch?

For the simple reason that if one is thin, one has no waistline and flexibility is taken for granted. I have deliberately kept a little bit of paunch to show that a stout septuagenarian can be very agile. You have to give me credit that even this paunch is no barrier for my doing everything. The paunch has not come in the way of my remaining unsurpassed in the field of yoga.[2]

Q.- Can you live up till a hundred through yoga?

Birth and death are not in our hands. But the space between birth and death can be definitely moulded by our will power, perseverance, persistence and tenacity to maintain what has been learned and sustained. It is not a question of whether I live for a hundred years. My only desire is, I should be as good in yoga and other things till my last moment as I am today.

Q.- What is your most terrible memory?

Pains, aches, the tear of the tendons, tear of muscles in my early practice are among the terrible memories.

---

[1] Actually Achārya Rajneesh's father had taken a few lessons from me in the late sixties. He found a tremendous improvement and relaxation during the course. I helped him to solve the problems that he was facing during meditation. At that point of time Rajneesh's father mentioned to me that his son should learn yoga under my guidance in order to get rid of stress, high blood pressure, diabetes and tremendous fatigue and exertion. He, in fact spoke to Rajneesh who said that one day he will come when he gets the time. However that did not happen.

[2] In fact, he does not have a "paunch" because of eating. It is rather a tremendous over exertion. He is the only one who has taught continously for almost sixty-eight years. His teaching process is unique and therefore effective, he performs *āsana* and *prāṇāyāma* during the teaching process several times along with a commentary in order to convey the accuracy. Again he goes to the students personally and fixes them in the proper position. This kind of exertion brought about the puffing of the abdomen. He was not only a tuberculosis case but had suffered from rickets which went un-diagnosed and untreated. He came out of it only with yogic practice.

One other terrible memory that stands out is the yoga demonstration before the International Conference of Doctors for Cancer in 1952. I was asked to give a lecture-demonstration but the late Dr. Khanolkar, the then President of the Conference, told me on the stage that I should not speak at all. This was the terrible experience. It was the conference of doctors. All of a sudden, he asked me to cancel the lecture and demonstrate the *āsana*. It would have made no sense by just demonstrating the *āsana* one after the other, without giving any background of the subject. I had travelled to Mumbai all the way for this purpose. Again, he gave me only ten minutes to demonstrate. But fortunately it went on for fifty-five minutes as the delegates insisted I showed more. Though I was prevented from explaining the science and beauty of yoga, after, say thirty minutes, I asked them to permit me to speak. When the President permitted me to speak, I explained the value of yoga, continued my demonstration, and stopped even though the delegates wanted more and more. Thirty-three scientists from all over the world were present.

Q.- There is an allegation that you are particularly violent towards the women in your class. Is it true? Please clarify.

People mistake my intensity for violence. It may be a rumour spread by my yoga colleagues or professional colleagues to frighten people not to come to me. I am neither violent nor softhearted. For your information, I may tell you that I am not an attractive person. The women are attracted to my art and my character. That is why I have more than sixty percent women as my pupils and more than eighty percent are family members of the womenfolk in the class. If I was violent, then the women students would not have come to me and would not have sent their family members to my classes.

Firstly, I am certainly a very strict disciplinarian. As far as the practice of *āsana* is concerned, accuracy, awareness, perfection, attention, faith and devotion are my demands. In demanding these qualities in practice if you call this violent and rough behaviour of mine towards the pupils, I do not know what to answer. As far as women are concerned normally they do not expect roughness from a man. My demanding nature for yogic discipline appears as rough or violent for you, the media people and not for them. Do not mistake my sincerity for violence. I am not a propagandist but a very religious practitioner and teacher.

Q.- Do you believe in *Guru dakṣiṇā* apart from fees?

It is better to collect fees and live with a clean conscience. I stick to the fees even though they call me a commercial man. *Guru dakṣiṇā* should not be unlimited commercialism in the name of divinity. *Guru dakṣiṇā* is commercialism coated with divinity.

Q.- Would you ever wear a suit?

I was wearing pants and shirts up to the age of sixty. After sixty, to respect age, I changed to simple *dhoti*, *jubba* and *shawl*. I wear this dress even when I go abroad. I walk on streets like a proud Indian, wearing *dhoti* and *jubba* and a long red mark on my forehead as a mark of the auspiciousness of each day.

Q.- What do you remember most about your trips abroad?

Quite a few significant occasions.

(a) My appearance in London University in 1960 to give a lecture-cum-demonstration before the academic elite. Yehudi Menuhin introduced me to the distinguished audience. My knowledge of English was very poor then. But I was thrilled when all clapped for minutes admiring my presentation.

(b) In 1963, I appeared on BBC in a programme, "Yehudi Menuhin and his *Guru*".

(c) In 1971, when I had a tremendous unbearable backache that made it impossible even to stand or sit. In spite of it I gave a solo lecture-cum-demonstration in a well packed Westminster Hall, in London, for three hours.

(d) In 1978, my lecture-cum-demonstration at UNO to present before the community of nations, the cultural heritage of India.

(e) In 1980 at the capital of Swaziland, Southern Africa, I gave a lecture-cum-demonstration in unusual costume. In a hurry, while travelling to the city, which is about fifty miles away, I had forgotten my yoga costume. I took a bed sheet from my hotel, cut it in the form of *langot*, and gave the demonstration before 600 people. There was enthusiastic and non-stop clapping when I narrated the story of my historical underwear.

(f) Last but not the least, my demonstration in Tokyo, Japan, in 1981. The hall was filled to capacity and there were thousands of people, who went on and on clapping for each of my *āsana* presentations and never allowed me to stop until they had forced me to do all the *āsana* as they are in my book *Light on Yoga*.

Q.- Can yoga be taught through television?

Yoga cannot be taught through T.V. But it is possible to ignite interest towards yoga by presenting the subject along with the demonstration of *āsana* and *prāṇāyāma* educatively, attractively and accurately, as they should be done in the truest sense of the terms.

Q.- Would you ever become private adviser to some important politician? Please give reasons for your answer.

Politicians with prejudices and ambitions will not take advice from yogis as the yogis are straightforward. Hence the question does not arise at all. But there is the danger of the yogis being used by politicians for their political ends.

Q.- Give us the golden rules to perfect health.

Character building and culturing of the cells through yogic practices is the golden rule for perfect health. The unison between the cells and the individual leads to perfect health where body, mind and soul work with 100% co-operation and concord.

A CONVERSATION WITH *GURUJĪ**

The afternoon sun slants oddly into the cavernous library. The air is hushed and composed around our dear Gurujī. *His dynamic and energetic stance is relaxed, but there is a certain quiet alertness in his* 'āsana' *as he sits sedately, on his furred chair. This is a rare opportunity – to catch* Gurujī *by himself, when he is in an expansive mood – ready to talk; and the words flow like a mountain stream.* Gurujī *has been talking about consolidation, repose and his increasing detachment from the effort of teaching yoga. The struggle in one sense is over.*

Today, hundreds flock to see and learn his art, to imbibe his rigorous discipline, hoping that some shade of their guru's *greatness will cast its spell benignly on them. In his discourses and also as he stalks around in his classes, he is drawn increasingly into himself. It is an inwardness that has resulted in greater clarity, simplicity and conviction. Today as we sit to talk, I marvel at his wit and sparkle. He is not easy to 'catch'. His abrupt, sometimes brusque manners, harsh interjections, unexpected chuckles made the interview a challenge. Energetic, intellectually full of vigour, characteristically witty, devastatingly ironic, warm, and engagingly frank,* Gurujī *is always the impresario. Ultimately, his presence transcends all that is written about him.*

Q.- *Gurujī,* you have been termed a 'violent teacher'. How do you feel about this epithet?

My 'violence', as they call it, is really my sincerity and integrity and my intensity of purpose. It is a merciless mercifulness. Unless I appeal to the fire in you to get the spark with the fire in me, how will you learn? *(A statement typically paradoxical.)*

---

* By the late Neela Karnik. December 1988. Published in the *Souvenir Book* of the 70th Birthday Celebrations, reprinted in *70 Glorious Years of Yogacharya B.K.S. Iyengar* and in *Yogapushpāñjali.*

Q.- You have often spoken of your perseverance, trials and triumphs in the path of yoga and of the influence that this struggle has had on your practices especially in the evolution of the dynamics of your poses. How must your students, who rely so much on your book *Light on Yoga*, understand this? Surely a perfect pose may be utterly 'hollow'.

Oh yes! *(He chuckles impishly).*

Many of my sincere students try to imitate me. It has the wrong kind of effect. I convince them to be creative, not imitative. Imitation too has to be a path to convert into one's own and originality makes the practice lively. Each *āsana* is a manifestation of a mental working. I speak of my yoga as an art and I use my body as a painter would use his canvas or a musician his instrument. *Yogāsana* are not prototechnics. The quality of spirituality is inherent in each body. If the body is the mirror to the mind, the *āsana* will reflect that self-awareness, consciousness and deep intelligence – it will be an act of the mind on the body and self.

Q.- But *Light on Yoga* is a teacher's book. It concentrates on the techniques of the *āsana*.

(Typically, Gurujī *interrupts me. Impatient, he is miles ahead and has anticipated my questions and objections.)*

If I had to write it again, I would write it quite differently.

(What a revelation! As I gasp in astonishment, Gurujī *gently talks about one of the most difficult and challenging phases of his life, which culminated in the idea of* Light on Yoga*).*

The book was written when I felt the need to convince people of my authenticity and sincerity. I had no *guru* at that time for the kind of task I had to perform – to carry yoga to the people at large. I had to evolve my own techniques to teach. Now, I am proud of this fact. You see, there is no book on yoga prior to *Light on Yoga* giving the detailed techniques. After all what do techniques stand for: they stand as an essential ingredient to reach the precision, which is nothing but the taste of divinity. Techniques are a part of an attempt to reach the Ultimate.

However I was always convinced that *āsana* was an essential part of the eight aspects of yoga or the *aṣṭāṅga yoga* as Patañjali calls it. It could not be differentiated or separated from other aspects of yoga. Yet, I worked to bring out how the body, that is the instrument of the soul is trimmed to convince them to see the truth behind *āsana sādhanā*. To project my *āsana* as a totality, was the challenge of the '30s and '40s. I faced these boldly by rigorous practice and minute attention to detail. It was *svādhyāya*. My body was the book and my mind and awareness was the keen avaricious pupil who could not learn enough. Even my limitations helped me learn.

Later, I also learnt that mathematical precision, calculation and skilful presentation are the essence of this art. It is what culminated in the *āsana* in *Light on Yoga*. The understanding, the struggle, the dynamics, were the hidden contexts that forced the precision of the *āsana*. Then I developed... The *āsana* came because I followed the principles of other aspects of yoga in totality. I involved my entire self – physical, emotional and intellectual. The entire body became the base for meditation. Each *āsana* for me acted as meditation. The body is a temple. The *ātmā* needs a clean place to live in. That is why the book shows a detailed technique for the dweller of the body to live contentedly. The book will have the limitation of a book and my pupils as well as my readers must realise this. When I am teaching you, you realise how I involve you in your own culturing of body and mind. Don't you feel that you are evolving emotionally, intellectually and spiritually when we both communicate in the art of learning the subject. Now this could not be put in the book; it is implicit in my technique.

Q.- How would you change the book?

I would include the finer things as well. For instance, how to penetrate the *pañcakośa*,[1] how to balance the *pañcabhūta* – the five elements of the body – how to channel the *pañcavāyu* which bring about the changes in you. This is a subjective transfer. It cannot be given as a rule.

Q.- Do you feel it is easier to teach now than earlier?

Yes. A lot of the earlier tension has eased; problems like how to teach yoga en masse or how to teach women or very young children or the effort I had to make to prove that yoga had to be part of the syllabi in an educational curriculum, are no longer acute problems. More people accept it, probably because it is fashionable. I don't know. Now the struggle is very different, wrong things are propagated more easily than the right things. By this I mean that a teacher, more than anyone else, has to teach by example. One cannot grow spiritually without moral or ethical awareness. My ethics make them aware of their ethics. That is my way of teaching. If I am sometimes blamed for this, well, it is for the good. One must take a broader view and look at the good of society.

---

[1] For further reference see *Aṣṭadaḷa Yogamālā* vol 2. "The Dual Function of *Āsana*", "*Āsanajaya* – a Search for the Infinite" and "*Āsana*: Physical, mental or Spiritual Practice", "*Yogāsana*: A search for the Infinite in the Finite", "*Yogāsana* – To yoke the Body-Mind to the Self", "The Grace of Consciousness in Āsana", "*Āsana* – Cosmic and not Cosmetic", "*Jñāna* in *Āsana*: Experiential Knowledge", "*Saṁyama* in *Āsana*".

Q.- Were there any failures in your life? Did you feel exiled from the grace of your art at any time?

(A shadow passes over his eyes and for a moment his ebullience is stilled, as he recollects the days of frustration when nothing would move with the fluidity of motion and joy.)

Yes, there was a distinct period of barrenness or turbulence... In 1944, the year of my first failure, when nothing was moving within, I felt 'stale'. My practice was still hard but it was coming from my will, my ego. There was no inner harmony, it was important but it was missing. My presentation was 'soulless'.

(When Gurujī *speaks with such sensitive self-reflectiveness and anguish, who can say that his yoga does not reflect the inner life?)*

In 1958, it was the onset of giddiness, it affected me whatever I did. There wasn't anything but tenacity in my practice. My horizons went beyond pain into the clear light of knowing. That is how I evolved. I am self-taught in this way... the evolution of this intelligence and my awareness of a language, where does it come from? I am a sentimental man and I have faith in my subject... a faith that bathes the soul. I believe it comes from there. Then in 1977, I had two accidents, which I felt negated all my progress in yoga. I was at a zero stage.

(I felt the prickles crawl along my back as I imagined this man of vitality and optimism facing the abyss of zero. How did he begin to recover? Where did he look for that spring of regeneration?)

I had torn the muscles in both shoulders, my spine got twisted and had lost its alignment; each *āsana* was painful. I vowed not to cut my hair until I had regained some of my former skill and strength. Then came the long, arduous and almost clinical analysis – the ABC of *Trikoṇāsana.*[1] It was a form of meditation for me. In the process, I developed a masterful technique for teaching this *āsana.* I had recovered. God gave me the pain, you get the benefits.

(A smile flashes in a mercurial moment his mood changes from the sombre to the bright.)

Q.- *Gurujī,* in your classes you have students of different calibre, how do you teach them all at once? Each student understands and applies what you teach in his or her own way, according to the kind of *sādhaka* he/she is. Is this something you do consciously as a teacher or is it inherent in the art of yoga itself?

---

[1] A video cassette of the same name is available.

It is in the teaching. I had to evolve a method and then a language. The subject is highly esoteric and it was riddled with misconceptions; a large part of my teaching was to clarify certain ideas for myself and for my students. It was a highly educative process. I had compassion and I learnt from each kind of student: the mild *(mṛdu)*, the average *(madhyama)*, the keen *(adhimātra)* and the intense *(tīvra)*. I tried through identification with them, and internalising their weaknesses in me I learnt. I have taught great intellectuals, but I have also taught great duffers, eh!

(Gurujī *laughs heartily, remembering no doubt, some uproarious situations. He has taught scientists, philosophers, businessmen, housewives, professionals and even men of faith – Christian priests, Muslims and Jains. He has communicated the philosophy of yoga in the language of each one's faith. Truly remarkable! He is generous with his art.*

He says, "Even if a totally unethical man develops a bit of ethical quality, I will have done my duty. That is why I teach according to their capacity... When I teach children, I teach according to their nature. I have to become a child. So I learn from everybody. There is a quality of innocence that one must take from a madman and a quality of courage from the wise man.")

Q.- Recently, you have been talking more and more about renunciation in practice. What does it mean? Have you invested this term with your inimitable interpretation?

"Renunciation in practice" was my answer to a lot of people who wondered why I continued to practise even after I have achieved what I wanted. But by 'renunciation', I mean freedom of the self. When one stops thinking of the 'effect' or the fruit, it is a deep, inward experience. It is not meditation as the term is used today, which is more a kind of sedative, a drug, which does not allow full spiritual growth. *Dhyāna* is electrifying. Through it one withdraws from the periphery to the core. This very journey from the periphery to the core is *vairāgya*. There is a detachment from the effect and attachment to the Soul. One has to transcend the *tri-guṇa – sattva, rajas and tamas* – while practising.

Q.- What kind of an art is yoga? Music or dance or dramatics being emotional, how does yoga qualify as an art?

(Gurujī *looks thoughtful, but is never at a loss for words.)*

Though yoga has a scientific base, when it is put into practice, all of one's skill is needed. The *citta vṛtti nirodha* is a very subtle thought that has to be dealt with in a subtle manner; it has to be revealed, the inner through the outer. Each *āsana* is a delicate balance, a harmony between the inner and outer, the mind and the body. Though it begins with a physical vehicle, the body, it is taken to the level of the soul. Creatively, there is sublimation, the gross emotions like anger, frustration, despair, are all sublimated. One goes beyond mere feelings or emotions. All arts have science *(śāstra)* and art *(kalā)*. The *ānanda* (bliss) expressed and experienced in a fine artistic state or aesthetic divine state is art.[1]

Q.- What expectations have remained unfulfilled?

(Gurujī *chides me for using the word 'expectation'.)*

The word implies worries and anxieties that I do not have.

Q.- How do you see the future of yoga shaping?

My friend, yoga is as old as civilisation itself. Once it was pure and uncontaminated. But since men will take from this great repository of wisdom according to their natures, it may be tainted; it depends on us. Our myths have taught us the co-existence of good and evil, pain and happiness. That is how we experience them and we measure them, whichever dominates our lives. But once a *sādhaka* has had a fragrance of pure *ānanda*, he will hanker after it, become a seeker of the divine. There will be upheavals but no void or barrenness. Just as everything in nature lies dormant for the rain, light or grain of sand to regenerate, so too there is a time to create a pearl from one's *sādhanā*.

As you all know, I see the future of yoga to be very bright. The credit for this goes to you all, for the simple reason that you all formed the Light on Yoga Research Trust. This is now getting generous public support, by way of advertisements and donations. This has given me great hope that the beneficial effect of the work, which I started 55 years ago, seems to be bestowed permanently on future generations. If not for this hope and confidence, I would tend to be pessimistic, even though I am not a born pessimist. While you generously credit me for starting the Trust, I feel that the efforts and continued support have ensured its sustenance and growth. With the Trust, the great yogic switch has been turned on by you all. I would like to express my gratitude to you all, though you are my pupils.

The brightness of yoga is going to enlighten further not only through the Trust members, but also through all my countless pupils spread all over the globe. We could collect data through

---

1 See *Aṣṭadaḷa Yogamālā*, vol. 1 – "Is Yoga Art, Science, Religion or Philosophy", and in vol. 3 "Yoga and Dance".

them and go in for new methods and research, to study the actual changes taking place while in the process of doing, rather than the evaluation of results. The present-day yogis are only doing the conditioning of the pressures and stresses 'before and after'. Our Trust should not commit this mistake but study the changes in the nervous and circulatory systems and the changes in the brain while the structural adjustments are made in the body. If this is presented in a scientific manner through the Light on Yoga Research Trust, I am certain that yoga is going to take a permanent place in the scientific world as a discipline of great utilitarian value to the human race.

Q.- What are the concrete steps that need to be taken to preserve the pure form of yoga?

As an individual, without help and support from anyone, I built up this art and made people of different intellectual levels to taste and enjoy the fruits thereof. It would surprise you to know that I have taught yoga to people from all walks of life: sweepers to postmen, policemen to administrators, musicians, dancers, writers, lawyers, doctors, sportsmen, politicians and philosophers. Craftsmen like carpenters and others have also been my pupils. In fact, I have taken this art to people in all trades and professions, all round the world.

I consider that one of my greatest achievements has been the formation of the Light on Yoga Research Trust. This Trust must provide stipends to genuine students interested in learning, teaching and propagating yoga. If, after a good training, these students could be absorbed as yoga teachers and sent to villages to teach and spread this art, I am sure that yoga would have a concrete bearing not only on the urban intellectuals but also on a large number of innocent, rural masses. The villages will then become beautiful health resorts.

Governments all over the world are spending millions for research on diseases and drugs to make unhealthy people healthy. But alas! No Government has woken up to the need to keep healthy people healthy. Hence, I consider that this Trust has a tremendous challenging responsibility to offer the means, not only for the unhealthy to turn healthy but also for the healthy ones to remain healthier for ever. I would be more than gratified if all of you could continue your support to the Trust to fulfil this dream of mine. I would consider this as a concrete step for a great leap forward.

GURUJĪ ON *PRĀṆĀYĀMA**

Gurujī *was hardly sixteen years old when he went to Mysore to study yoga. During that time, he was under the* guru's *tutelage for a very short period.* Guru *T. Krishnamacharya was concerned more with very vigorous and intensive practice in* āsana.

Being a sick person by birth, the practice of merely the āsana *made him weak. He had no strength even to stand. The lungs were inexpansive. Even the normal breathing was a strain. However, circumstances forced him to teach yoga, and he did so.*

Naturally, at that time it was not possible for him to do prāṇāyāma. *His* guru *was unwilling to teach, perhaps because of his structure of the chest, which was narrow and collapsed. When his* guru *visited Pune in 1940,* Gurujī *asked him about* prāṇāyāma. Guru *Krishnamacharya gave him just an outline of* prāṇāyāma. *He said to do deep inhalation and to hold the breath and to do deep exhalation. This was the victual that was available to* Gurujī *on which he built up the whole empire of* prāṇāyāma.

Knowing this very well, I approached Gurujī *for the interview, which I thought worthwhile for every student of yoga. I am sure that this will guide those who are on the path of yoga.*

Q.- *Gurujī,* you have already mentioned that you had to face a lot of problems to start with *prāṇāyāma.*[1] I have a few queries here.

You said that whenever you sat to do *prāṇāyāma,* the negative thoughts used to overpower you to give up the practice of *prāṇāyāma* for the day after a few trials. Can you talk about these "negative thoughts"?

Patañjali clearly mentions that *prāṇāyāma* is practised after the mastery of *āsana.* A practitioner has to gain stability, strength and courage to proceed towards *prāṇāyāma.* In my case, though I had

---

* An interview by the late Neela Karnik on the occasion of the author's 70th birthday – December 1988 – first published in *70 Glorious Years of Yogacharya B.K.S. Iyengar – Commemoration Volume.* Light on Yoga Research Trust, 1990.

[1] See *Aṣṭadala Yogamālā*, vol. 1, pp. 62-65.

practised *āsana*, there was no guidance from my *guru* about which poses and in which way the *āsana* have to be practised to proceed towards *prāṇāyāma*.

I used to get totally exhausted with the practice of *āsana*, which made my ribs, intercostal muscles and lungs literally numb; therefore I had lost the sensitivity for proper respiration.

My *guru* had already instructed me to do deep inhalation, retention and deep exhalation. This made the situation worse since I was not given any technical instruction. Fortunately, I, having a strong will power, did not decline towards depression. There was a strong inclination to tread on the path of yoga. In my case, the weakness, lack of strength, instability of the body, which Patañjali explains as *aṅgamejayatva*, or unsteadiness of body and irregular as well as laboured breathing, caused the problem. Therefore, for me it was not the negative thoughts but the physical inability to withstand the practice of *prāṇāyāma*. The shallow breathing was creating hollowness within the body, which was creating shakiness in the body, fear complex and breathlessness. Perhaps there was a big gap between "knowing" and "doing". My *guru* had already put an idea in my head that the breathing should be deep, therefore I knew that I have to take a deep breath. This is a "knowing" part. But it was not happening, I knew that I was not "doing". There was a huge gap between the idea and practice. This gap did not make me negative but restless.

Fortunately, my practice of *āsana* kept me restlessly on the practice track. Therefore, I used to feel, "If not *prāṇāyāma*, then let me do *āsana*."

Later, when I started teaching, I came across many sufferers who had taken to the practice of *prāṇāyāma* without having any background of the practice of *āsana*. Such people suffered with headache, bleeding nostrils, eccentricity, mental imbalance, amnesia, insomnia and what not. I consider myself lucky in this sense because though I used to lose the battle, the "inner fire of hope" never extinguished. In a way the practice of *āsana* protected me.

Q.- *Gurujī*, you have mentioned to us once that you used to do a lot of back extensions and that caused the failures in *prāṇāyāma*. Is it so?

I do not attribute this failure to my wrong practice of *āsana* but to my overdoing them more than my nerves could take. From the day I was taught backbends, I had overexerted myself in backbends; I realised that it was on account of my hours of practice of my backward extensions that my body gained suppleness but not the power of resistance. If I kept my spine up straight by force in order to do *prāṇāyāma*, my chest would become taut and breathing would be heavy and laboured. So I began to sit taking the support of the wall. This released the tension of the muscles of the chest but I could not sit longer.

My chest muscles used to become sore. Therefore, I had to open my mouth to breathe after one or two deep breaths. Then I had to wait for a few minutes to take another two deep breaths. I was restless throughout. After three or four breaths, I was feeling heavy in my head.

It is true that I was paying more attention to back bends as they were spectacular. In 1958, for the first time, I made up my mind to do forward bends with chronological timings like back bends. The forward bends were giving more excruciating, sore pains than back bends. This sore and dull pain continued even after the practice for hours. The pain was of such a nature that I felt as if someone was hitting my back with a sledgehammer. This pain from forward bending made me live with pain, but in due course I overcame the pain and I do them with timings once a week even to this day.

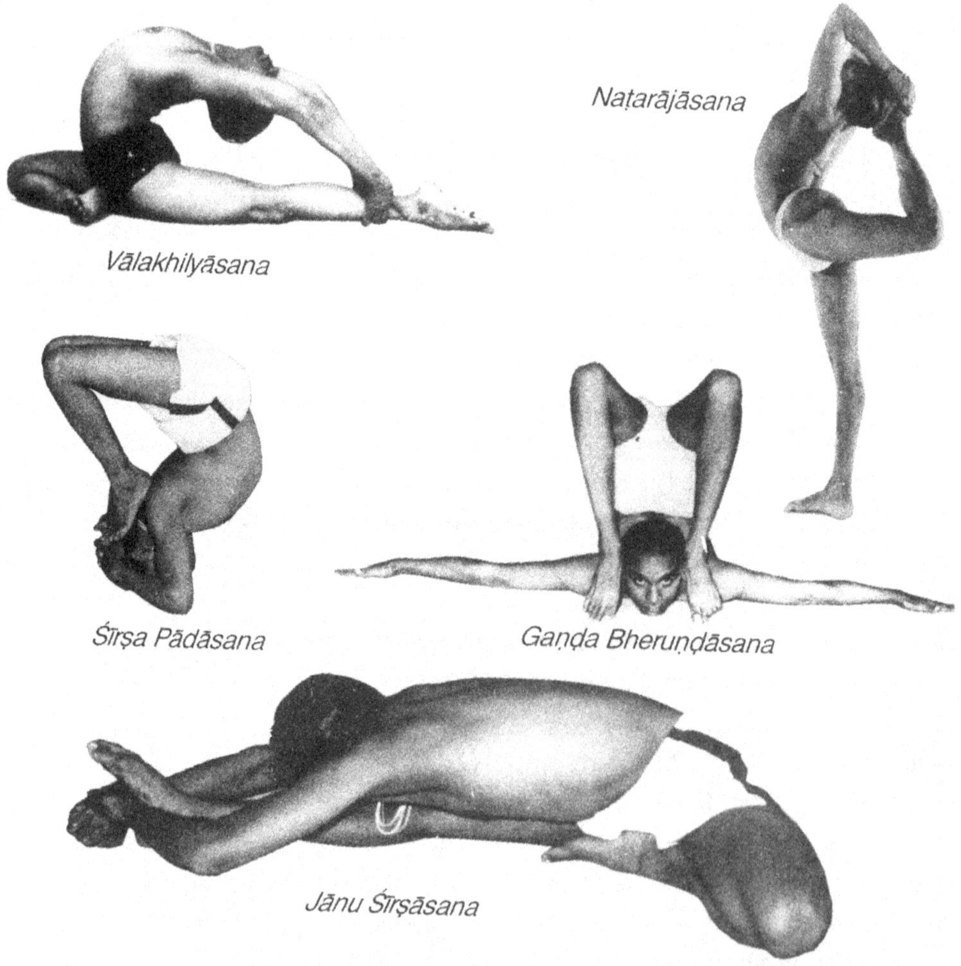
Naṭarājāsana
Vālakhilyāsana
Śīrṣa Pādāsana
Gaṇḍa Bheruṇḍāsana
Jānu Śīrṣāsana

Plate n. 23 – The spectacular back-bends and forward extensions in *Jānu Śīrṣāsana*

Forward extensions such as *Jānu Śīrṣāsana* began to help me keep the spine erect while doing *prāṇāyāma*. I learnt from this experience that back bends strengthen the inner muscles of the spinal column while forward extensions develop and strengthen its outer muscles. I could sit well and use the inner and outer muscles of the spine to run parallel to each other while doing *prāṇāyāma*.

This taught me a lesson that forward bends, back bends and lateral movements of the spinal muscles ought to be developed to tone the muscles of the spine as they act as a base for good *prāṇāyāma*. I realised how a balanced practice of *āsana* is required to do proper *prāṇāyāma*.

All these failures taught me many things in the art of teaching *prāṇāyāma*. Though it is essential to learn from a master, as a teacher was not available to me, I learnt the methods in the art of practice of *prāṇāyāma* by chance. The credit and merit of my repeated struggles, failures and successes, culminated in 1980 with my book *Light on Prāṇāyāma*[1] that will act as a living *guru* for a long time. Every yoga teacher claims that if one is out of mood or dejected, the practice of *prāṇāyāma* helps to overcome that state of mind. You can never do *prāṇāyāma* with an upset mind. That is what I learnt. Sometimes I used to feel fresh in the practice of *prāṇāyāma*, while at other times it was bringing a moody state and tension because I never knew how to relax the brain in inhalation or the art of grip needed in the process of exhalation.

However, with all these hurdles in my practice, I say emphatically that I had a strong determination to continue. The determination made me to face successive failures very courageously. Therefore, there was no negativity on my part but restlessness due to failures.

Q.- *Gurujī*, you talked about your determination. Now how much of this *prāṇāyāma* learning was determination or did you feel a predisposition for this innate art within you? How far did you have to surrender to that force?

Of course, there was a predisposition, which was perhaps unknown to me; otherwise, I would not have tried the same again and again as well as day in and day out. Determination was the outcome of my disposition and inner tendency.

It was not a complete negative attitude of surrender but a will just to do. You can say that I surrendered to this inner hidden predisposition but my will power forced me to have strong determination. Both helped me to progress further.

No doubt, I had one thing in my mind. That was, how to make myself fit to teach *prāṇāyāma* for group classes. Though I agreed to take *prāṇāyāma* classes, finding that I could not explain well, I changed them into meditation classes by explaining the mental effects of *prāṇāyāma*.

---

[1] Published by Harper Collins, London.

I tried to explain methods of *prāṇāyāma* that I was doing. But the right words were not coming. I had said sometime back[1] that when I failed in *prāṇāyāma* I took to *trāṭaka*, in which gazing is done. The practice of *trāṭaka* helped me to explain meditation by progressing from active, non-blinking of the eyeballs towards passivity of the eyeballs and eyelids with closed eyes. I took precaution that my pupils did not suffer with the problems that I had to face after *trāṭaka* such as burning sensation, day blindness, headaches and tension.

While I was explaining the passive sides of the *trāṭaka*, I was acting at the same time as a teacher and as a pupil. If one part of my intelligence acted as a *guru*, the other part acted as a *śiṣya* (pupil). So, I was a *guru* and a *śiṣya* at the same time. This made me think and to use words carefully so that the learners could get the points right. I also used to work on myself using the same words to see the reactions. Often, I constructed words according to my experience and changed my stance in group classes. Through actions and observations I understood the ascending and descending energies of my intelligence and learnt the art of surrendering the intelligence and will power from the seat of the head towards the seat of the heart, which you call conscience. Soon it helped me to teach the techniques of *prāṇāyāma* better and better. That is how I learnt to practise and teach. My early failures were because of lack of guidance as well as my own weakness.

As the challenge came to me to teach *āsana* in 1936, similarly the challenge to teach *prāṇāyāma* came to me from pupils in 1970. In those days, when I was running group classes of *āsana*, many of the yogis criticised me saying that *āsana* could not be taught on a mass scale. I was a pioneer to introduce *āsana* in groups in 1937. Similarly, I accepted the challenge of teaching *prāṇāyāma* in group classes and gained confidence as I went on teaching. Until then I was under the impression that *āsana* could be taught to many at the same time, but not *prāṇāyāma*. After years of experience, I learnt the art of seeing many doing at the same time and could observe the mistakes at once. I codified the sentences needed in general for public or what you call the open classes and slowly developed to impart subtle points of explanations that people could take with ease. This is how I learnt the art of practice and art of teaching *prāṇāyāma* simultaneously.

Q.- *Gurujī*, as you have told us, in most of the other systems, normally *prāṇāyāma* is taught mechanically, in as much as they sort of count down inhalations to a time schedule; they say, one, two, three, four. Whereas you have concentrated more on the physiological and the psychological aspect of *prāṇāyāma*. So how did you develop this technique? Some teachers recommend the practice of *prāṇāyāma* first, then *āsana* while you emphasise first practice of *āsana*.

---

[1] See *Aṣṭadaḷa Yogamālā*, vol. 1, p. 63.

It is true that most people recommend *prāṇāyāma* first. I feel that one has to make the inner body healthy, clean and free from blockages through the practice of various *āsana* and prepare the body for the life force circulated in the body that is generated from the practice of *prāṇāyāma*. Otherwise, the generated life force or vital energy will not only be wasted but prone to be injurious. Hence I prefer the body – the temple – to be clean and healthy for the life force to move freely without obstructions.

It is a fact that all textbooks speak of the ratio of inhalation, exhalation and retention, whereas Patañjali does not speak of the ratios but of depth, subtlety and precision. If one concentrates on counting the numbers looking at the movement of the second hand of the watch, then the practitioner is only interested in attending to the numbers and not attending to the movement of breath within the body, reaction of the fibres and the reaction of the cells. Even muttering the *mantra* while doing *prāṇāyāma* may become a *japa* and not *prāṇāyāma*. If one is doing *prāṇāyāma*, one should be totally absorbed in the fineness of inbreath, outbreath and naturalness of retention without causing any stress in the cells of the brain or unnecessary disturbances or jerks to the vital organs and nerves.

Everybody will have his own capacity of inhalation, exhalation and retention, which cannot be forced by using the will power on lungs or brain. One may count the numbers or chant the *mantra*. The *mantra* also will have a certain meter, certain length, which could be long or short. How can one chant the *mantra*, even mentally, in order to equal the length or duration to the duration of inhalation or exhalation or retention? Obviously, one hurries up either with inhalation, exhalation, retention, or with *mantra japa* or with counts. And then both the breath and *mantra japa*, or the counting, go in an unrhythmic way.

Suppose, the lungs cannot hold to the prolonged inhalation – *pūraka* – or exhalation – *recaka*, what does one do then? One pays attention to complete the *mantra* rather than paying attention to the qualitative approach in the process of inhalation or exhalation. In such cases, inhalations may be prolonged, while exhalation period may be short or vice versa. For many, concentration is not on *prāṇāyāma* but on the *mantra*. This way, one loses the factual practice of *prāṇāyāma*. Many would be more particular to finish the counts or the *mantra* while doing *prāṇāyāma*. In that case, it cannot be termed *prāṇāyāma* but *mantrāyāma*. Therefore it is better to keep the brain as an instrument to witness and observe the smooth flow of inhalation and exhalation. Better to watch the interruptions occurring even from inhalation to exhalation. One should check the unknown occurrences of interruptions, and feel and see that the smooth flow sets in. Similarly, in retention, learn to retain the first grip, which is free from the stress factor, throughout with stability. If that stability loosens, then it is better to let go the breath, rather than holding the breath with strain.

How did I develop this technique? I too was under the impression that the *mantra* has to be used as measurement of time, as others are. But soon I realised that this makes the mind to rush the *mantra* creating fluctuation. The mind and the breath both go on hurrying, and there begins an inner clash. In order to stop this rush and hurry, I preferred to watch my breath and mind in order not to fluctuate in the process of practice. This gave me a key point to learn and proceed gradually with confidence.

Prāṇa is life force, commonly known as bio-energy. We are made up of five elements. If the element of earth is the foundation, the element of ether is the distributing element. Element of air acts as a piston in the form of inhalation and exhalation to fuse the remaining two elements, water and fire, through which energy is generated (because of their opposite qualities). This is *prāṇāyāma*.

Q.- *Guruji*, here I want to interrupt you. When you are talking about *mantra japa* or the forced prolongation of breath or the role of elements in *prāṇāyāma*, what about those who, having no background, jump on the practice of *prāṇāyāma*?

I do agree with you, since *prāṇāyāma* is a fascinating subject, people do get attracted towards it. The mysticism attached to it is one more reason. As I said earlier, I have seen people getting deranged because of lack of strength in the nerves to bear the energy it produces. The container needs to be stronger to hold the content, otherwise the content breaks the container. The body is the container and energy is the content. In order to make the container stronger to hold the content, one needs to do the practice of various *āsana*.

The practice of *āsana* makes the inner body respond to *prāṇāyāma* properly. In the performance of *āsana* the conative and cognitive actions are involved to a great extent. A beginner always wants to go with conative and cognitive actions. So if he begins to do *prāṇāyāma*, his mind goes on the movements. That is conative action. Conative action exerts the nerves but prepares the body for the correct movements and actions. Gradually he begins to judge his conative actions through the cognitive awareness. He questions himself, "Am I doing rightly? Am I exerting unnecessarily? Can I remove wrong efforts?" He polishes his actions. That makes the respiratory, circulatory, nervous and glandular systems function properly and in coordination. In the practice of *prāṇāyāma* one needs to keep conative and cognitive actions aside. You cannot jerk your body. You cannot exert your muscles. You cannot force the mind to remain quiet or suppress the senses. One has to train the muscles of the body, mind and senses to become quiet or subdued through the practice of *āsana*. Otherwise they rebel. Those who do *prāṇāyāma* without having any background of practice of *āsana* may invite physical, psychological and mental problems because of the wrong stress put on the muscles, nerves, senses, brain and mind due to the wrong, jerky, aggressive, indiscriminate movements of the breathing action or respiratory action. In such conditions the practitioner will invite mental problems much more than physical problems.

In my case, my weak body was the obstacle. I did not suffer from distress, dejection, despair or derangement when I failed to do a right method of *prāṇāyāma*. There was no dereliction from my side. In fact, I did try *prāṇāyāma* practice every day in spite of failures. I was saved from all such problems because I was cautious and practised *āsana* when I could not do *prāṇāyāma*. I learnt from my mistake that I should keep a balanced practice of *āsana*. Therefore, even now, I ask the beginners to concentrate on the practice of *āsana*. I ask them to prepare themselves with the practice of supine postures, inversions, forward extensions, backward extensions and lateral twists, so that they are well prepared on the physical, psychological and mental levels.

The practice of *āsana* brings them closer to their body, nerves, senses, breath and mind, igniting the awareness. First of all, the *sādhaka* should be out of stress, strain and anxiety. Their very nature and outlook of change, therefore they are well prepared for *prāṇāyāma*.

I do not ask them to prolong their breaths with exerted will power but with subdued will power. Smoothness and delicacy are maintained. Therefore, there is no chance of harming themselves.

Q.- *Gurujī*, knowing your apathy to book knowledge, it often surprises me how did you evolve the terminology? *(Laughter.)*

Words never came to me at all. Even today, I fail in my words, but I never fail in actions and in corrections. The practical subject, when practised honestly, does not need too many words. See even Patañjali has limited words in his work on *Yoga Sūtra*. Having practised yoga uninterruptedly with devotion, I have cultivated and cultured myself, my cells, my body, my mind and that cultured practice revealed words for me to say exactly what I want to convey. Book knowledge sometimes does not convey the real meaning of the practice. It remains just the idle amplification or assemblage of words or verbal exuberance. This does not happen with Patañjali. He chooses the words so that they convey totally and completely. For instance, if you take the words, *kāla, deśa* and *saṁkhyā* of Patañjali,[1] the word *saṁkhyā* has many connotations such as number, precision, minuteness, reflection and deliberation. So yoga, *prāṇa* and God are inexplicable, and at times they are explicable on a very limited level. When certain words strike, they have to be completely moulded and blended in

---

[1] *Bāhya abhyantara stambha vṛttiḥ deśa kāla saṁkhyābhiḥ paridṛṣṭaḥ dīrgha sūkṣmaḥ* (*Y.S.*, II.50). *Prāṇāyāma* has three movements: prolonged and fine inhalation, exhalation and retention; all regulated with precision according to duration and place. For more details see the author's *Light on the Yoga Sūtras of Patañjali*, part II.

the practice. If they are blended in practice, these words become factual words. Having used those words directly in practice, they have a direct force that conveys the right meaning to the practitioner to do it correctly. And that is how I got the words.

Q.- *Gurujī*, though practice of *prāṇāyāma* is very personal and subjective, can we ask you to share some of your experiences with us? Is there any special feeling, special experience or such that you could share with us?

Actually, for me *prāṇāyāma* acts as *bhakti mārga*. I see the incoming breath as a universal force entwining my system and my releasing breath in the form of exhalation is an act of surrendering myself to that cosmic force.

As long as one is not regular in the practice of *prāṇāyāma*, one is not going to be charmed by my words. In one sentence I say that practice of *prāṇāyāma* takes my intelligence towards my very core of being and keeps me non-egoistic for a long time. I had visions of light, vision of my Deity and it has made me move towards the simplicity of life.

If you all watch your *citta* at the time of *prāṇāyāma* practice, you experience the quietness and sublimation of it. From this stage, you surely advance towards higher consciousness.

Q.- Are you avoiding describing your experiences?

When I have explained my experiences, how can you say I am avoiding? The effect of *prāṇāyāma* is dependent on one's individual practices. I do not want you to go to a dreamy state by describing my experiences and I do not want to misguide you either. I already said that I had visions but my experiences will not help you much to progress. I do not want to boast about my experiences. However, I want to help you people showing the proper direction for you to experience the feeling of closeness of your mind, intelligence and consciousness to the seer or the Self.

As I told you earlier, I knew nothing about *prāṇāyāma*. I began to think of the first breath a newborn child takes, how the child cries and why the child cries and so on. The child cannot take breath rhythmically. Therefore, it cries. The child cries in the same way as we gasp for air. You make the child cry by pinching, hitting or turning it upside down. Though the child can cry naturally, at the time of birth, pinching is done probably for the child to cry, which may relieve the pressure. The pressure of liquid accumulated in the lungs is forcibly released so that air may go in.

Similarly, we gasp to take away any load on the lungs. When we do *Sālamba Śīrṣāsana* on the ropes, our brain becomes empty like animals in sleep. Animals can remain immobile for a long time. Often, the movement of the limbs will not be visible. Like a gorilla hangs from a tree, I do *Sālamba Śīrṣāsana*[1] on the rope. It makes one's brain very passive and breathing becomes automatically slow, deep with unconscious retentions in between. The brain becomes instinctively quiet in rope *Śīrṣāsana*, as animals instinctively remain silent. This way I deaden my brain like a log of wood – insensitive. In *prāṇāyāma* too, often this state is felt in which the body becomes like a log of wood. Sometimes, I have done *Sālamba Śīrṣāsana* very frequently without ill effect, except the sensation of being like the log of wood. Some of my pupils tried like me and got fever, which persisted for days. Some got dehydrated.

This state of feeling came to me during my practices of *prāṇāyāma*, particularly at the time of *kumbhaka* – the retention of breath. I was foolishly holding the breath thinking that my *kuṇḍalinī śakti* may arise as was said by many authors in their books. My practice of *kumbhaka* was creating hardness in my brain, which became like a log of wood. In *Sālamba Śīrṣāsana* too when one stays longer than the brain and skull can take, the brain becomes heavy, dull and feels like a log of wood. This experience taught me to be cautious while doing *kumbhaka*. In place of egoistic retention, I learnt to be humble in *kumbhaka*. It also gave me indications that wrong practice of *prāṇāyāma* affects the practitioner faster than wrong practice of *āsana*. I developed irritability, restlessness, shakiness and discomfort. As I began to practise carefully without jerking the brain or the body, slowly these uncomfortable feelings began to fade and calmness, quietness, stability in the body, endurance in the nerves took their place. The practice of *prāṇāyāma* became inspirational.

Subjectively, each practitioner has to study each inbreath and outbreath, moment to moment, to keep a steady flow. It triggers the life force to be active in the body. A feeling of pleasantness and presentness is felt. One's mind does not waver between the past and the future. If one feels an exhilarating sensation in inhalation, invigorating sensation in retention and complete passivity of brain in exhalation, it is a good sign. If one feels restless, drowsy, empty or dull, it is a sign of wrong practice of *prāṇāyāma*. If the exhilarating and invigorating sensation is lost, one should not hold the breath. This is the guide for you all. I advise you all to follow with caution, confidence and clarity. If the exhalation after *kumbhaka* gets disturbed, lessen the time of *kumbhaka* to enjoy the physiological and psychological quietness. Observe the fragrance of inbreath, outbreath and also the placidity of the mind at the time of retention. If the spine collapses, one has overstrained, or if one goes into a swoon, it is wrong practice. Don't go into a swoon or dreamy state. Do not wait for special experience to come. The spiritual feelings or divine experience have to come on their own.

---

[1] See plate n. 8

Q.- Thank you very much, *Gurujī*. Most of us feel a little consoled, some of us feel inspired by the fact that even *Gurujī* has had his ups and downs and sometimes has found prāṇāyāma routine and felt reluctant to do it. But that was a very, very long time ago. We have to see *Gurujī* as he is now, and *Gurujī* has truly inspired many of us to start struggling, even in *prāṇāyāma*.

Prāṇāyāma stimulates the peripheral nerves, semi-voluntary nerves and the central nervous system. As *prāṇāyāma* has to be done with judicious intelligence, each inhalation begins with the central nervous system triggering into the peripheral nerves and each exhalation begins with the peripheral nerves going to the central nerves. In retention all the three systems get electrified.

Inhalation commences like the rolled leaves opening out, enters the centre of the body and spreads through the bronchioles towards the air cells of the lungs. Similarly, the inner body grips the cells to release the breath in exhalation. It is a wonder to observe this relaxation. As compared to this just observe your normal breath, there is a tension in the brain. Naturally, the known deep breath is a tremendous strain on the brain. But why *prāṇāyāmic* breathing keeps the brain free from stress and strain is that the brain is made to remain as an object or as a thing and hence it gets quietened while doing *prāṇāyāma*. This makes the central nervous system function better.

In our yogic terminology, these major nerves are called *iḍā*, *piṅgaḷā* and *suṣumṇā*. *Piṅgaḷā* or *sūrya nāḍī* means the solar plexus, which has access to the sympathetic nervous system. *Candra nāḍī* represents the parasympathetic nervous system, controlled by the hypothalamus of the brain. It is called *iḍā* or lunar plexus. Balancing the flow of sympathetic and parasympathetic nerves is the job of the *suṣumṇā*. It represents the central nervous system. So *suṣumṇā*, which is the central nervous system, is the storehouse of energy, the storehouse of the nectar of life. Practice of *prāṇāyāma* produces this nectar for it to be stored in the *cakra*.

In *prāṇāyāma*, one should remember that one should not bloat the abdomen in inhalation or in *kumbhaka*. Also one has to observe the *bandha*. If *bandha* are not followed properly, stress is felt in the brain and strain is felt on the diaphragm, the lungs and on the heart. If the core of being is brought in contact with the frame of the body in inhalation, lifting and holding the very self in *kumbhaka* and moving the intellect from the skin towards the core of being in exhalation, then it is a spiritual *prāṇāyāma*. Just inflating or deflating the chest is not *prāṇāyāma*, but purely a physical deep breathing. Hence, *prāṇāyāma* is the most difficult and monotonous subject, but at the same time it is also fascinating. Accept the monotony, as it is a natural process in *prāṇāyāma*. At the same time taste the fragrance of breath, as you taste food with the tip of your tongue. If you fail after a few cycles, be happy that you did at least two, three or four cycles well. Even if you have done two breaths with attention, tasting the fragrance of breath from intelligence, I say you have done good work.

Don't worry, nor say that "I did not do more than that." If it continues to three breaths, consider that you are a blessed one on that day, because you did one more. If you do four, then say that you are doubly blessed. That is how you have to learn *prāṇāyāma,* accepting the failures also. There are going to be failures in *prāṇāyāma.* Even for me – don't think that I could do *prāṇāyāma* very accurately every day. I also faced failures. Even the food affects the practice. If you have not digested the food, you fail while doing *prāṇāyāma.* If you have not slept well, your *prāṇāyāma* gets affected. Naturally, one can't say that one has to get the *prāṇāyāma* as one did yesterday. I say, do not get disturbed or perturbed by these shortcomings. Give room for these weaknesses and try to get the best; when I say the best, don't compare that best to what you have done – to yesterday's best. Out of the ten breaths you did today, find out how many were really good breaths for today. And if you do that way, I am sure you will master *prāṇāyāma.*

– *Thank you,* Gurujī! *It is very valuable advice.* –

IYENGAR THE ENIGMA*

Yoga and Health *talked to the great* haṭha yogi, *Mr. B.K.S. Iyengar, when he visited Brighton recently.*

It was with some trepidation that I went to meet B.K.S. Iyengar, the internationally known yoga teacher and author of, amongst other works, Light on Yoga.[1] *Mr. Iyengar, whose brother-in-law and* guru *was the esteemed Krishnamacharya, has a reputation of being harsh and aggressive, of being 'too physical' in his approach to yoga, of manhandling his students, of being egotistical. In short, he had some reputation to live down. Luckily for me, I was not going to have my* āsanas *scrutinised but just to talk and to try to discover what this man was all about. Over lunch, my impressions of him were of a warm, kind and considerate person who loved being with his students. He had a good sense of humour and made everyone – including me – feel at ease.*

I was intrigued by the hearsay that he 'ignored the spiritual' and that no meditation was apparently taught in his classes. So I kicked off with a 'biggy'.

Q.- Mr. Iyengar, what to you is the goal of yoga?

You know, if I create a *goal* in the field of yoga for my practice, I may be caught up in that word 'goal' or 'achievement' and lose the benefits that come unknowingly from my practice. On the contrary, I want to know where and how far yoga *takes* me, rather than having a set plan. The aim of everybody is to experience the Self, and if you ask me I too have the same goal, and if you question me further, "Have you experienced your own Self?", my answer will be that I cannot put my felt feelings into words. Yet I say that I *live* in myself without using my conscious mind.

In the early days, I had a simple ambition of having a place for me to teach. But I was getting no help from any corner. My only reason then was I wanted to prove that yoga has something to give to mankind. I used to take on challenge after challenge, and then I had to fight within myself to find a solution. I used to ask myself: "Will my encounters to these challenges

---

* Interview by Colonel D.I.M. Robbins, O.B.E., M.C., published by *Yoga and Health*, 7/1/89.

[1] Published by Harper Collins, London.

happen or not?" It was my fear that they would not. But I religiously devoted to yoga, I worked using all my time for the practice of yoga and I am contented in its success.

I keep myself open to receive the knowledge which comes through my practices, rather than blocking myself and saying, "No, I want to experience only this". I know that I need not go in search of the Self; it exists in itself – there is nothing beyond the Self except the Universal Soul.

I have been doing yoga for fifty-two years. Something has to be a key in order to develop and that became my philosophy. Now I have taken this aspect of yoga – *āsana* and *prāṇāyāma* – to see whether it could give the real essence of yoga in totality, and by using it as a springboard, whether I could reach to a higher level – and therefore by the grace of yoga, it has taken me! People say, "Oh, *haṭha yoga* is a physical thing", but it has lifted me to this extent and I want to be faithful to that which has lifted me up – I could not discard it now. The amount of finer points that come when I am doing the *āsana* is amazing: for example, even the bottom part of my foot sends a message to bring my consciousness on it. My body intelligence takes me back to see the weaknesses, so I re-adjust the posture in *āsana*. I just love it. This is the amazing quality I am deriving from my *sādhanā*. I feel the existence of my consciousness from the bottom of my feet to the crown of my head as one unit with life and vigour. There is a tremendous fullness in whatever I do – so I am happy and contented with that fullness. I can feel the existence of my Self entirely. What more do I want?

Q.- Other *gurus* talk about the state of *samādhi*...

It is because *samādhi* is only a state where you experience the absorption of body, mind and soul as a single unit. But from *samādhi* we have to reach a higher and subtler state called *kaivalya*. The Self cannot be divided – so can I be in that undivided state? Can my mind surrender to that which is ever stable and steady?

Q.- I understood that the way to reach this 'undivided state' was through meditation – yet you do not appear to teach meditation in your classes. Why is this?

No, that is a mistake. I prefer to say that the focus of attention, when it is uninterrupted, is meditation. When I do the *āsana* I expand my consciousness into every cell of the body. *Āsana* means the fusion of intelligence and consciousness, equally and evenly into every part of the body. When the water of a river is flowing smoothly embracing the banks without any ripples, you say that the flow is smooth. Similarly, while one is in an *āsana* the intelligence flows from the median inside touching gently the banks of the body without any dualities, sensing beautiful experience. That is how *āsana* done by me is to be done by all. Hence, for me this way of observation and reflection is meditation. There is a tranquil flow, a tranquil experience of action, and the effect is one hundred percent clarity. This is my true awareness – I am aware everywhere. Do you mean to say that closing the eyes, sitting in a corner, is meditation? Or is it to live in fullness, without any oscillation?

First of all, know well that while practising any *āsana* there is a postural adjustment in order to spread the intelligence and bring the *prāṇa* to balance well in the vital body. In order to look within there is a withdrawal of attention from the objective world and the focus of attention is concealed inside. This leads further to have attentive awareness, without any divergence or interruption. That is what I do as well as teach. Why should I be bothered by people whose only aim is to attack, criticise and call my practice physical yoga? For me as a practitioner it is an experience from *yama* to *samādhi*.

My students never say that I do not teach meditation. You should know meditation is part and parcel of action. Maybe I may not be teaching the so-called meditation, where one just sits, closes the eyes and does nothing, feels nothing, which makes one dull and stupid.

Q.- I am intrigued that in your teaching you place a lot of emphasis on the skin. Why is this?

Mr. Iyengar explained that the skin is an organ of perception – one that receives, rather than acts. If the flesh overstretches in an āsana, *the skin loses its sensitivity and does not send a message to the brain. In the West, we tend to overdo the stretch in our impatience to get it right, and in doing so we lose our sensitivity.*

Medical science speaks of efferent *nerves, which send messages from the brain to the organs for them to act, and* afferent *nerves, which send messages from the skin and organs to the brain about what they perceive. Perfect understanding between the nerves of action and the nerves of knowledge is yoga.*

I say that while practising yoga, there should be a space between the end of the fibres of the flesh and the end of the fibres of the skin. A space between receiving the message from the organs of perception and the message returning to the organs of action. If you are conscious of that, it is meditation; usually we leave no space because we feel we have to act immediately. This is not meditation.

To someone who, like me, has not practised haṭha yoga *the Iyengar way, this degree of refinement in awareness seems inconceivable. He goes on to explain, in* The Tree of Yoga:[1] "The mind exists in the entire fabric of man. When you reflect on the action produced by the flesh in an

[1] Published by Harper Collins, London.

āsana and when you create an equal balance everywhere, it is *dhyāna,* contemplation. It is *dhyāna* in the flesh, *dhyāna* in the skin, in the mind and in the intellect. There is concord and unity in all these four. When you reach this state of balance, there is oneness. There is awareness through your whole being from the skin to the self and from the self to the skin. Unfortunately, in meditation as it is often practised today, we go in the name of meditation into loneliness and emptiness. Emptiness is not meditation."

Apparently, Mr. Iyengar made the discovery about the importance of putting the consciousness into the skin when he realised that he was not gaining as much as he should from his own practice. When he began creating this new awareness, everything fell into place.

Yes – no books explain this. When I began yoga I was a boy of fourteen or fifteen, and I used to look at all the yoga books and study the positions of the *āsana.* Then I thought, "How is it that ten books are giving different varieties? Which is the correct one"? Then I started experimenting on myself. For example in *Sālamba Śīrṣāsana,* if I do not keep my shoulders parallel, I watch my knees and I study what happens to the rest of my body. And if I keep them parallel, how do my knees align with each other and my feet get the grip? If I set a discipline for my shoulders then my knees too have to keep discipline. If I drop my right shoulder, my right knee turns outward and obviously the foot also turns outward. This showed me the correct way of doing. Then I used to question myself what happens if I imitate someone else's pose? The imitation of a wrong pose used to show the difference immediately, I could see the imbalance, feel the pain and the feel of adverse effects.

Today, I say that I know the 'well' of an *āsana* and the 'ill' of an *āsana.* Having done both, I know the good and bad of each *āsana;* my practice has given me excruciating pain but has also given me the highest satisfaction. That's why in a class, if somebody does something wrong, I know that the person will suffer with pain exactly in a particular area. If the *āsana* shows any adverse effect, I know where the practitioner has gone wrong. This swiftness in correcting the wrong of the students brought me the title of a violent yogi, a hard taskmaster and so forth.

My intense and honest practice of yoga awakens my urge and compels me to correct the practitioner for his own benefit.

Q.- So your teaching is adapted for each individual.

In ten seconds I can see about forty people's mistakes, whereas some teachers cannot see one percent of their mistakes. I have taken four hundred[1] people at a time, and I have caught 100-200 mistakes. My eyes go so fast! Seeing quickly is the beauty of my teaching. If I teach, say *Tāḍāsana,*

---

[1] The author has taught 1170 people in Crystal Palace, London in 1993.

I will not look at the face but at the toes and foot. If the foundation is wrong, the entire posture is wrong. So I focus like that; that is how I learnt – how to look into a person's *āsana*, how to see a person's mistakes.

At this point, Mr. Iyengar used Mira Mehta, Secretary of the Iyengar Yoga Institute in London, to demonstrate Tāḍāsana, *the standing pose. It looked perfect to me – but the master was not satisfied. Some refinements, barely visible to the non-initiated like me, were necessary.* "You see? This inner heel is short; that inner heel is long – you can see the lines from the edges of the heels. Now I will correct it. If you observe, this part is nearer the floor, is it not? *(If you say so...)* Still she is not touching well – she is not touching this edge; she is touching the opposite side. Bend your knees! Open the foot! Walk on the foot – now put this foot down first, and then do that foot. Now what happens? Can you see it? Can you see the thickness here? Now, this is the first time she has had inflammation.

(There was the minutest tinge of pinkness above her middle toes.) Now stretch here, pressing back, keeping that on the floor. Lengthen, now move the skin away." *And so it went on, for a good five minutes; the technician observed, adjusted, challenged the student, getting her full concentration until:* "Ah, at last she has it – that part of the skin has touched the carpet for the first time! This is intelligence's success."

Tāḍāsana: In this example the students Right foot was corrected

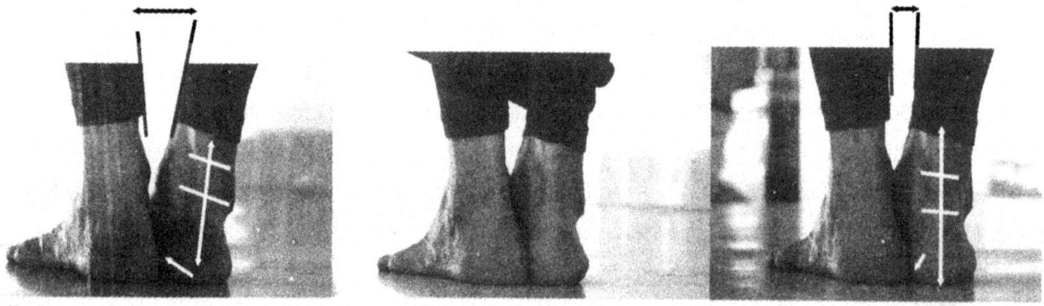

Before adjustment.
Lines are showing:
Angle at the back of the heel
Direction of the skin on the inner heels

Being adjusted by BKS Iyengar

After the adjustment.
See the change in the angle on the back of the heel

Plate n. 24 – Success of the intelligence (correcting *Tāḍāsana*)

Mr. Iyengar chuckled with delight. He and his students had achieved perfection, and he was full of joy. I could understand why his intensity is interpreted as impatience, aggression even. He sees a problem with a clarity that is incomprehensible to most people – and he is anxious and impatient to put it right, for the student's benefit and for his own satisfaction.

So you see, this is my way of teaching. How much of my intelligence has to work? How much do I purge my very self? Now, without meditation, what could I do? When I meditate, people don't understand. What I do is known to me, because I meditate in a posture. People see only the outer impression. They do not know what is going on inside me.

Yoga is movement. You never stop learning. I work constantly in my own practice and in my teaching. I never miss my daily practice and every week I do almost all the *āsana* mentioned in my book *Light on Yoga*.[1] If I see a person's problem I imagine the same problem in my body in order to watch and I see how the person reacts and how they resist. I imitate the same stiffness. Now I assume that I am that person who is suffering. For two days or so I will observe so that I can see the structure, behaviour, everything – so I create the same psychological barrier in myself. I'm like a madman, totally restless – until I get to that point, that solution to the problem. And then I'm transformed, one hundred percent sane once again. People call me mad because I yell at them sometimes, but we must reach that point of transformation.

[1] See the author's book, published by Harper Collins, London.

VISION IN ART*

Simon Buttonshaw is a painter, designer, surfer, and yoga teacher. He is a student of Shandor Remete, and he studied yoga at the R.I.M.Y.I. in Pune in August-September and October of 1988. He lives with his wife and two children in Bellbrae, Victoria, Australia.

Q.- From studying the *Vedas* and the *Upaniṣads* I can see that in ancient times the understanding that the form and the posture were able to embody the Absolute was there, and then it seems like that understanding got lost. And that seems fundamental, that if art is real then the Absolute can quite easily enter into the *form.* I want to know your feelings and opinions on this, because it seems to me that this is where your contribution is most unique. It's that the truth of the *āsana* has been rediscovered and re-established. It's not so much the artistic expression as something much deeper than that, the archetype of the posture itself.

I have several quotations here that express what I'm talking about:

"As is the realisation of *Brahman*, such is the knowledge of form. With this knowledge, the artisans manifest *Brahman* indirectly, in the creation of form, enjoying it as an ancient wisdom." *(Vastusūtra Upaniṣad)*

"Setting the limbs along proper lines is praised like the knowledge of Brahman" *(Vastusūtra Upaniṣad)*

That struck me as fundamental to the way you practise and the way you teach. And the idea here, from the *Kena Upaniṣad,* "Brahman is the ear of the ear, the mind of the mind, speech of the speech, life of the life (breath), the eye of the eye". So again there's no denial of the body and senses. The *Kena Upaniṣad* also calls for perfection in all parts of the body, speech, bearing, sight, and for the strength of all the senses, for the sole purpose of not being cut off from *Brahman.* Even in the *Ṛg Veda:* "Every form is an image of an original form".

---

* Interview by Simon Buttonshaw, Published in *Yoga '90. The Second American Iyengar Yoga Convention,* San Diego, California, pages 26-29.

As God exists, the soul exists in the entire frontier of the body, does it not? Diffusion or expansion of the soul in its own frontier is the body. The soul, which is ever present, has the identity in the body, in the senses, in the mind and at every cell of our body. Keeping that the soul exists everywhere, I practise the *āsana* that way. So I don't really think that yoga has lost this concept.

- You haven't. No, no! But it has been lost. -

No, you can't say that. You see, art is like the spokes of a wheel, which move down and up and again up and down. It does happen in any art, because the decay or stagnation sets into the minds of the people. Even intellectual decay sets in. So there will always be a pause or stalemate in between the periods of evolution and growth. But as long as the creativity exists in the cosmos, the fragrance in the art cannot be lost. Creativity is an ever-continuing process; art too gets re-generated and re-produced. I believe in this.

- Yes. But sometimes it takes people of great vision to reinstate... -

This is true. God exists in the moving material as well as in the non-moving material. Just think, without His existence and His will the leaves would not come out from the branches of the tree. He is the seed. His existence is not cognisable to our mortal organs of perception. Some develop that extraordinary quality to see His presence. Similarly, his *śakti* (power) as creation continues and guides one or the other who has the power to think correctly for recreating the art. Hence, nothing gets lost. Only it may appear as a new dimension but this is all based on the previous insights and study.

The important point is, art is of two types. One is called *bhogakalā* – the art of appeasing the pleasure of the body and mind, and the other is *yogakalā* – the art of auspicious performance to please the spiritual heart or the Self.

For instance, if you take the *āsana*, I don't think that you will find anyone thought of presenting from the soul as I have presented in *Light on Yoga*. Each fibre, each cell presents from its source – the Self. You do not see the presentation of the *āsana* in physical form but from the elegance *(lāvaṇya)* of the soul.

- No, that's what I was trying to say. -

It's like sculpting my own body using my intelligence and consciousness as hammer and chisel. Due to constant practice, I learnt at a later stage exactly to strike at the right place. It took me long years to learn. Many people do the *āsana* but they don't understand how each and every part of the body has to be connected to the Self. As an artist would draw thin lines, thick lines, faded lines and often rubs them to get the better finish, similarly we have to work our own body in presenting the *āsana*. *Āsana* can be presented properly if they are done in that way of thinking and acting. A photographer only concentrates to take a good profile but does not care to know about the profile of the finger, profile of the palm, profile of the foot, profile of the spinal vertebrae. Whereas the yogi has to see each and every minute part of the body since it has a profile of its own. And this is known as *viśvarūpa* - all pervading, in all *āsana*. It should be done like *Brahman* engulfing his frontier – the body.

Until one works like this, one cannot present the *āsana* in the yogic *kalā*. We develop compartmentally, no doubt, but when all the compartments are rhythmically put together, then it becomes a whole. Though that wholeness takes a long time for any artist to develop, know that it certainly becomes the holistic or the spiritual art.

Q.- Yes. But I think there's something unique to yoga where the development is more homogeneous than it is in other arts...

Homogeneity is a necessity. As you use different colours, different types of pencils, what about different types of joints, different movements of the joints, different behavioural patterns of the muscles? How do they have to be toned? As an artist, how do you tone your own work? So also we have to tone each and every part involved. We have to tend the self, we have to tend the body in all its aspects. Do not conclude that there is homogeneity in yogic practice. It is far from truth. You have to work with emphasis to bring out the core of the being to be present in each and every pore of the body. Hope you understand this.

Q.- All too well. But you must admit that this awareness has not been presented for a long time.

You are right. It was not presented for a very long time. And the minute I did show the difference between the existing presentations and my own, everybody started calling me an artist, not a yogi. Without the glimpse of the philosophical insight one cannot become an artist. If that philosophical background and touch is not there, one cannot become an artist. Philosophical thinking goes together with the art as well as the artist. But a scientist may not be a philosophical person because his job is only to analyse. Here we have to make an effort to find out whether what is heard or said coincides with the *sādhanā*. It's no doubt a big problem.

Art is very difficult. When I practise my art, I think of the *āsana* in such a way that there is equal power of resistance in each motion. If there is no resistance in the body and the *āsana* just comes, it has absolutely no life in it. As Shakespeare said, "To be or not to be", we must say, "To do or not to do", and at the same time to know when to do and when not to do. Exactly at what time it has to be done, at what time it has to be undone. Which part should be done, which part should not be undone in order to get that feeling of homogeneity is essential to note in the *sādhanā*.

- So this necessary tension for creating... -

It's internal. In yogis it's mostly internal. That makes it difficult for others to understand. For example, take the knee ligament. There are the knee ligaments inside as well as outside. Suppose I want to do *Padmāsana:* that curvature of the ligament on the outer edge and the inner edge should not vary at all.

By thinking this way, that's how I learned. The ligaments move like a pencil line. They must both move like thin pencil lines. While practising we have to see whether this thin line is short or long. Is it going in the right direction demanded by the body or its right construction? Or is it going a wrong way? We need to question ourselves.

Q.- So what is the balance between will and surrender, then?

Both are necessary. Discretion is the only needle in balance between will and surrender.

- And you need that razor's edge... -

Yes, will and surrender are like moving on the razor's edge. Will can be aggressive. When will becomes aggressive, then you have to learn to make the will to surrender, so that aggressiveness is nullified, do you follow me?

- All too well. -

The will power can be of two types – positive and negative or educative will and destructive will. When the will power transgresses its limit, then surrender has to be brought to surface. Because will does not work on every part at the same time. The will makes one part to take the load and do, that's all. But the interactive corrections have to come from the other end also. One has to activate the negative parts and pacify the aggressive parts, to bring harmony between will and surrender as well as in body and self. You are an artist, you are a creator, you are creating, you are producing an object. The object reflects again back to you to say whether your way of thinking was right or not. Without looking into the object, you cannot correct it.

– It's an undeniable mirror. –

As a creator, one has to reflect subjectively the will and surrender in the *āsana* practice – like a pencil, or ink, or a pen, or a brush...

– As a tool. –

Yes. But beyond the action of the will, the real action of the will has to come from the object, that is the body. For the yogi it is the body. For you it is the paper and the colour. So if that produces homogeneity, then there is a contented satisfaction, and in that contented satisfaction you see the surrender.

At times you also fight with the will, saying why am I not getting it? Do you follow?

– Oh, yes. –

So that is how – when to surrender to the will, or when to subdue the will, when to subjugate the will – has to be understood. Will alone cannot make any person perfect.

– So the softness and the surrender have to be there. Softness, yes. –

Q.- And when you work with the *āsana*, is it a process of seeing the posture internally and exposing yourself to that?

How can I see only the *āsana?* If you look at the roads of New York, they run straight. In Japan, the roads go circularly and zigzag. In art, do you have to take only one or do you have to take both?

– You take both. –

Similarly you have to think. But one cannot depend on the body, as there is consciousness and also the soul, which is known as the seer. Is that consciousness ever-present on that spot, where I am dictating the movement? I may be dictating the movement but my consciousness may not be present there. So, I also attend to the consciousness to be present there, when I am dictating the terms for movements.

– Is it the degree of awareness? –

Yes, it is the degree of awareness on each and every part. If the fruit is ripe everywhere, the colour is different. If the fruit is half-ripe, you see the change in colour in patches. Similarly, in the *āsana*. If the consciousness is present everywhere, the *āsana* is fully ripe. You might have done it with the will, but did you feel the consciousness existing at the same time? Suppose you are doing *Vṛśchikāsana*, scorpion pose. You may place your foot on your head, but is your consciousness existing in every cell, creating room when you are doing it? Is your foot communicating with your self? Is it communicating with the other foot, right foot with the left, left with the right, the inner foot with the inner foot of the other one, or the outer foot with the outer foot of the other one? Or the bottom shins, top shins, are they sending messages in which direction they have to be moved? This understanding doesn't come by will. It comes only by reflection.

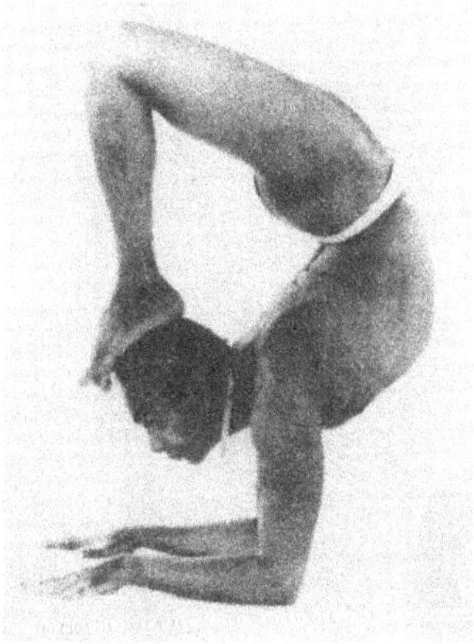

Plate n. 25 – *Vṛśchikāsana*, scorpion pose

Reflection comes only when you look at the object, the body, in a total sense: how the body is doing it. The body has to become the object for the soul. The body becomes an object. So there is a tremendous intellectual awareness within oneself, which is a moving force. Can I bring this same life in that object of the soul, which is the body in presenting the *āsana?* Do I exist only in my head, or do I exist only in my heart? Do I exist everywhere, even at the top end of the small toe? Is my consciousness there equal to that of my head? Is my will there equal to that will which is created from my brain?

– In this respect I think yoga is a unique art. In every other art, they're specialised in one sense. –

Yes! For example even if you stretch your hand, now draw a line. You may say your arm is stretched straight. But the line you draw from the middle of the arm shows that the arms are not stretched straight. The line will tell you whether they are properly divided or they are unequal. See the line.

– Oh, yes. –

This seeing helps one develop the art in one. It also guides you how to see and adjust and then to see again. Even if I go wrong – I am stretching my arm over the head and look at the division on my hand. If that division is not accurate, it means something is wrong in what I'm doing, or in drawing the line. I draw the *āsana* and the *āsana* draws me, follow? What I am presenting when I do a pose is like a drawing.

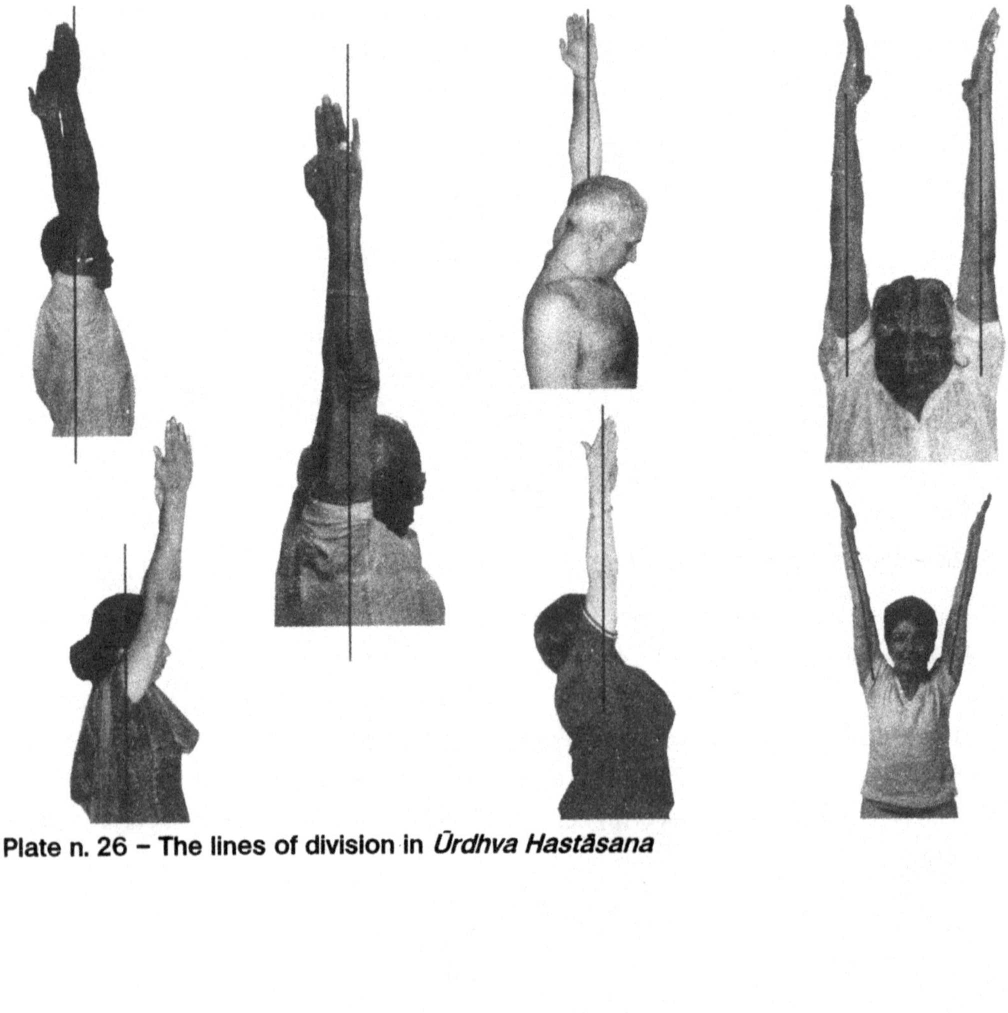

Plate n. 26 – The lines of division in *Ūrdhva Hastāsana*

- Oh yes, very much so. -

I am drawing the life force as I would draw a line on a piece of paper. On paper you can play, but can I play on my body? If I can play there on the paper I should also learn to play here on a live body. That's how I became an artist in my own way.

Q.- It seems to me, *Gurujī,* when I read the *Veda,* that these men were poets. They were visionaries.

Yes, they were not only poets but they were seers who saw divinity everywhere, in every thing, in animate and inanimate, organic and inorganic things. Somehow or other, it was lost. As I said, stagnation comes because of this insensitivity. Then naturally the intelligence fades. Even when it fades, people say that is their zenith but the zenith is much higher, although they can't see it. They don't observe.

- Because they hold wherever they are. -

Yes, that's why the art dies. But by chance, somebody is fortunate enough to come along and rework on it...

- More than fortunate, I think, Gurujī. -

(Laughing) So that is why Patañjali says you have to start with the original books, like the *Veda, Upaniṣad,* or any original texts. We have to analyse what has been written. We have to think it over, put it into practice and find out whether it goes parallel with what we find in the original sacred books. This is my way of thinking. We have to stop the oscillations of our own intelligence, then put them directly into factual form.

Q.- I have always heard that you are a revolutionary, and yet I find you very deeply grounded in *Śāstric* authority.

I have to be. How can I be otherwise? I have not broken the tradition. But I am a revolutionary at the same time because without departing from tradition, I look for the original way of seeing it. Many things have been lost. How do I come back to the origin, I study. So I have to think, also, what is the meaning given by others. And then, I keep their thoughts or ideas aside and think subjectively.

Suppose I did it with my own awareness, my own intelligence, how much can I find out without depending on those who have already given their experience or thoughts? This brings purity and originality.

As an artist you too need to find out. The predecessors have given their notions. You must look at them, study them. But since you haven't experienced them, you have to forget and start subjectively verifying. Their knowledge is objective for you. So think in this way, "Let me look with my own fresh mind, fresh eye, and see what type of understanding I get." Then you can balance your experiences with their experiences, and see where these two meet. Where they meet you can build up a new thing. So that's known as evolution.

– *Still very much grounded in tradition.* –

Without the background of words and works, how can we progress? Obviously we will be nowhere. We are all dependent on our parents and *guru*. All our parents are dependent upon the grandparents. So it is a continuous process. You cannot deny that. That is the foundation. You cannot say there is no foundation. Tradition is a base that builds up, for us to be firm inside as well as outside. There won't be emptiness inside; there won't be emptiness outside. So you see with a new way of looking. Without that background, you cannot see.

Q.- You need the firm support of tradition.

Can you quote anything that is not dependent on tradition? Here it means sacred books. It was written centuries ago. But you also have to look at it and see how does it stand for today. You have to think that way also.

Q.- Even as a painter I've done that. It's worked for me as a painter. As a painter my art is developed but as a yogi my art is very primitive. The disparity is difficult for me to live with.

Everybody grows from crudeness to refinement. But the advantage is that an artist can understand the artistic feelings, artistic approaches of the other art. Every art inherits the traditional touch. You as an artist can't expect the artistic touch to come fast, because the way of seeing, the methodology is different, the adaptation is different. But later, as you begin to appreciate both the arts, you see how they can mingle together. That's important for an artist to see, where the arts meet.

– I think they can meet in a wonderful way. –

That's what we have to see. So if they do not meet, then it's not art at all. There is no homogeneity; there is no harmony. Art has to have harmony. Somewhere it has to meet, subjectively as well as objectively.

– It's no small job. –

No. Certainly not. Art cannot be learned with ease. It cannot be learned by chance. It requires tremendous orderly behaviour, in one's mental attitude.

Q.- One other thing that I feel is unique in your yoga is that there is a profound respect for individuality. This intrigues me. I think it's marvellous.

Yes.

– In most so-called yoga there is a complete denial of this. –

As we said before, God exists everywhere. So respect has to be given where respect is due. Even where one has to treat mercilessly, that does not mean one has shown disrespect to the soul. An artist who has evolved shows respect to the soul in seeing whether he can help the other person also to that level. It may appear crude to observers, it may appear aggressive, but for the individual, the person involved, it is something necessary. Because he feels that when chances are available, if the budding artist does not pick up, an opportunity is lost. In the initial stages, that does pain the artist. That is the way one has to work and I work that way. Respect has to be given. This is a type of respect to show for the budding students what is right, so that they also could come up to that level. The artist should not suppress the other artist or look down upon them. That would not be the life of an artist at all, though many in the world today do that.

Q.- I watched you teaching the class last night. Everyone had told me you were very aggressive. But I watched, and you were never aggressive with the person, only the nonsense in that person.

(Laughs) That's true. That's what people don't understand.

Q.- It seemed to me that you had more respect for the person than they often had for themselves. It was very moving.

I only show aggressiveness for the dullness in their work. You have to do that.

– It's a great skill, not a common thing. I had one art teacher a little like that. He would come up and slash my canvas. –

(Laughing) Yes, you are right.

– ...but he was my favourite teacher. I learned so much. –

How many musicians of old have broken the musical instruments when the students played wrong? How many people have hit so hard that people have lost their senses of perception? How many painters have thrown the paint on a painting when it had gone wrong? I don't do such things. They should be happy that there is a man who is aggressive but who is not destructive, don't you think so? *(Both laugh).* Because I know that if I ruin somebody, then they won't come up at all. Because here we play, not with the outer thing but the very subjective thing, the very human being and his existence. The body is the object of the soul. So if something happens even to a knuckle that means this fellow cannot create tomorrow *(Laughs).* So even though the words may appear crude or aggressive, when I touch them, the way I touch, they understand how constructive I am, how accurate I am.

Q.- Your birthday celebration committee would like to use some photographs of you teaching to illustrate a presentation they are doing on *yama* and *niyama*.

Yama and *niyama* what? In every word we say we have to live like that. *Yama* and *niyama* are not separate from human beings.

– That is apparent in the touch, in the look, in the directions you give, in the way you describe the āsana. *–*

You can't just take the words in their old meanings, *ahiṁsā* means non-violence, and so forth. How many teachers are there who say, "Don't smoke", and they smoke themselves. Even those who call themselves 'divine' do smoke and drink. So, I do not agree with this double standard of behaviour. At least, let us be ethical in our vocation. If I am a teacher, I have to follow the ethics of teaching. If I am a practitioner, I have to follow the ethics of practice.

– This is another area where yoga as art is unique. –

That's what I'm saying! So if I am an artist, I have to follow the ethics of art in order to present properly. Suppose I am doing an *āsana* that is good, and the student doesn't do it the same way, am I supposed to say, "Never mind, it will come after one year, so continue." That would be unethical. I would be breaking my *yama* and *niyama* in the name of teaching. I have to be on the spot to say, "No, it's wrong; it should not be done that way." So if people call this frank opinion aggressive, then what can I do? They don't understand that I am following *yama* and *niyama* in the teaching. You have to follow a certain path.

Suppose you are driving a car. If there is a red light, and you pass through, what happens? You are caught and fined. Aren't you? So you follow the ethics of the road. So don't you have to follow the ethics in each and every part of yourself?

If your painting goes wrong or unaesthetic, then it is no more art. As an artist says that he wants perfection, I too say so. Imperfection, wrong practice, half-done, half-heartedly done, is unethical practice according to my understanding.

TRANSFORM *SĀDHANĀ* INTO A DIVINE PRACTICE*

Q.- Sometimes in the class you ask students if they come to do or to learn. Can you speak about the art of learning?

When people say, "I am doing", it is a mechanical repetition without perception, without observation. Whenever the *sādhaka* practises, he or she should keep the mind attentive and look within the body in the practice of yoga to observe, absorb, adjust and readjust, to see that either side of the body, the nerves, the organs, the joints are kept rhythmically in a steady concordant position along with alignment. If such things are not observed, then it is known as "doing", where the body movements take place without the involvement of the mind, whereas life is dynamic, so the *sādhanā*, either in the *āsana* or the in-breath and the out-breath or the meditation should be dynamic. If anybody says they are not dynamic, I think their understanding is very poor.

The flow of intelligence in the body should be made to be viable for feeling. Like fluid, the intelligence moves in the body from position to position, as we re-adjust the body from *āsana* to *āsana*. So the learner cannot just do the *āsana* without bringing the intelligence to function. His intelligence has to equally observe how the joints, the muscles, the cells have to be placed, maintained and retained in a certain required position (as each *āsana* has a different angle and shape). For this he has to bring his intelligence to study the flow of it in the body.

If you don't understand what I mean by intelligence, I would say the sensitivity in the body that is felt by the mind is the intelligence. Even sensations have to be aligned. Through this felt sensation you have to find out where the sensation is and where it is not. This is the function of the intelligence. Then to bring the sensation where it is absent is to make the intelligence to flow there. You need to trace in your practices such insensitive areas and 'intelligise' them. Then, bringing the intelligence into the insensitive areas, it has to observe the sensation whether it is equal or not. The *sādhaka* then studies its flow and readjusts the *āsana* to bring the equanimity in the flow of intelligence on either side of the body. That requires not only total attention but also total penetration.

---

* Interview by Christian Pisano, on 8th June 1990.

When you are doing the *āsana*, you have to find out where the intelligence and the body meet. The meeting of these two has to be accurate in each and every cell of the body, synchronising the length of the intelligence (sensitivity) with the length of the extended muscles, or the cells, without deviation, division or differentiation. There has to be the synchronisation of sensitivity between the *āsana*, body and mind.

One who does studying all these is a learner. He learns while he is acting and doing. He does not just do. He does in order to learn. So this is the difference between a "learner" and a "doer". A learner observes moment to moment what is going on in his cells, in his body, in his mind, and brings back life in the different parts of the body while staying in the *āsana*. A learner is an introvert, a doer is neither an introvert nor an extrovert. A doer does the *āsana* according to the mould of his body; whereas a learner does by transforming the body to fit into each *āsana* and through this he develops finer intellectual quality.

Everybody is a doer in the beginning. So I say, in the beginning you have to go on repeating over and over again to develop the memory. Through that memory you develop by looking and thinking and gaining a logical understanding of what and how you should do. Do not use memory just to repeat mechanically, but make use of it to guide you to re-educate in moulding the body, mind and intelligence. Use the memory as a threshold to develop the power of intelligence to further penetrate the inner body. Do not practise to reproduce the experience of yesterday.

As I said, life is dynamic. Life is also motion. It is moving. As it is moving you have to know that in each *āsana*, new healthy cells grow and new chemical actions take place in the body. This way we have to keep a watch as the changes take place in our blood system as well as in the physiological and psychological systems. The blood group may be the same, but the quality of the blood changes according to the purificatory methods we adopt in our practice. Hence, yoga is not only a clarifying system but also a purifying system. One has to work in each *āsana* where one cleanses, purifies, absorbs and filters. Each *āsana* filters the cells in the body. The impurities are thrown out. The cleansing takes place. When the cleansing takes place, then the process of filtering also takes place. *Āsana* practices cleanse moment to moment as the body and mind get polluted or disturbed due to food habits or ways of thinking, living and relationships. These things change the mind and they change the cells too. Hence, regular practice is essential as they have to be filtered and purified again and again. The practice of *āsana* has to be more interpenetrative in order to re-filter the system every now and then. By this, the blood is purified. The cells are purified. When the blood and the cells are purified, the mind too becomes quiet and meditative. Even the nerves and brain are drained of impurities and oxygenated. Learning while doing includes the process of sensibility, sensitivity of touch, intelligising, vitalising, placing and spacing of the cells. In the doing process you do not attend to all these things. Hence, the doer's mind remains outgoing whereas the learner's mind goes inwards.

Q.- People have often criticised you saying that you just teach two limbs of yoga, *āsana* and *prāṇāyāma* and that your approach is mainly physical. But in your teaching you never made a difference between a so-called physical and spiritual yoga.

In order to educate oneself, one first learns the alphabet. Later one may become the master of the chosen subjects. So also it is possible that by first undergoing the physical way of *āsana* practice, one in course of time acquires the knowledge of the real.[1]

It is simply onlookers who speak of me that way. They see only verbal expression and carry wrong impressions of me and my yoga. For real practitioners *(sādhaka)* it is *sādhanā*, whereas for onlookers it is "verbal expressions". Hence the criticism.

Body is a part of the mind, mind is a part of the body. These are interconnected and interwoven. Similarly all the eight yogic aspects are interconnected and interwoven. When I teach *āsana* or *prāṇāyāma*, I involve implicitly all the other aspects of yoga. If one has not observed the subtlety of these things in my teachings, naturally one demarcates. Take *Adho Mukha Vṛkṣāsana*. If one stretches one arm fully and the other arm is not stretched fully, yet one balances, it means *pratyāhāra* and *dhāraṇā* is not followed.

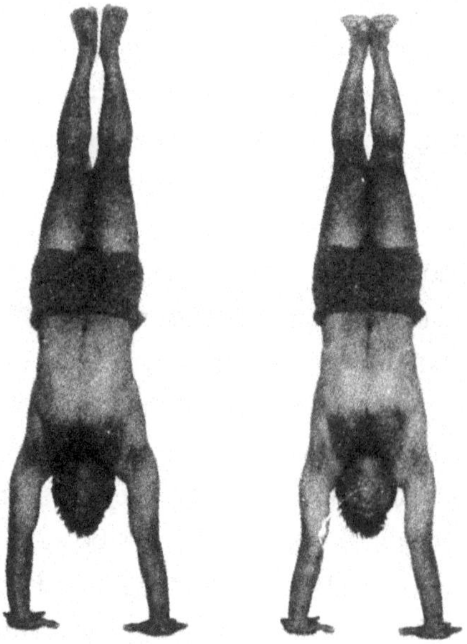

Plate n 27 – *Adho Mukha Vṛkṣāsana* (wrong and right)

[1] *Abhyāsātkādi varṇānām yathā śāstrāṇi bodhayet /*
tathā yogaṁ samāsādya tatvajñānam ca labhyate // (Gheranda Samhita, I.5).

There is imbalance in the *āsana*. Equanimity is yoga. Equanimity means to bring alignment and alignment means introduction of discipline in that *āsana*. One has to watch the mounds of the palms, the knuckles of the palms, the back of the fingers of the right and of the left; equal stretch and lift of the legs. Do we pay attention to see all these points and stretch equally?

- Most of the time no. -

That means there is disparity. Disparity is not yoga. Yoga brings parity – oneness. Then is it not "doing" again for correction? People do not understand that *yama* and *niyama* are involved in each and every cell while doing an *āsana*, or *prāṇāyāma*. How many people exactly place their finger digits on the nostrils to do *Nāḍī Śodhana prāṇāyāma*? They may block the right and open the left without proper rhythmic pressure to allow the breath to flow smoothly. Do they study how much the passages have to be kept open? Do they think about how the skin of the finger should be, how the skin of the nostrils should be, where the passage has to be and how the passage should be to control it? Skilful intelligence and action has to be developed in order to know where and how to keep the digits of the fingers. Then one has to watch where the breath is moving. Are these not the commandments of *yama* and *niyama* to be observed while doing *āsana* or *prāṇāyāma?*

If the breath is flowing into the inner portion of the nostril and you keep the finger anywhere on the outer part of the nose, is it *dhāraṇā*? Just blocking without knowing where the breath is touching, is it *yama* or *niyama* or *dhyāna?* Blocking one side of the nose fully and keeping the other side fully open for inhalation, can you call it *prāṇāyāma?* Secondly, when you are closing, are you sure that you are exactly maintaining the closure without disturbing the septum? If you begin to study all these, then you know not only *yama* and *niyama* but also *dhāraṇā* and *dhyāna*.

- We don't even think about it. -

That is how people, without knowing, say it is just physical. When you do *Paśchimottānāsana* have you seen whether all the five toes are properly aligned and toes of the right and left feet are touching and moving in the same direction? How many people observe the extension of the bottom of the feet? If you don't pay attention to such things, where is the truth *(satya)?* Tell me. Is *satya* just keeping your leg straight and banging the head down? When you take the head down, you do not know what happens to your arms, from which fingers you grip more and from which less, which foot you grip, which foot you do not grip, which part of the body moves and which part does not move. One shoulder blade may be active and the other dull. It is also called *Ugrāsana*. Why did they call it by this name, one has to ponder on it. Does one observe all these things? They only advise one to do yoga softly and slowly. If yoga is to be done with softness, then why does Patañjali use the word "code of conduct", *anuśāsanam?*Has he advised you to do as you like according to your comfort? Tell me, is it Patañjali's yoga? See the first two *sūtra.*[1] Is there any respect for that word *anuśāsanam?* A code of conduct has to be followed with full dynamism whether one is walking, sitting, standing. *Anuśāsanam* is code of law, law of the human system. As there is a code of law in society, there is a code of law for a human system. The body, the cells, the mind, the organs of action, the senses of perception, have to behave according to the code of yogic discipline. Misinterpretation has brought this subject to ridicule.

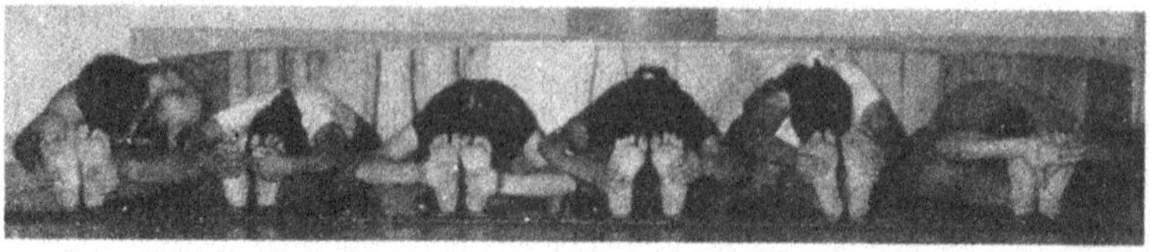

Everybody practising with differences in hand grip and shoulderblade action

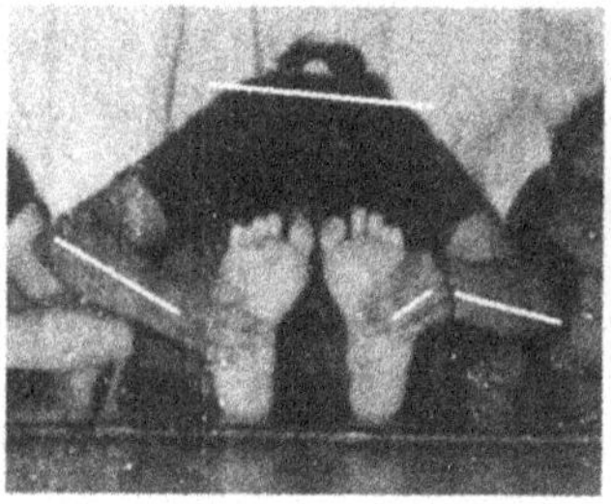

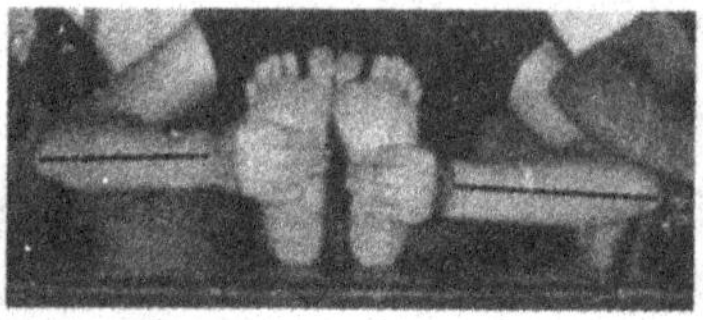

Differences in shoulders, arms and hand grips

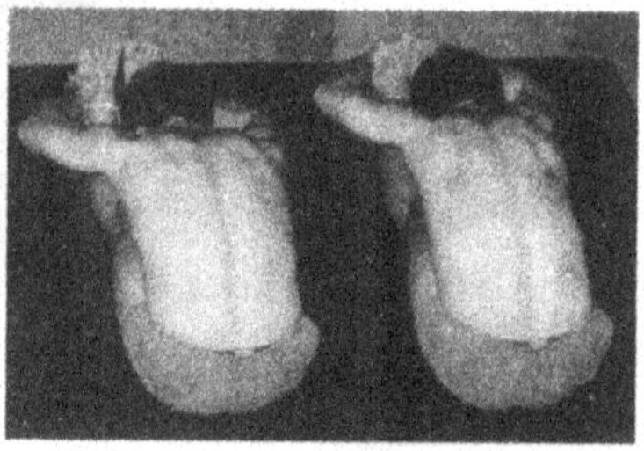

Spinal extension and shoulder blade action changing with the different hand-grip

Plate n. 28 – *Paśchimottānāsana* observed and unobserved

For example, I was just reading *Gheraṇḍa Saṁhitā* translated by Śrī Chandra Vasu.[2] In the foreword, he says that *samādhi* can be obtained by the purification of the body through *āsana*, as certain *āsana* induce certain mental transformations. For this, one has to observe the feelings that take place as well as the transformation taking place in the mind in each *āsana*. In one *āsana*, you can be more active, or you can be more passive. Suppose I am standing in *Tāḍāsana*,[3] I have to study my intelligence. When I do *Śīrṣāsana*,[3] I study what type of stability in intelligence comes. With these experiences, I introduce the principles of *yama*, *niyama*, *pratyāhāra*, *dhāraṇā* and *dhyāna* in *āsana* and *prāṇāyāma*.

Here, you are made to be within yourself, which is nothing but *svādhyāya*.

- The study of the self. -

---

[1] *Atha yogānuśāsanam*, now begins an exposition of the sacred art of yoga (I.1), and *yogaḥ cittavṛtti nirodhaḥ*, yoga is the cessation of movements in the consciousness (I.2).

[2] Published by the Theosophical Publishing House, Adyar, Chennai, 1933.

[3] See *Aṣṭadaḷa Yogamālā* vol 3, plates n. 27 & 28

Is not the body part of the self? Is not the mind a part of the self? In deep sleep, does the mind function? If it is in function, how can you say that you had sound sleep? If the mind was there, then you should have known what was happening around you in sleep. So there must be something superior to the mind and the mind is subordinate to that. When the body is subordinate to the self, the mind is also subordinate to the self. What is the use of differentiating the body and mind when both are subordinates? How can one speak of mind control when there is no body control? For a *yoga sādhaka*, both have to go together.

Can you express anything without this body? So this body, according to yoga, is given to be used for fruitful means and self-knowledge. The practice of *āsana* and *prāṇāyāma* makes the body and mind worthy,.when practised the way I am saying.

It is not for my critics to decide what I teach. I am interested in those who come to me, how I convert each action, each thought from the physical and mental levels into a spiritual action and thought.

Q.- The other day you were talking about people who proudly say that they just have a spiritual practice like *mantra yoga*. But is it not true that they still have to use their tongue, which is connected to the body? Some advise candle gazing...

Yes, you may say that you are gazing at a candle, and that you are doing it as a spiritual practice. Is gazing connected to the body or not? You gaze with your eyes and your mind is brought there, isn't it? When you do *Paśchimottānāsana* bodily and your mind is brought into *Paśchimottānāsana*, then what is the difference between the gazing at a candle and doing *Paśchimottānāsana?* When you do *Uttānāsana* you gaze at your toes. Does it not become a spiritual practice as long as the mind does not wander in the *āsana?* The moment the mind wanders, the attention wanes, cells become dull. You bring back the awareness and the potency comes again in the intelligence to be stable. Whether *mantra yoga*, *tantra yoga* or the practice of *āsana*, whatever it may be, the practitioners have to use their body and progress only with these means. Don't they? In my case *Paśchimottānāsana* or *Uttānāsana* becomes my *tantra* and *mantra*. Then why call it physical?

It is a great challenge, but that is how you have to learn. You have to bring the intelligence, which is superior to the mind. Yoga teaches us to refine the intelligence more and more to take us to the subtle and subtlest part of consciousness. *Āsana* and *prāṇāyāma* can't be neglected because the moment you neglect them you have neglected a part of your soul.

Today everybody is using the words that yoga is wholistic and holistic. What are these words? When the body transforms itself to be wholly with the soul, it is not only wholistic but also holistic. When you are doing *Tāḍāsana*, if you are attentive from the bottom of the foot to the head, without oscillating your intelligence in your body, what is it? The consciousness is existing evenly, that means that consciousness is not divided, it is steady, it has not deviated. The moment it has deviated, you forget, you forget the *āsana*. If you bring the absoluteness, what happens? The totality comes. If you do all the *āsana* in totality, it is divine. Is it not? You are in a state of divinity.

At that time even the search for the soul is not there, do you know that? Because you feel its presence, then it wanes and you want to get to that waxing again. Patañjali has used the word beautifully that the feeling of *ātmabhāva* disappears the moment the *ātman* surfaces: *ātmabhāvabhāvanā nivṛttiḥ* (*Y.S.*, IV.25).[1]

When you do not get an *āsana* correctly, but thereafter it comes suddenly, can you measure that elation? Does this elation come from the mind or something else?

- From something else. -

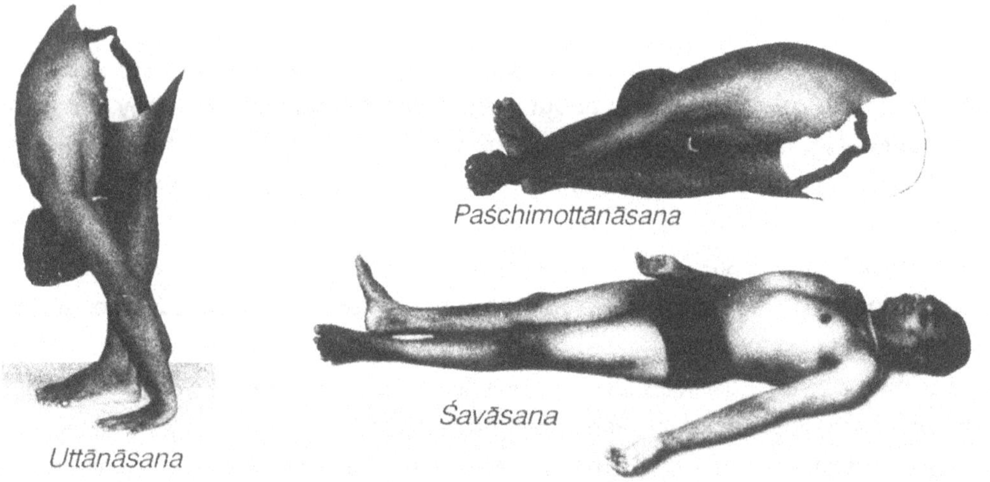

Plate n. 29 – *Paśchimottānāsana, Uttānāsana* and *Śavāsana*

That is how the *āsana* practice has to get involved. So you need to make your brain like a layer of skin. When you do *Śavāsana*, are you aware of your skin?

- No. -

See whether you can make your brain like that. The wrong word used is hibernation. In *Śavāsana*, is it hibernation?

[1] As long as one is ignorant, he considers that the body, mind, consciousness are the soul; therefore the distinction remains. When all these are purified, the sense of separation disappears and *ātman* alone is felt.

- No, it is passive. -

Becomes passive, does it not?

- Yes. -

So find out whether you can retain that passivity which is rhythmic in the body. Can that rhythmic passivity be built up in the brain? See whether you can keep your brain as an object. The leg does not look at the leg; the arm does not look at the arm. Similarly watch whether you can learn that the brain may not look into the brain in *Śavāsana*.

You can see how the words are simple but how difficult they are to put into practice. To keep the brain in that passive and peaceful state without psychological fluctuation makes *Śavāsana* spiritual. The brain is always psychological though it is a physiological object. It doesn't want to remain quiet. We say the mind is not quiet. It is the brain that is not quiet. That's why the brain is called intelligence of the head, whereas the region of the heart is known as intelligence of the mind. The intellectual stability from the brain and the emotional stability from the mind, both have to be developed through yoga so that both lose their independent existence. They become one without showing any disparity and that is Self-realisation.

Therefore, in any *sādhanā* you undertake, you need to introduce the element of spirituality because no *sādhanā* can be done without the body. The human life is meant for *sādhanā*. So you have to begin any *sādhanā* with the body. The mind has to get involved and ultimately, it has to bring together the head and heart, intelligence and emotions, i.e., *jñāna* and *bhakti*.

This is called Divine Practice.

YOGA – A PATH FROM PHYSICAL TO SPIRITUAL*

Bellur Krishnamachar Sundaraja Iyengar is one of the world's foremost teachers of yoga and author of Light on Yoga, *the widely translated best seller on yoga.*

At the age of fifteen, his brother-in-law, T. Krishnamacharya, a well-known yogi at the Mysore durbar instructed him initially. Soon Iyengar was forced to start on his own in Dharwar and later Pune. Despite years of hardship, privation, he persisted and kept experimenting and refining his practice towards perfection. In 1952 the violin maestro Yehudi Menuhin became his disciple and in 1954 he introduced Iyengar to the western world. Today, Iyengar's pupils literally number in millions in over 160 centres scattered over all parts of the globe. He has had fifty-five years of experience of using yoga against disease.

Assistant Editor Vithal C. Nadkarni journeyed to Pune, to Ramāmaṇi Iyengar Memorial Yoga Institute, to interview the master on a wide variety of topics including yoga and therapeutics; yoga and miracles and esoteric practices, during two sessions spread over two days. Excerpts from the interview with one of the undoubtedly forceful and accomplished personalities of our times.

Q.- Let's start with your approach to yoga.

Yoga is a *mokṣa-śāstra*, the science of emancipation and liberation. Yoga is the path that cultures the body and senses, refines the mind, civilises the intelligence and takes rest in the core of our being.

It is unfortunate that many people who have not penetrated the depth of yoga think of this spiritual path to Self-realisation as being merely a physical discipline and the practice of *haṭha yoga* as nothing but a kind of gymnastics. But yoga is more than physical. It is cellular, mental, intellectual and spiritual. It involves man in his entire being.

---

* Interview by Vithal C. Nadkarni, assistant editor of *The Times of India Group of Magazines*, Mumbai, 2001.

Q.- Is that why Svātmārāma, the author of the celebrated manual on yoga, calls *haṭha yoga* the ladder to the heady heights of *rāja yoga* in the very first verse?

Precisely. Those who approach yoga intellectually say *rāja yoga* is spiritual and *haṭha yoga* physical. This is a gross misconception. Do they know that the last chapter of Svātmārāma's *Haṭhayoga Pradīpikā,* known as *Samādhi Nirupaṇa,* speaks on the state of *samādhi* or union with the Supreme Soul? And what is the end of *rāja yoga?* It is also *samādhi.*

Q.- Can you briefly explain the eight limbs of yoga that help you to achieve this goal?

Yoga is traditionally divided into eight aspects called *yama, niyama, āsana, prāṇāyāma, pratyāhāra, dhāraṇā, dhyāna* and *samādhi.* These can be divided into two tiers:[1] external – *bahiraṅga* – and internal – *antaraṅga. Yama* and *niyama* are social and ethical disciplines, *āsana* or posture and *prāṇāyāma* or breath control are the external – *bahiraṅga* – practices whereas *pratyāhāra* or withdrawal of the senses leads the aspirant from the outside to the inside, to the understanding of the Self.

The other three limbs are the inner ones – *antaraṅga* – which include concentration *(dhāraṇā),* meditation *(dhyāna)* and absorption or dissolution of the mind *(samādhi)* in the Universal Self.

Q.- This Indian way of looking at the body is obviously different from the way western science looks at the human body.

The essence is the same. An Indian body is the same as the American or Italian one. Indian anatomy is no different from the Western one. Both have considered the body as the temple of the soul and hence it has to be kept pure and clean. At the same time hedonism was recognised by both eastern as well as western philosophers.

Maybe the words are different and the symbols to describe universal processes too may differ. But we must not get carried away by words that are used in different countries.

---

[1] See *Aṣṭadaḷa Yogamālā,* vol. 1, *"Yoga and Dharma",* p. 163; vol. 2, *"Kṣetra-Kṣetrajña Yoga",* pp. 200-201. See also *Light on Yoga, Light on Aṣṭanga Yoga* and *Light on the Yoga Sūtras of Patañjali.*

Q.- Let's take an example: the way *āyurveda*, the Indian science of healing, looks at the body and the way yoga approaches the body.

In a way, you are right. Yoga and *āyurveda* look at the body from different angles. Yoga has gone a step further than *āyurveda*. Unlike western science, *āyurveda* has gone beyond the bones, muscles and vital organs recognising the vital energy that plays the great role.

Yogic science has penetrated further to find out the inner storehouses of energy where the confluence of physical, mental, intellectual, spiritual, cosmic and divine energies takes place. These storehouses are known as *cakra*. Through the practice of yoga the flow of energy is traced in the visible and invisible or known and unknown channels in the body known as *nāḍī*.[1]

The aims of yoga and *āyurveda* are almost the same. Both are concerned with Self-realisation. The only difference is that yoga adopts a psycho-spiritual approach and *āyurveda* uses a physico-physiological one. The cause of diseases, according to yoga, is the fluctuation of the mind, or *citta*, on account of the three *guṇa*, namely *sattva*, *rajas* and *tamas*. On the other hand, in *āyurveda* diseases are caused by imbalances in the basic constituents of the body. Western science has recently started tracing the role of the mind. They have to take support of yoga and *āyurveda* in order to know the depth of the mind.

Q.- What are these constituents?

They are the five basic elements: earth, water, air, fire and ether. The first element is earth, which is the ground for the production of energy. When the energy has been produced, its distribution requires space which is given by the element ether. The other three elements, namely air, fire and water, act, react and interact with each other in order to produce the energy. As we need an empty vessel to cook food, similarly, earth is the vessel, the open space is ether, and air, fire as well as water are the elements which contribute their energy to produce vital energy in the human body. Besides the elements, *āyurveda* emphasises *rasa* (chyle), *rakta* (blood), *māṁsa* (flesh), *meda* (fat), *asthi* (bone), *majjā* (marrow) and *śukra* (semen).

Q.- *Āyurveda* also speaks of the three humours of the body, does it not?

Yes. They are called *tridoṣa*. And they are known as *vāta*, *pitta* and *kapha*. These are also viewed as the principles of air, fire and water as they manifest themselves in the physiological body using the

[1] See *Aṣṭadaḷa Yogamālā*, vol. 2, pp. 174 - 193, and *Light on Prāṇāyāma*, chapter 5, *"Nāḍīs* and *Chakras".*

element of earth and ether. Basically the earth and ether elements are mixed with water, fire and air. According to *āyurvedic* theory, imbalances or disequilibrium of the *tridoṣa* lead to disease, which causes the disturbance in the elements.

Q.- Can you give an example of this?

If you have an imbalance because of an excess of the earth element, you get constipation. Similarly, if there is an excess of the water element, you get dropsy and so forth. For instance, take arthritis, which is a very common disease all over. In this, the *vāta* is vitiated along with the other two, *kapha* and *pitta*. The lubrication, which is the main work of *kapha*, deteriorates and the joints of the bones – the earth and ether elements – get affected. The aches and pains, the swelling and immobility, are the result.

Q.- Where does yoga fit into this scheme of things?

According to the science of yoga, the disturbances in the vital elements occur because of the imbalances of the three *guṇa* or tendencies.

– Again a triad? –

Yes. You can find the three qualities of body and mind in each individual's behavioural patterns. And they are described as the qualities of *sattva*, *rajas* and *tamas* or illumination, dynamism and inertia. According to the yogic point of view, these qualities of nature disturb the mind, which in turn disturbs the functions of the body, which are dependent on *tridoṣa*. That's how *āsana* and *prāṇāyāma* are introduced in yogic science and methodology. These two aspects connect the body and its innumerable parts with mind together in order to develop an integrated intelligence.

Q.- So there is no need to take medicine?

Yes, provided one does the practice of *āsana* and *prāṇāyāma* in the manner it is required or demanded.

In yoga, you have to generate your own energy to combat the disease. This requires tremendous will power. Since not many people possess such potency, they are advised tonics and vitamins which restore the harmony of the elements and humours and expel the irritants and infections and so on. On the other hand, the 'vitamins' you need to maintain yoga are faith, courage, boldness, absorption and tremendous memory to understand exactly what is happening in us today, what happened yesterday, the day before yesterday and many days ago, with an uninterrupted awareness.

Q.- That sounds like something from psycho-neuro-immunology. Both stress and eustress or positive stress and happy emotions are said to release their own chemicals such as adrenaline and endorphin. These in turn have profound effects on the state of our body. A sort of a deeper intelligence of the body-mind.

Patañjali did not forget psycho-neuro-immunology. He projects aptly in one *sūtra: maitrī karuṇā muditā upekṣāṇāṁ sukha duḥkha puṇya apuṇya viṣayāṇāṁ bhāvanātaḥ cittaprasādanam* (I.33).[1] One needs proper, healthy and effective emotional deliberation and deliverance. The outer world, the society, the people and environment, being the objective world for the subjective being yields the experience of happiness, sorrow, virtue and vice. However, everyone as a subjective being has to have emotional deliberation in the line of friendliness, compassion, gladness and indifference towards these various experiences.

Well, you should not be surprised at all. Every physical action has a chemical counterpart and vice versa. Even the various states of mind and the various emotions have this dimension. What yoga does is to develop a tremendous sensitivity to feel these changes and even modulate and tune them.

Q.- If I understand you correctly, you begin with the physical body at the very foot...

Āyurveda starts with the body. Yoga starts with consciousness. But the basic principle for both is the same. In the *Upaniṣad* we read, "One who is a weakling cannot have the experience of the soul".[2] Thus, the body is the vehicle for the evolution of each individual. For any righteous action *(dharma sādhanā)*, health of the body is the foundation.[3]

---

[1] Through cultivation of friendliness, compassion, joy and indifference to pleasure and pain, virtue and vice respectively, the consciousness becomes favourably disposed, serene and benevolent.

[2] *Na ayam ātmā balahinenalabhyaḥ.*

[3] *Śariram ādyam khalu dharmasādhanam*, Kālidāsa.

Think of yoga as a factory built to make a certain product. Suppose the factory also produces useful by-products, you can sometimes forget the original purpose for which the factory was built. The side effect of yoga is health. It's not the main purpose. The main purpose of yoga is emancipation and freedom from sorrow.

Q.- Can we talk about the by-products? For instance, the practice of yoga is supposed to endow the yogi with miraculous powers or *siddhis*. Are these real? They account for the greatest confusion and fascination people have for yoga.

This is very interesting. Patañjali in the third chapter of his classic, *Yoga Sūtra*, talks about the 'wealth of yoga'. He has given the so-called super normal powers in thirty-five aphorisms connected with the progress, the wealth of the practitioner. These deal with the kind of feelings the *sādhaka* gets. This answers the first question you put, as Patañjali gives thirty-five indicators or sign posts on the royal road of yoga. If you have any of them you know that your *sādhanā* or practice is on the right path.

But unfortunately people forgot and they gave it a mysterious type of meaning. In a way the *siddhi* are also by-products, whereas *yoga sādhanā* for the *yoga sādhaka* is meant mainly to recognise and realise the very soul, the core of his being.

Q.- It is very fascinating that you should say this. Because the famed yogi-poet of Maharashtra, *Śrī* Jñānadev, said something very similar seven hundred years ago. He says in his classic commentary on the *Bhagavad Gītā* that doing yoga is like climbing a very steep mountain, after hanging on the cliffs by the skin of your teeth. And once you reach the summit of equilibrium it's like walking on a meadow, with no sense of duality, nothing more or less. Of course he also gives vividly metaphoric descriptions of the *siddhis* in the sixth chapter of his *Jñānadevi*.

The Lord says in the *Bhagavad Gītā*,

Yogasthaḥ kuru karmāṇi
saṅgaṁ tyaktvā dhanañjaya
siddhyassiddhyoḥ samo bhūtvā
samatvaṁ yoga ucyate (II.48)

Oh Arjuna! Perform the duties by establishing your mind in yoga. What is this yogic mind? The mind that remains detached renouncing the attachments, remains even-tempered in success and failure. This equilibrium or equipoise of the mind is yoga. With *siddhi* the sense of achievement flourishes and the ego get nourished. Then where is the state of equipoise? Therefore you need to reach that summit which is higher or above the *siddhi* and that is *samādhi*, where the duality vanishes.

Q.- Then what happens to the *aṇimā* and *garimā*[1] and the various powers that you are supposed to acquire?

That's all enticement to drag one away from the path of emancipation and liberation. Nature, with its three constituents, is like that. It would not yield the harmony so easily. The *triguṇa* create imbalance in the mind similar to *tridoṣa* in the body. It wants to see if this person is able to retain his mental poise throughout. If you are caught in *siddhi*, you are caught in *rajoguṇa*. Obviously the *sattvaguṇa* remains in the background.

Q.- I want to ask you about the theistic view taken by yoga. Is it necessary to believe in God, to practise *Īśvara praṇidhāna* as the fifth *niyama* or the rule of yogic conduct requires you to do?

If you read the *Yoga Sūtra* carefully, Patañjali begins by advising surrender to God. As he realises that this state is not possible to one and all, he suggests various alternative means to achieve the state of self-surrender to God. Having said this, know whether you believe in God or not. There is a Power which cannot be understood by the conscious mind. That Invisible Force touches and fills peoples' lives. We have read about a sinner becoming a saint and a saint becoming a sinner. How does this happen? You have to believe either that you can bring about the transformation in you or there is some Greater Power that intervenes to cause the transformation.

– But is it necessary to invoke a mystical God for this?

As the very definition of yoga is to bring the individual soul to unite with the Universal Soul, there is nothing wrong in thinking of God. Patañjali explains God as a unique entity who is eternally free from afflictions and unaffected by actions and their reactions or by their residues. This explanation

[1] *Aṇimā:* the capacity of making oneself infinitely small. *Garimā:* the capacity of making oneself heavier.

is not mystical but practical. Yet, can't you practise yoga without having to believe in God? It is not a question of faith but of the inner refinement. If you can refine yourself without bringing the name of God into the picture, who knows, as you get refined, your present view may change.

Q.- Is it not possible to do yoga, as they do in the West, without recourse to the mystical side; as a purely physical science?

No. Those days have gone. If you had asked me this question thirty years ago, I might have agreed with you. But today a revolution has taken place and they have changed. Let me narrate a personal experience. A yoga teacher has been suspended for six months for his sexual misconduct in one of our foreign centres. And he was censured by the community for another six months. Is this not a value revolution? So even Westerners cannot treat yoga merely as a physical science.

You see, it is not the question of acceptance of God or not. Normally, when we question anyone about whether he believes in God or not, we reduce God into a material thing. We reduce God to matter; therefore the question of belief arises. To believe in God, we need to believe in ourselves first. As the Universe that is beyond our reach is unknown to us, so the entity God which is beyond the reach of our consciousness is unknown to us. Our consciousness, the *citta,* has limitations. We need to open the horizon of consciousness to see the other entity, "God". Patañjali knows our weaknesses, that our consciousness is caught in *vṛtti* and *kleṣa*; therefore, we in general and our consciousness in particular, cannot conceive God. If consciousness gets purified, then the existence of the Cosmic Force, i.e. God, can be felt.

Patañjali undoubtedly refers to *Īśvara praṇidhāna* but keeping the path equally open for the theistic and the atheistic. When he mentions *Īśvara praṇidhāna* in *niyama*, he refers to it after *śauca, santoṣa, tapas* and *svādhyāya.* He wants us to cleanse our body, mind, intelligence, I-ness and consciousness first in order to have *Īśvara praṇidhāna.* Even while referring to *kriyā yoga,* he wants *tapas* and *svādhyāya* to be followed in order to cleanse the *karma* and *jñāna,* so that *bhakti* arises from the pure state of consciousness. While referring to *sabīja* and *nirbīja samādhi,* he again keeps *Īśvara praṇidhāna* as the end. First he wants the practitioner to develop faith, vigour, right memory and profound meditative awareness with intense and severe practice. Patañjali wants the *sādhaka* to surrender his *sādhanā* to God *(Īśvara praṇidhāna)* so that he subdues his ego consciousness and in its place develops humbleness.

This is how he wants the practitioner to convert himself from an atheistic state of consciousness to a theistic one, knowing very well that the unevolved consciousness will deny the Highest and Greatest Entity.

So do not think that one can invoke God that easily with this underdeveloped state of consciousness. God is mystical to those who are still at the perverse level of intelligence. The mysticism ends when one's intelligence and consciousness evolve totally.

Q.- What about western science? How is it reacting to yoga?

Very positively. Some of my pupils are working in hospitals for the mentally retarded, and some are working with AIDS patients. We have had some promising studies where the T cells increased with the practice of yoga. But the problem appears when the patients do not continue with their practices regularly. For example, another patient of H.I.V. has maintained T cells without falling back.

Undoubtedly, the Westerners have started accepting the fact that the mind like the body needs a healthy and positive approach.

Q.- What was the regimen you gave to these patients of AIDS?

Since it is the failure of the immune system, one needs to work to ignite it. Obviously, I worked first at flushing the whole system. Basically, it is invited because of a wrong and unethical way of living, therefore I had to improve the blood circulation from the navel to the generative organs. Since the innocent people too get affected, I have to give the list of *āsana* in order to improve the overall function of the body.

Q.- What *āsana* did you prescribe in therapy?

Mainly, I concentrate on inversions such as *Sālamba Śīrṣāsana, Sālamba Sarvāṅgāsana, Halāsana, Setu Bandha Sarvāṅgāsana, Uttāna Padma Mayūrāsana.* Later, I add some backward extensions such as *Dwi Pāda Viparīta Daṇḍāsana, Ūrdhva Dhanurāsana, Laghuvajrāsana, Kapotāsana.* Often I have to change the sequence symptom wise since the immune system deteriorates, and I have to see from what problems they suffer.

For instance, if they get pneumonia, I give stimulative *āsana* such as head balance – *Sālamba Śīrṣāsana* – and shoulder balance – *Sālamba Sarvāṅgāsana* – for the longer periods where the patients have to stay minimum fifteen minutes to forty-five minutes so they recover. When they have tremendous fatigue, I give them supine *āsana* such as *Supta Vīrāsana, Supta Baddha Koṇāsana, Matsyāsana* and so on.

When they suffer from poor digestion, I give them forward extensions such as *Jānu Śīrṣāsana, Paschimottānāsana, Ūrdhva Mukha Paschimottānāsana* I and II, and so on.

Basically, I see that they do not get tired and fatigued. I see that they do not get profuse sweating. My main concentration is on digestive, circulatory and reproductory systems. Yoga gives them physical strength and moral courage so that they can strengthen their immune system.

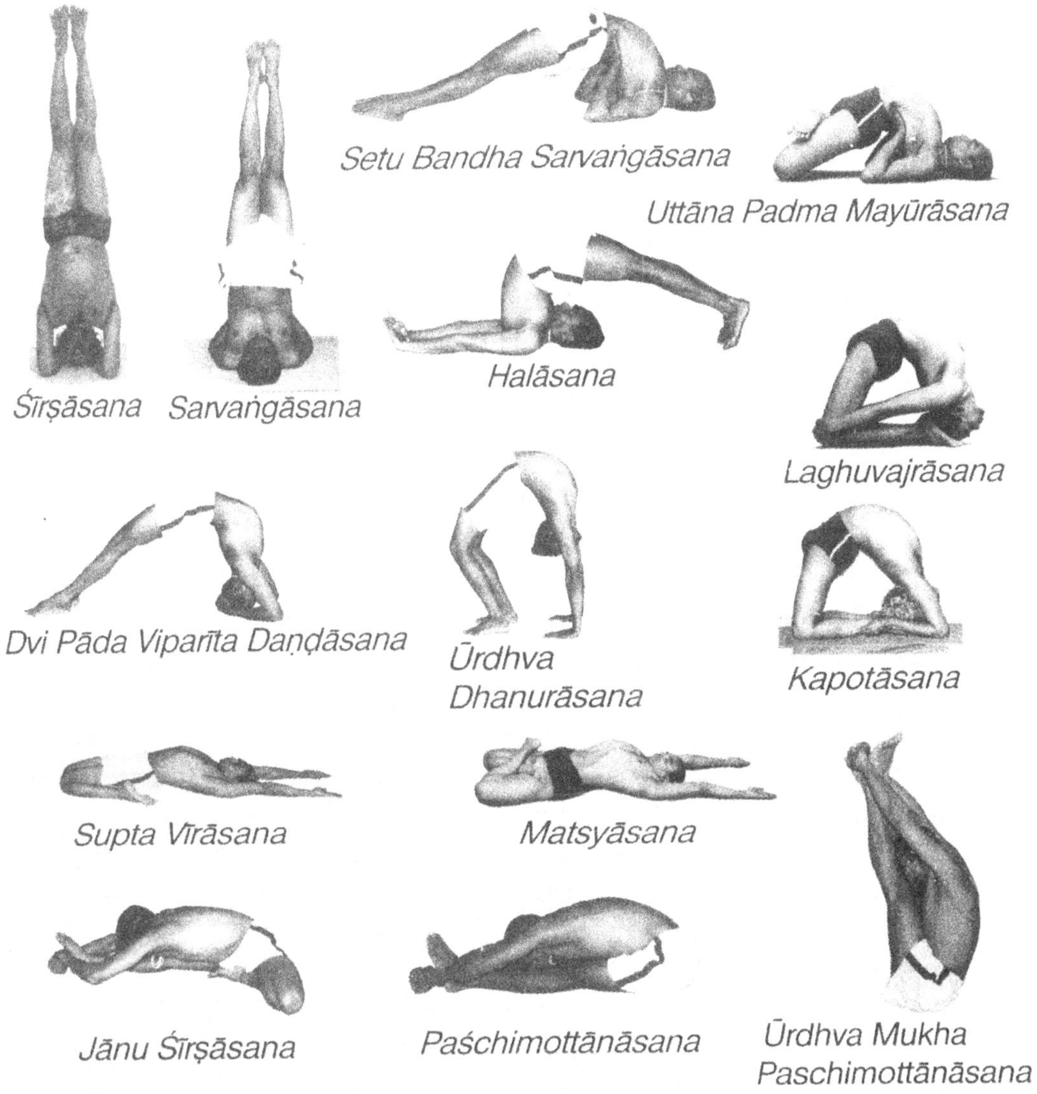
Setu Bandha Sarvaṅgāsana
Uttāna Padma Mayūrāsana
Halāsana
Śīrṣāsana
Sarvaṅgāsana
Laghuvajrāsana
Dvi Pāda Viparīta Daṇḍāsana
Ūrdhva Dhanurāsana
Kapotāsana
Supta Vīrāsana
Matsyāsana
Jānu Śīrṣāsana
Paśchimottānāsana
Ūrdhva Mukha Paschimottānāsana

Plate n. 30 – Various *āsana* to bring relief

Q.- What about effects of techniques like meditation for fighting drug abuse? Have you had any experience in this growing urban problem?

Know that one should not only work on the mind of a person but also on the nervous and circulatory systems, which are also most important in drug abuse. Yoga was tried by some pupils of mine fifteen years ago in England to wean children away from drugs. And they were strikingly successful. But due to some politics, the programme was stopped and the children went back to drugs and the police caught them. The kids told the police, there is no yoga so they feel their lives are empty and monotonous and so they went back to drugs. While making them do *āsana*, I make them to look within the functioning of the body which is nothing but meditation techniques.

Q.- Can we talk about your experience in popularising yoga in the West?

When I first went to England in 1954 I had only two students. Today hundreds of thousands practise my method. I have taught hundreds of thousands of people. I have not travelled to Argentina or Brazil or Uruguay or Chile, but you will be surprised to know that many are following my method in these countries.[1]

– That's what we would like to know! –

My book has been a bestseller in the USSR, too! They have begun from a purely practical angle. This most philosophical and artistic yoga – which is one of our heritage, must, therefore, have a tremendous strong foundation. It may put you into the yogic net and then keeps on propelling you onwards and forwards. The changes it causes manifest permanently in your life. I need not sell this subject to you as you are the judge of how yoga made a difference in you. See, I have been doing yoga for fifty-five years. The effect of this is not so much on me as on my son and daughter. My son is forty years old. You should meet him. He had a very severe accident a year ago. He has lost the use of his right arm, the sensation has just returned after one year. We are expecting some more improvement. You should see his tranquillity. Neither he nor I were disturbed. There was no emotional upheaval. I expect the coming generations to have a better orientation.

Q.- Now you are beginning to sound like Maharshi Mahesh Yogi who says he can achieve world peace through meditation alone!

[1] Now my centres are there and good teachers are carrying on teaching yoga as taught at the Mother Institute at Pune.

I am sorry, I do not claim that. Please know that I am not talking about peace. I am talking about the culture of mankind. I am not talking of the bodily changes or mind changes but on the increase of the *sattva guṇa* or the illuminative intellectual quality.

Q.- You went to the USSR recently. What was the response to your work there?

I think they can be a better bridge between the East and the West for yoga than our own interface with the West directly.

- Do elaborate. -

Their emotional balance is like the Easterners. But their way of thinking is like the Westerners. They are very hospitable, very traditional and at the same time very revolutionary. I was the guest of their Government last November. I think they are definitely looking for spiritual life, for unalloyed joy.

Q.- Did you have any contact with their medical scientific fraternity?

The medical people came to the conference. You'll be surprised to know that my *Light on Yoga* has been in circulation there in a cyclostyled translation! Because yoga was a proscribed subject there until last year. Because of my (samizdat) status, I was widely known to the Russians. And they presented me with this xeroxed copy.

(Shows a large red book bearing the translation and photographs of his poses).[1] This was a conference on alternative medicine sponsored by the Health Ministry and the Sports Council there. When I gave a demonstration they filmed it. I am told this three-and-a-half hour film is circulated to the various institutes and Universities.

- Amazing. -

Q.- Tell me how do you manage to do poses at this age of seventy-two which boys of sixteen would find taxing to the limit?

---

[1] See plate n. 34.

Well, I do them. Of course I have to do them, don't I? But let me confess, the body is rebelling. My body says, "give me rest". It's very interesting: there was no physical fatigue until three years ago. But now I feel as if the body refuses to accept that vigorous action. And I have to struggle. So I am on the threshold. It is easy for me to leave. But if I leave, where do I live? Where do I end? I still practise for three-and-a-half hours a day.[1]

Q.- What about your *gurujī*? Isn't he over a hundred years old now and the French government was to make a film on him?

Yes, they did. My *gurujī* is no more. He died fourteen months ago.

Q.- How? Of what?

Maybe his age that kept him in bed. He was in coma for some days before his death. Similarly Krishnajee in the end required so many tubes and catheters for breathing, for eating as well as for urination etc.

That's why I'm doing yoga. You know, death has to come majestically. Because I know if I let go of my practice, I am creating dull cells in the body. I am taking the example of J. Krishnamurthy and my *gurujī*. The body says, "Don't do the practice". But the mind says, "No. Don't listen to the body". And I try to my optimum. If I don't, a certain pessimism will come upon me after a certain age.

Q.- Is there any hope for us?

That's why I am showing you by example! This body has to be kept healthy till the last moment. All great people said, "I am attached to the body". But I say, even a dull man is not attached merely twenty-four hours to the body. In old age the mind becomes petty and listens to the body language and gives up *sādhanā*. So I am trying to keep the body and mind alert and active. If I surrender to the dictates of the body, then I am in the wilderness. That's why Patañjali defines yoga as *citta vṛtti nirodhaḥ* – curbing the tendencies of the mind, which affects the body, and body language negates the mind.

---

[1] The author has not stopped practising till now.

During the ageing process it is essential to follow the rules of keeping the body healthy so that the mind is free from attachment towards the body. That is the peak of time when one has to practise, perhaps more than ever, to keep the mind away for it to be detached from the body.

So there is a hope not only for you but also for others to keep the body intelligence alert and active so that the mind also remains positive and alert even in ripe old age.

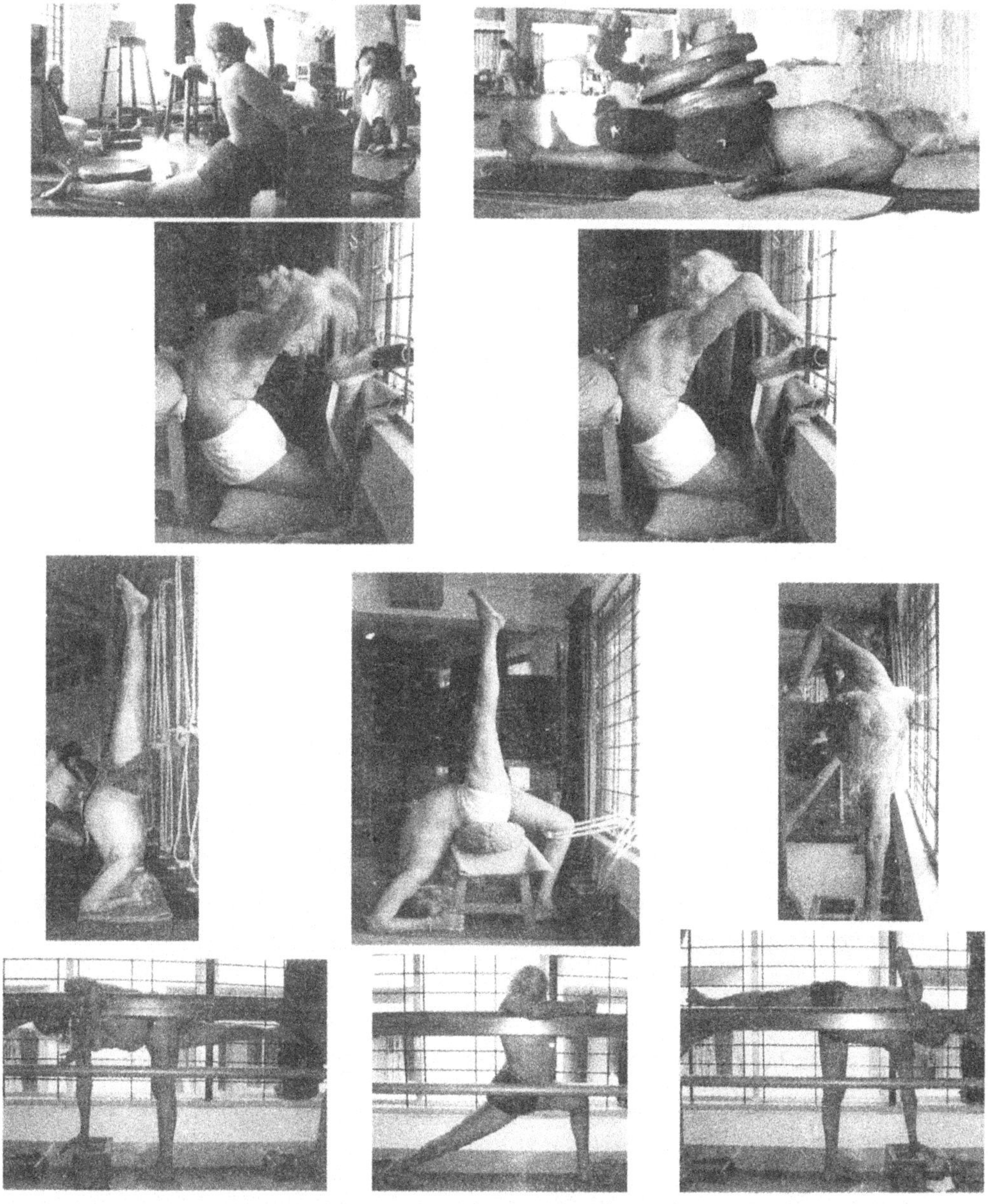

Plate n. 31– Pictures from the authors current practice (2004).

THE PATH OF YOGA*

Yogacharya B.K.S. Iyengar is one of the truly great contemporary yoga masters. He is renowned and respected all over the world for the depth and refinement of his study, practice and teaching of yoga. His dedication to his art has inspired teachers and students on every continent, and sparked a light which illuminates the study of yoga in all corners of the globe.

We are honoured to publish the following interview with Mr. Iyengar, which was conducted by Margot Kitchen of Calgary on Thursday, July 5th 1990 at the University of Alberta in Edmonton during the Canadian Iyengar Yoga Conference. It was transcribed and prepared for publication by Jennifer Rischmiller and Shirley Daventry French.

– Welcome, Sir. –

Thank you very much.

Q.- Perhaps we could start at the beginning with a definition of yoga. What is yoga?

The traditional meaning of yoga is to unite the individual soul to the Universal Soul, which is rather abstract and difficult for the common people to understand. So the simple definition is that yoga is to uplift the body to the level of intelligence of the mind, and then take the vibrant body and intelligence of the mind, to come in contact with the serene spirit within.

Q.- Yoga has escalated in the last decade or so in the West. Why? What are we searching for?

---

* Interview by Margot Kitchen of Calgary, on 5th July 1990. Published in *Victoria Yoga Centre Society Newsletter*, December 1990-January 1991

The simple reason behind this is that all the technical growth and material comforts that developed in the West did not bring mental peace or physical freedom. When I began taking yoga to the masses, a large number of people began practising. They experienced some kind of freedom of the body and lightness of the mind. This created interest to continue practice in order to find out and experience something which can be like an eternal bliss. As far as the material benefits are concerned they felt that they have reached the zenith, which must not have brought that unalloyed bliss which they were expecting. But the restlessness in them was there. Yet having tasted physical and mental lightness, they turned towards the Eastern methods that deal with the ways of living and also for the sight of the Self.

Q.- Popularity, though, can sometimes damage the true nature of a subject. Has this happened to yoga in your estimation?

It is true that the individual ego plays tricks and instead of making the subject known the practitioner wants to make himself popular.

Well, it is true that such things do happen, for the simple reason that the pride sets in, though we try to improve ourselves physically, morally, mentally, intellectually and spiritually. In many cases, name and fame take the upper hand and not the subject. Some forget the essence for which they practised; they jump to the idea of becoming popular like film actors or actresses. The personality cult is built up. When the person goes in for glories, damage does happen to the subject, however true and real the subject may be.

Q.- People have many misconceptions. For example, is there any religious dogma attached to the practice of yoga?

The meaning of religion is realisation. Realisation of one's own self gets involved at a certain stage. In this state religiousness plays a role and not a selective sectarian religion. I again repeat that the moment virtuousness begins to work within, one aspires for realisation of the real, which appears as a religious deed and not a religion in a denomination or in a colour.

- But it is spiritual as opposed to a religion. -

It is wrong to assume that spiritual is opposed to religion. All religions preach, "to know thyself." When religion preaches to know thyself, how can they oppose each other? All systems that help in self-culture have no denomination as a religion. The quality of religiousness gets involved when one strives for self-culture.

In fact spirituality and religion are not opposite polarities. Religion is that which uplifts the human being and leads towards the realisation of the Self. One does not advocate religion for animals! But religion is stipulated for human beings. Firstly they break the rules of law and secondly, being intelligent, they are made to be conscious of their duties.

Every human being has the right to find the ultimate purpose of his existence, which is nothing but Self-realisation. This very thought is religion itself. Religion is nothing but controlled and conditioned regulations on life. Religiousness is the essential quality of any religion. Hence, there should be no difference between religiousness and spirituality.

Q.- Ah, one myth dispelled! But there are other myths! I think a lot of people associate walking on coals and pretzel-like behaviour as the aim of yoga. That is not the aim. What is the true aim?

Yoga does speak of such powers. But these are not the aims and ends of yoga.

Exhibitionism should not be viewed as the end of yoga. The aim of yoga is to develop humility with perfect intelligence. According to Patañjali, one has to purify the intelligence through the continuous practice of yoga to such an extent that the wisdom of yoga goes on progressing without building up arrogance.

One can exhibit such achievements but can one exhibit humility or wisdom? The moment you exhibit humility, humbleness or wisdom, it is no more humility, no more humbleness and no more wisdom. Yoga is meant to sublimate egoistic powers.

– People are afraid of change. –

This is true. The fear is that they confuse transformation with change. The change is quite different from transformation. If they distinguish, then 'fear' never exists in their minds. Change is momentary but transformation is permanent.

Q.- Can people practise yoga as you have described and still live in our western society as a householder?

It is difficult to transform soon. In fact, the transformation is like the process of evolution, which occurs slowly. Human life has two aspects. We use the terms *bhoga* and yoga. *Bhoga* is to experience and enjoy the sensual pleasures and yoga is the auspicious state of the union with the Ultimate Supreme Soul.

One should know that, even if one wants to enjoy the pleasures of the world, one should have good physical and mental health. Without health one can neither enjoy the fruits of the world nor think of God. So from that sense I think there is nothing wrong to begin yoga to have perfect health and mental harmony. As you go on practising, the inner transformation takes place to move from good to better and from better to the best.

Man has several aims in life. All aims are capsuled in *dharma, artha, kāma* and *mokṣa,* meaning; right living, making money, love and freedom. Wealth and lust are placed by our sages within the banks of *dharma* and *mokṣa. Artha* and *kāma,* which lead towards *bhoga,* are placed between the banks of *dharma* and *mokṣa* and hence are a guide to the householder to experience and enjoy *bhoga* within these two banks. When one lives within the banks, that transforms a householder to go ahead after fulfillment of *bhoga.* He does not indulge in *bhoga* alone.

In order to have fulfilment of these aims of life, the sages have divided the span into four aspects, known as *brahmacaryāśrama, gṛhasthāśrama, vānaprasthāśrama* and *sannyasāśrama.* These four aspects are like supportive shelters to be taken to fulfil the aims of life and are placed between two banks of spiritual aspects. In *brahmacaryāśrama* you study and educate yourself under the guidance of a *guru* to know the meaning and depth of life. Here the foundation for spirituality is laid. In *gṛhasthāśrama* you fulfil the inborn tendency of pleasure seeking, which is natural for everyone to enjoy the wealth and passion (*artha* and *kāma*). But these two are placed between the banks of yoga. In *vānaprasthāśrama* you train your self to withdraw from enjoyments and entanglements by completing the responsibilities of a family bondage. The period is like a threshold where you train yourself to have an inner transformation from enjoyment to emancipation, from bondage to freedom, from evolution to involution.

This understanding in practice goes beyond the thought of West or East. As music does not divide East and West, yoga does not differentiate between East and West. The aims of life are common to all whether one is an Easterner or a Westerner and hence the *āśrama* type of life-style is applicable to one and all.

– So one does not have to live in solitude. –

Not at all. I am a householder with six children and grand children. It is not the environment that is important but the attitude in the mental frame. It is possible for one to remain in Piccadilly

Circus or anywhere downtown and be peaceful. A man in a cave with serene surroundings may be having cloudy thoughts in his inner mind and be restless. How do we know whether he is serene or turbulent?

Q.- Is it so those of us who are staying in society just have it a little more difficult perhaps?

I think, it is the frame of each one's mind. It may be difficult staying in society. But please note that it will be difficult for those who live in the caves. If the mind is prepared, then it is not difficult. Our intellectual exposure is always to the external world. Practice of yoga turns the mind inwards. It is interesting to know that the moment one does yoga, the direction of the mind goes inwards. One gets cut off from the external world at least for the time being. Is it not something good to be in contact with one's own body, mind and self? Hence, I think it is possible to do yoga in the middle of a town, in a crowded place or anywhere while leading a family life.

– So you can be in contact with your own mind, your own self, and be at a cocktail party. –

Yes. The cocktail party may be a social side of the life, but looking inward and being with oneself is an essential side of life. When you go to a cocktail party, you follow certain mannerisms. When you have to be in contact with your own mind, you need different manners and yoga teaches that only.

Q.- There are many interpretations of yoga that have come to the West. How do we discriminate and find the true practice?

It is very interesting because the fundamental principles of yoga are often beyond the known. I wrote a book on yoga to which I gave the title *Light on Yoga.* Somebody else may write a book and they call it, say, *"Yoga for Enlightenment".* The titles differ but who knows, the same contents may be put differently because the origin remains the same though one twists and turns.

The yogis with knowledge and understanding, gave us four pathways for Self-realisation: 1) path of action, 2) path of knowledge, 3) path of love, and 4) the path of yoga. This path of yoga, (as you put the question before,) gradually got polluted to such an extent that each one started calling it different names, like *mantra yoga, laya yoga, rāja yoga, haṭha yoga, tantra yoga, tāraka yoga, kuṇḍalinī yoga* and so on. These things came later, but yoga has one meaning, i.e. to associate oneself with one's own higher Self. Only the definitions vary: one book says control the mind, another book says control the body first and then the mind so you will be one within yourself. Another may say in order to have the union of the individual soul to the supreme soul, one has to purify oneself. But the aims of all the texts on yoga are the same.

We have been given arms and legs to follow the path of action – *karma mārga*. We have been bestowed with the intellectual head to think and follow the path of knowledge – *jñāna mārga*, and the seat of the spiritual heart, emotional centre for affection and love – *bhakti mārga*.

Compassion, friendliness, do not come from the head, they start from the heart. So these three paths are given to us by God to develop purity in action, purity in intelligence and purity in love. In order to develop purity in action, clarity in intelligence and true love without lust, the fourth path, yoga, was discovered as an instrument to develop these qualities. From this, yoga became the fountain for the other three paths. These were the only paths given by the sages of yore, but to name them differently is the choice of an individual.

Q.- There are many books on yoga that are available nowadays. Does one need a teacher?

No doubt all subjective knowledge needs the help of an experienced teacher. But there are lots of books. Writing books has become a fancy to many for fast fame in life. As you put the question about the purity of the work – a good book is better than a bad teacher! If a good book is available, then I would have to say it is a better guide than a bad teacher, as good teachers are rare.

Q.- Then the next question has to be, what are the qualities of a good yoga teacher?

I would not say only for a "yoga" teacher. The quality of a teacher is that the teacher has to study the calibre of the pupil. The teacher has to climb down to the level of the pupil and gradually bring the pupil from that standard to his standard. If the teacher can do this, then I say he is a top class teacher.

Q.- There are many "India returned" teachers. Is it necessary for one to go to India to be a good yoga teacher?

If a good teacher is available here, there is no need to go to India to learn. If you cannot get a good teacher, as they are rare products nowadays, then it is worth going to India; not just going and coming back as "India returned" without getting the best from the teacher.

Q.- So the student must be very discriminating, ask questions, compare and not just accept the first "India returned" teacher?

Yes, definitely. What has happened is that yoga being a subject from India, if a teacher announces, "I am India returned," then people think, "Oh, he has gone to the source." So this illusion should not be created regarding the "India returned" teachers, just to build up their egos and fill money in their pockets.

- The word guru has been used indiscriminately here in the West...-

The word *gu* stands for darkness and heaviness, *ru* for lightness and knowledge. One who removes the darkness of the pupil and enlightens with the light of knowledge is considered as a *guru*.

Q.- Sir, you are called *gurujī*. When is it appropriate for one to call you *gurujī*?

People never called me *gurujī*. I have been teaching yoga since 1936 and people started calling me *gurujī* only a decade ago. Even today people call me Iyengar, some people call me Mr. Iyengar, but those who experienced the light that came to them through learning started calling me *gurujī*. I don't tell them to call me *guru*. They call me *guru* because they experienced the light.

- So it comes from the heart? -

From their heart, it means some light has come to them, otherwise they would not have called me *gurujī*. Yesterday some people addressed me as Iyengar. I never asked them why they are calling me Iyengar without even adding Mr. We are just dust in the eyes of God, but if a student feels that I have the light and calls me *guru*, it's his right. As I say, *guru* is a rare product.

- Yes, that's true! -

Out of two thousand million population, I don't think anyone in this field has drunk the depths of the good and the bad of each posture or each breath as I did. My own practice gave me the enlightenment and I pass on the light to others who come to me.

Q.- Do you have an understanding of why you have become so revered throughout the world?

Perhaps, for the simple reason, I think, of my sincerity, integrity, honesty and dedication to the subject. I do not pretend and do not demand unless I have understood myself.

- Yes. I have read that your early life was very difficult. -

Yes. The difficulties of life put me on a righteous path.

Q.- Would you tell us how you came to be on this yogic path?

In the early days, I had a tough time. I could not find even one meal per week. I was living on water. I don't know what made me do yoga. I had no interest to do yoga. I was suffering from tuberculosis; I had no health at all. There was no penicillin available in those days. So my sister's husband, who became my *guru*, said: "Why don't you do some *āsana* for gaining health?" I thought, instead of living a parasitic life, why should I not try? I tried but did not regain health for nearly five or six years.

In India, in the thirties, women were not mixing with men, and if they wanted to learn they were not willing to learn from a grown-up man. When I was only sixteen years old, the women-folk told my *gurujī*, "We don't want to learn from you or from any of your senior students, but we'll learn from this young boy. We are interested in yoga and so solve our problems." So my *gurujī* had no other alternative except to ask me to teach. I said that I did not know anything. He advised me to teach whatever I knew. That's how life began for me and I developed. I had not mastered the *āsana*. I used to refer to lots of yoga books in those days. I had very little knowledge of yoga at that moment. All the books were filled without experience. I would look at the illustrations: they would write something, the figure was different. I said, this is not yoga. Then I took it up as a challenge.

I felt that these illustrations, which I see in the books, are not correct. In *Śīrṣāsana* some people keep their heads on one side, some to the front, some to the back. Some people throw their legs backwards, some forwards. Then I decided to experiment and find out for myself which would give inner serenity in the *āsana*. I started searching for serenity in each *āsana*, from restlessness to restfulness. All different styles of doing the *āsana* were making me restless, no matter which method I tried. Then in a flash, I would feel the restfulness. I struggled to find out how did I get this restfulness. This way I developed.

The colleges of Pune invited me to teach yoga en masse. In those days yoga was only taught on one to one basis and not at all for groups. I said to myself that I should teach one or fifty people at the same time. I was young and ambitious, and whatever chances came to me I accepted. Knowing very well that I did not know anything about yoga, the disease or the healing process, when the patients of different age groups with whatever diseases they claimed came to me, I said, "Let me try!" It was fortunately bearing fruit.

During my early yoga practices I was unhappy because I was not getting the expected results. I was restless, and felt like giving up. Within five minutes my inner voice would say, "Do it again, try again, try again." This voice, which was coming from inside, made me continue yoga. Though I was not attached to yoga, yoga was attached to me then. Now, I am attached to yoga *(Laughter).* That's how we two, yoga and me, got wedded.

Q.- I have read that at the beginning of this period of trial and error, when you were teaching you would take the pains of the students into your own body to help them better. How?

Yes. Even now, I do. If I see a person, the way he walks, the way he stands, I create that same kind of crookedness in my body and I walk. Then I understand that these are the muscles that need training and development.

– *But now, you just look at someone and act instantly.* –

Well, fifty-five years of non-stop practice! And lots of bodies that I have seen and touched gave me knowledge.

My fingers have touched between one hundred and two hundred thousand people. By touch, I can say what happens – my skin is so sensitive, my eyes are so sensitive, just by touching, the things reveal to me. You can call it insight.

Q.- You demand a great deal of your students and your teachers. In your own words you are an "intense" teacher. This is sometimes misinterpreted as aggressiveness or even violence, and I think it is time to dispel that myth.

My friend, firstly even Patañjali has categorised the practitioners of yoga, using specific terminology. He says there are four types of teachers and four types of students. Mild teachers, mild students

– *mṛdu*. Average teachers, average students – *madhyama*. Keen teachers, keen students – *adhimātra*. Intensively intense teachers, intensively intense students – *tīvra*. Now, if I belong to that quality of intensity as a teacher, then I want all my pupils to be intense. If I am mild, I will definitely introduce mildness. But I did not learn anything in mildness; I had to work so intensely that I realised it is only by intense *sādhanā* that it is possible to get the benefit of yoga, not otherwise. Remember that with that intensity, I had to keep my head free from tension.

Secondly, Patañjali is a disciplinarian. He himself is not a mild teacher. The word in the very first aphorism, *anuśāsanam* indicates this nature of his, which he has imbibed from his ancestors. Yoga is meant for all and its discipline has to be followed by all *sādhaka*.

Thirdly, as you point out that my intense teaching is taken as aggressive or violent, this also needs explanation. When a sculptor begins to sculpt or carve, he uses the hammer or chisel to break the stone or wood. In the first stage he is rough, but when he begins with fine work to refine it, he uses his hands very delicately. Similarly, I too use my discrimination. Qualities such as adamancy, fear, wrong habits, ego, pride, laziness, resistance, non-cooperation in pupils need strong hammering or chiselling, whereas when a refined touch is required I have to be delicate. If you ask the patients, when they are in pain or agony, they will tell you that my touch or correction in that *āsana* is soothing in the adjustment of the *āsana*.

So, do not worry about the words, 'aggressiveness' and 'non-aggressiveness' or 'violence' and 'non-violence' as framed by some. It may be professional jealousy. These words are the opposite ends of the same thread.

Q.- So when you are teaching and you touch your students, that is just to bring their consciousness to that area?

Yes. Consciousness exists everywhere, but it is hidden, dormant. So when we practise the *āsana*, we have to remove that dormancy of the consciousness, which is even at the bottom of the foot. If I say, feel the toe, consciousness rises there, otherwise it does not rise. So why not keep the consciousness in an even state through the entire body. That is for me intensity. To keep the consciousness not in compartments but in an absolute state of oneness in whatever *āsana* you may be in, demands intensity. Intensity appears aggressive sometimes, but intense is intense! *(Laughter)*.

- I'll quote you a lot because I have read your book Iyengar – His Life and Work *several times. I can remember you saying that a parent has to be stern, but it is done with love. That's what I understand from you. –*

That morning when I was in the class teaching, I told them that when I look at a person, if the brain does not take the message, I am aggressive with the brain, but I am compassionate with the body which is affected. If the knee is bad, I am sympathetic to that knee, not to his head. If I am dealing with the knee, your brain has to be cooperative with me. If you resist with rigidity that means the brain is non-co-operative.

- You've just struck a nerve. I remember that very well! (Laughter).–

Q.- I would like to talk a little about health and yoga. You have said that yoga is a way towards integration of body, mind and spirit. Where does our disintegration come from? We have spoken about that as far as the aim of yoga is concerned, but if you could elaborate a little more on how we got to this state of disintegration that we are in.

You know, health is dependent upon the cellular system because trillions and trillions of cells take birth and die in a split second. Our everyday life today is like a stillborn child. The delivery was healthy but the child was still. Similarly our cells, to a great extent, are stillborn cells. The practice of yoga, whether *āsana* or *prāṇāyāma*, is the gateway to see they generate full life and die after serving the needed ingredient of the body. I consider this supreme health.

The disintegration between the body, mind and soul arises out of ignorance or want of knowledge which Patañjali calls *avidyā* and integration comes only through understanding (*vidyā*). If *avidyā* (disintegration) is a non-healthy state, *vidyā* (integration) is a healthy state.

Due to *avidyā* it appears that the body-mind are a totally separate entity from the soul. The soul is the "seer", whereas the body, mind, intelligence, etc. are "seen" by the "seer". This identification, or the sensing of the seer and the seen as one, is the cause of all sorrows and pain. The disintegration is hidden in this identification. In other words, if we call them (seer and seen) as integration they mislead us because the characteristic of the seen is just the opposite of the seer.

By practising yoga we bring the understanding between the seen and the seer. With the practice of yoga the impure seen is made pure. Through its purity, only the seer is perceived. The identification of these two opposite entities is possible only when they are in a pure state – *śuddhisāmyatā*. However, the seen is in its impure state because of its outgoing nature, whereas the seer is always in a pure state. If the "seen" is purified, then there is evenness in the seen as well as in the seer. This integration in fact is a right identification though the seen and seer are separate entities.

Q.- So it is very important to the *āsana*. For someone who is not aware of yoga, how do they differ from other exercises? Can you explain?

Other forms of exercise work on the structural or physical body – the muscles and joints – but working on the peripheral parts is not the end of health, while the yoga practitioner concentrates on physiological organs, like the liver, the spleen, the respiratory system, the circulatory system and so on. He studies through various *āsana* how the liver or the pancreas work. By this one can understand the difference between other exercises and yoga.

Yoga works more on the physiological, psychological and neurological levels than on the physical level, and the yogis knew that the function of the structural body is as the base to act on the physiological, psychological and neurological organs to get the full effect. Hence, yoga builds up together the physical and physiological bodies, as well as psycho-neurological body. Unless these are attended to, one cannot go towards the self.

The physiological body is in between the physical body and the mental body. This body being the bridge between the outer body and the mind, it has to be cultivated and invigorated through proper blood and energy supply. Then the physiological body, with the cellular system, integrates the body and mind and evolves towards the self.

Q.- Have these aspects been recognised by the medical profession?

I think they have just begun; in a few years time you may hear about results from the good practice of yoga. For example, the scientists recognise now the importance of the principles of *yama*, or the ethical disciplines of yoga. They are explaining the bad effects of smoking and drinking, which were the part of the ethics of yoga. As they have accepted this part of yoga, who knows, soon they may also accept the chemical changes that take place in the brain when the *āsana* are done, which may be of great help to future generations.

The responsibility is theirs, and I request them to experiment and study by keeping their eyes and ears open. Unfortunately today, the scientists have their own dogma and they want the experience of the yogis to fit to their dogma. But keeping their eyes and ears open, let them study and see what comes of these practices.

Q.- So all your pupils, just by their example, can keep spreading the word?

For the present this is the only way left to the yoga practitioners. Recently in San Diego there was a pulmonary test of the yoga students conducted by some doctors. The result was that the pulmonary system of all the yoga students was healthy, because they blew out beyond their capacity. The capacity of their instrument was limited as the students could go beyond its measure.

Q.- What about cardiac function? The West is obsessed with aerobic activity, and the first question that I am very often asked is, is there an aerobic benefit to the practice of yoga?

I don't think so. The aerobic movements are strenuous. There are two types of exercises: one is irritative, one is recuperative and stimulative. Yoga is stimulative and not irritative to the nerves. There is a feeling that if you do jogging or aerobics, your heart starts pumping more and it supplies blood for the heart to function better. But at what cost? We advise *Setu Bandha Sarvāṅgāsana* where the cardiac nerve, which begins from the thoracic-dorsal spine, is made to exercise actively. That takes the blood towards the chambers of the heart from the other bank of the heart for the rhythmic function of the heart with no strain at all. It pumps the same way. I take cases where the blockage is great and today they are doing all the work even though they have reached the age of seventy. Today at my Institute in Pune, the cardiac patients have increased and the patients are improving progressively. I want heart specialists to take a lead to test these patients.

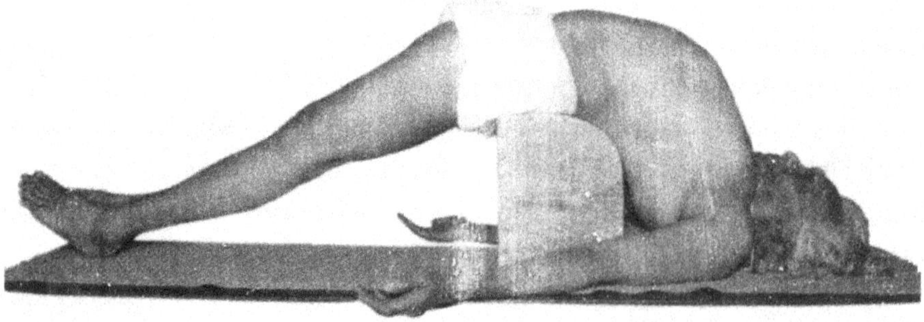

Plate n. 32 – *Setu Bandha Sarvaṅgāsana*

As a matter of fact, look at how many have practised yoga and experimented with it, whereas those experiments carried out by the practitioners of aerobics are only at a peripheral level, for instance, recording the blood-pressure and heart-beat, out-put and in-put of CO_2 and O_2, etc.

Has anybody experimented on *āsana* – how the energy is saved? Do they know the various ways of doing *āsana*? Do they know the language of the practice of yoga, which differs from healthy, young people to aged and diseased people?

–I hope it comes soon. –

I hope so. Today I have shown, Dr. French and Dr. Carruthers, here in Canada, how the neck traction and forward traction are available in yoga. They are completely logical and scientific.

– And practical! –

Q.- Would you give us some examples of specific medical problems that you have been able to help?

Many. I have worked with polio patients, cardiac patients, slip disc cases, depression, B. P. patients and so forth!

– Post-polio syndrome is something that has just come to light in the past few years. –

Yes. I have given life to the polio affected area. They walk now, they do not depend upon others. They ask whether they would become completely normal. I tell them that it all depends upon the range; but my job is to give them some control and self-confidence so that they can lead a natural life.

I have taken some heart cases; they even do inversions like *Śīrṣāsana* now. In the Institute I have handled more than a dozen cases and it took me two years to take them to do head balance. Please know that I didn't do that straight away. I tone their bodies and make them get confidence to keep their head down – forget about going to *Śīrṣāsana*. Some of the doctors who come from Europe and U.S.A. have seen them before and are amazed to see them in perfect condition. In addition to the heart problem, persons with Parkinson's disease could even interlock their fingers.

From the very beginning of my career as a teacher, I have treated unbelieveable cases of which I never kept the record. I am glad that they are leading a happy life.

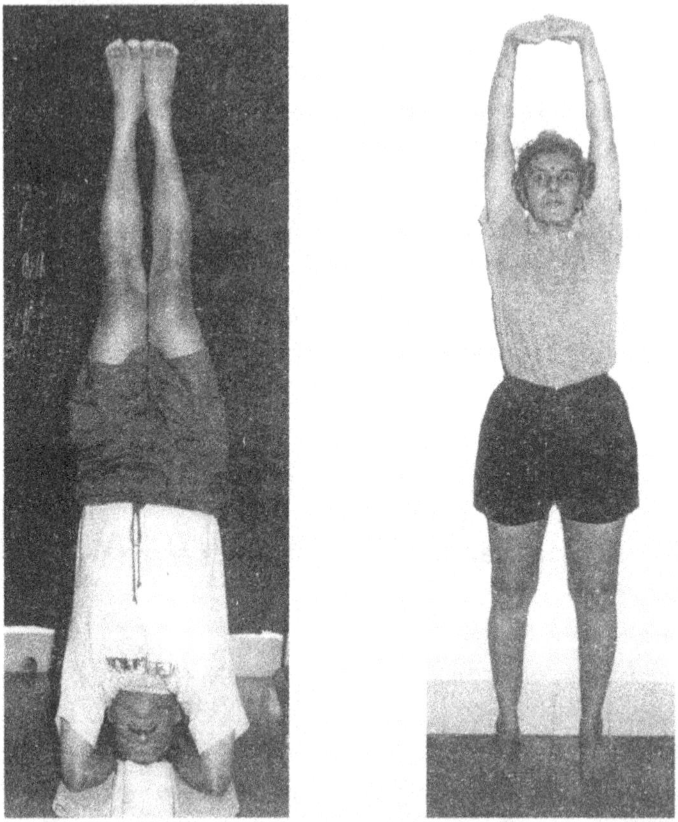

Plate n. 33 - A heart patient in *Śīrṣāsana* and fingers interlocking for a woman with Parkinson's disease

Q.- So you take these people and do a form of therapeutic yoga?

Yes, I have to do it to find out the depth of healing in yoga. Here, I will give you another example of my own daughter. When she was to deliver her baby, she was under the care of a doctor who comes to my class. The doctor told me that somehow the foetus was not moving to the centre, and as the time was up, the doctor wanted to go in for a caesarean. The doctor asked me to do something if possible through yoga. Today or tomorrow? That's all I said. She said, I'm not sure whether you can do it in one day, and I told her, don't do your class today, be with my daughter. Then I put my daughter in *Setu Bandha Sarvāṅgāsana*, which you all know. I moved the bench from side to side, without disturbing her in *Setu Bandha Sarvāṅgāsana*, keeping each time two minutes. Next

I made her do *Baddha Koṇāsana* in *Setu Bandha Sarvāṅgāsana*, and rolled the bench from left to right, right to left. Then I had my daughter stand up, and asked the doctor to examine her. The doctor said, it has come to the centre, and the doctor took my daughter to the hospital for delivery.

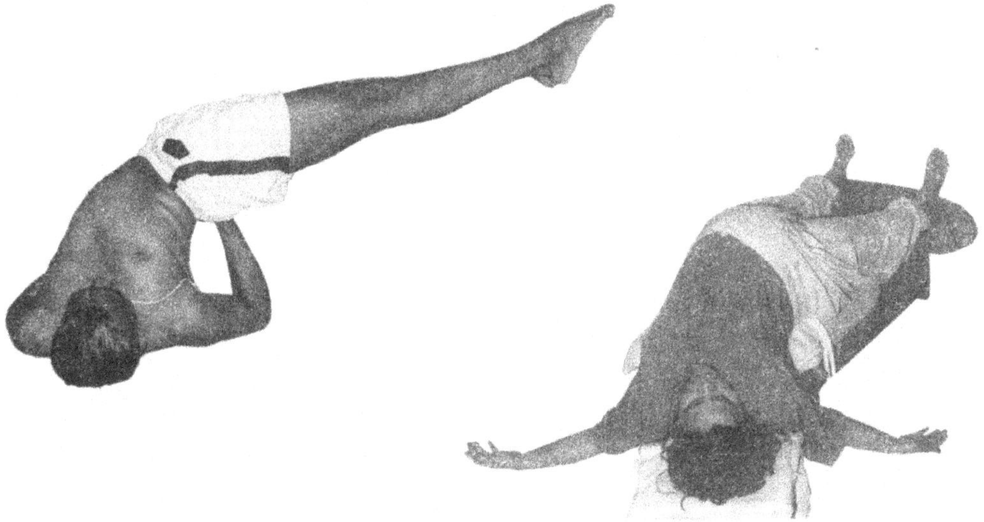

Plate n 34 – *Parśva Sarvaṅgāsana,* with the bench rolled side to side

Q.- That's a wonderful story. Have you treated any patients with AIDS?

Yes. One was in a very bad condition. He was from San Francisco. He was in Pune for one month, and I taught him. The first thing, perspiration stopped within one month. Water was just dripping from the body, and this stopped. The wetness of the generative organ was there, and for that I had to make him work very, very hard. Now, what was this wetness? It was untriggered or uncalled discharge of semen. I said to him, if you have will power it can be done, not otherwise. The person showed will power only for a few days, and from the periphery the generative organ began to dry out. He returned to the US, and the doctors when they tested him said that his T-cells have tremendously built up in his body, more than when an earlier test was taken, before he visited India.

In some of the hospitals in San Francisco, my pupils are teaching AIDS patients. There is a very interesting case in France also, where a man developed AIDS about six years ago. For the last five years he has been doing yoga. Last year he developed pneumonia; the doctors thought he would die. I had a telephone call from France. Having seen this patient while he was recovering, and knowing the defensive strength in his body, which was very good, I asked whether he had done a lot of back bends. I asked the teacher to find out whether he had devoted his time to back bends. The answer came back, yes he had. I immediately asked him to stop overdoing backbends and to do stimulative *āsanas*, such as head balance – *Śīrṣāsana* – and neck balance – *Sarvāṅgāsana*, one hour in the morning, forty-five minutes in the evening. He was asked to do no other poses. The doctor who was observing him every two or three days was very impressed as to how quickly his pneumonia went away. He asked his patient how this could be, and the patient told him, "My *guru* told me to do these *āsana* and I'm doing what he told me to do." Not only that but he couldn't eat any normal food for five years. Now, within six months, his diet is normal. Now he says, "I am normal."

I give you another example. An HIV patient from USA came to Pune for a month or so for treatment. As soon as the lady returned to the States, she went for laboratory tests, her "T" cell count rose by 80% from 160 to 280.

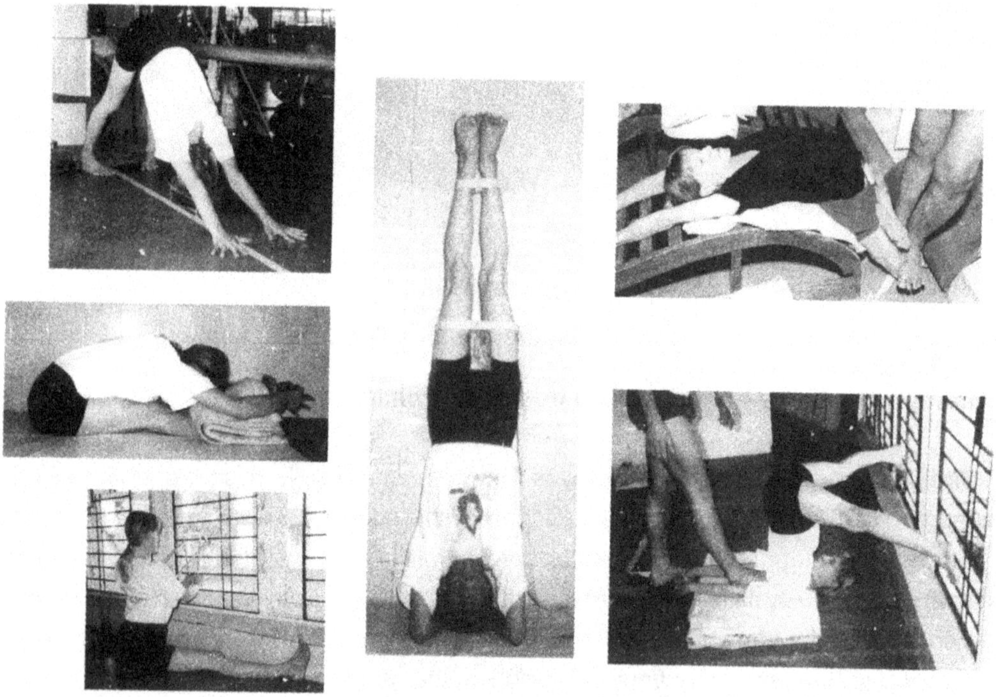

Plate n. 35 – Some of the *āsana* practised by a student with HIV

– A woman who is a friend of mine went to you in Pune with a respiratory condition, and she followed to the letter what you asked her to do. Now she is working with doctors in Calgary with people who have respiratory problems. It is very exciting; the doctors are amazed at the difference in the patients when they are doing the practice that you showed Erin. –

Yes, I remember.

– The practice you gave her was completely passive. It's amazing. –

I am teaching hundreds and hundreds of students, but the doctors have to change their way of thinking. They need to know the various approaches and methods that we have in yoga. There is one good thing, the change is now towards preventive medicine and alternative medicine. They are coming in place of conventional medicine. So at least, there is a slight change; people are realising conventional medicine is not such a help and are turning their minds towards alternative healing methods. I have attended two or three international conferences on the subject. I went to Russia on the same subject as a guest of the Russian government. Yoga was banned in Russia until 1988. It was only opened up last year, and the first conference was held by the government of USSR. When I went there I was surprised to see my book *Light on Yoga* in the Russian language, which was in distribution underground for practitioners.

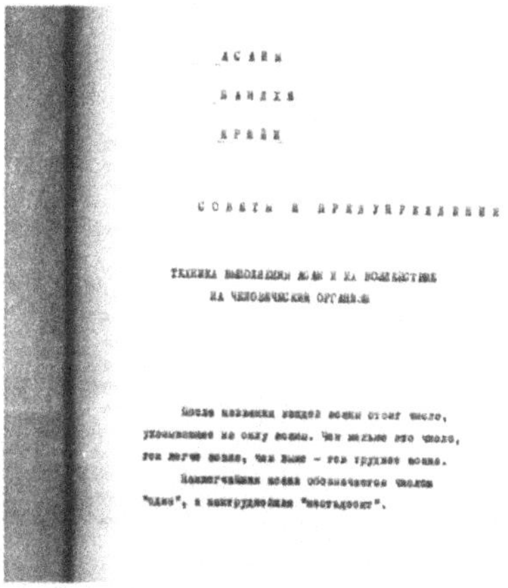
АСАНЫ

БАНДХИ

КРИЙИ

СОВЕТЫ И ПРЕДУПРЕЖДЕНИЯ

Plate n. 36 – Underground copy of *Light on Yoga,* in Russian

Q.- When you went to Russia, you went to a conference on health and preventive medicine. What did you do at the conference?

I gave a demonstration. I told them how yoga prevents diseases and increases health. Health is a dynamic process. As the cells improve, the body function improves and health also improves. Health is definitely dynamic, not just static. "I'm all right" is the expression of negative health. Negative health has been taught to us by the medical people. Nobody has taught the ways for positive health. To be free from diseases, aches and pains is not positive health. Yogic system doesn't allow calcification, nor allow the arteries to get blocked due to various positions of the *āsana*. Naturally health is gained by keeping each and every part of the body as it was when born, through yogic discipline. When there is a renewal of cells, renewal of energy, continuous flow of vitality, stability of mind, sharpness of intelligence, then there is positive health.

For example, take sports medicine. I have attended many sports medicine conferences. In one of the conferences the German doctors were impressed by my demonstration. Once I asked them, suppose a good athlete is there: he gets a cold, but has to run. What do you do? You can treat for the running of the nose, but his cold has sapped his vitality. Will you give the needed vitality? The pills are there, but do they build the inner strength? I took two or three athletes on the platform, and asked them whether they have a running nose. Some lifted their hands, and I put them in *Halāsana*. They said, "Now we feel the passage clear." After five minutes they came down and said, "We feel very light." I said, now they are fit to run as they got back the vital strength. Hope you understand how yoga can help sports medicine also.

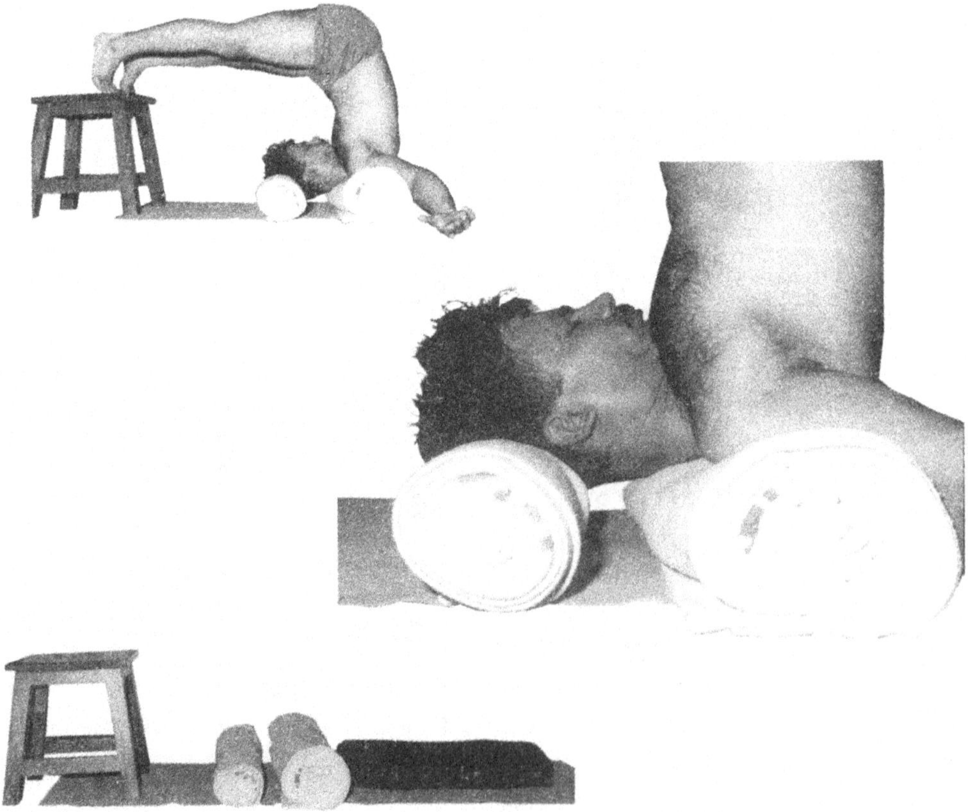

Plate n. 37 – *Halāsana* (half) to help clear the sinus passages

Q.- And hopefully it will influence athletes so that, rather than taking steroids for their outer strength, they will work on their inner strength and have an edge in that way.

You may not know that John McEnroe came back through Iyengar Yoga; this is what was reported in sports papers: "It's a very rigorous method but I practise Iyengar Yoga," he says. He does yoga for his backache. Now the test cricketers in India are all coming to Pune and undergoing training. They say their fielding has improved, their bowling has improved, their batting has improved.

In a way yoga is a better approach to gain inner strength and endurance rather than cheating and winning medals by usage of artificial steroids.

Q.- As you know, the Olympic Games were held in Alberta in 1988 and I had an occasion to talk to some of the coaches of some of the international teams, and they were using an aspect of yoga – they were using visualisation but they were not, as yet, using the posture. So that is where they need to be educated, to use the posture.

Another aspect that we are very involved with here is stress. Could you explain the ancient art of relaxation, *Śavāsana*, and how it could help us with modern stresses?

It is an interesting question. Stress comes by tension. Tension comes from the nervous system. When it comes from the nervous system, the energy which has to flow without disturbance cannot flow, and gets blocked. When you do the *āsana,* not to mention *Śavāsana,* like *Sarvāṅgāsana* or back arch, what do you do? You extend and expand the muscles of the body with these *āsana* for the energy to flow in the entire nervous system and the block that has taken place due to stress. In these *āsana* the energy flows uninterruptedly with no stress at all on the muscular and nervous systems.

There are many who think yoga means relaxation or meditation. When you say, "The use of visualisation," this concept is abstract. Often people think that yoga is a mental faculty. Similarly, *Śavāsana* for relaxation is again abstract as one does not become stress free or tension free so easily by doing *Śavāsana*. This is lack of knowledge on the subject of yoga.

Yoga practice is a concrete way to improve their skills in their performance. It could be in the body-level such as muscles, joints and bones. *Āsana* are done to bring sharpness, quickness, steadiness, strength and proficiency in their performance. It is done to eradicate slowness, dullness, laziness. It is done to recover from fatigue. It is done to freshen the mind. It is done to improve one's concentration and attention. Therefore yoga is a total approach in all ways. To improve these faculties, varieties of *āsana* and *prāṇāyāma* are there for athletes and players to cultivate a better performance. Unfortunately this concept is unknown to them. Hence, education needs to be imparted to the participants so that they derive the maximum benefit by a natural method.

Q.- The *āsana* could be the antidote to stress also?

Yes! The *āsana* can be done to get oneself free from stress factor. *Āsana* such as *Sālamba Śīrṣāsana*, *Sālamba Sarvāṅgāsana* and *Viparīta Karaṇi* make one release either the neuro-psychological or psycho-neurological pressure. When the nerves are stress free by these *āsana*, then the effect of *Śavāsana* is experienced at once. Please know that people cannot do *Śavāsana* when they are under stress. A person who knows how to stretch fully knows the art of total relaxation. A casual stretch brings a casual relaxation, so to enjoy *Śavāsana*, I say try to get the full extension and expansion in the system so that in *Śavāsana* it is extended and expanded like a river where the flow of water is uninterrupted by any obstacles. Keep your system in such a way that the energy in *Śavāsana* flows uninterruptedly and supplies energy. With stress we create a closure on the ends of the nerves. Yogic practice makes the nerves remain bottomless so that one can take any load. *(Laughter)*.

To know the technique of *Śavāsana*, I advise you read my book *Light on Prāṇāyāma*.[1]

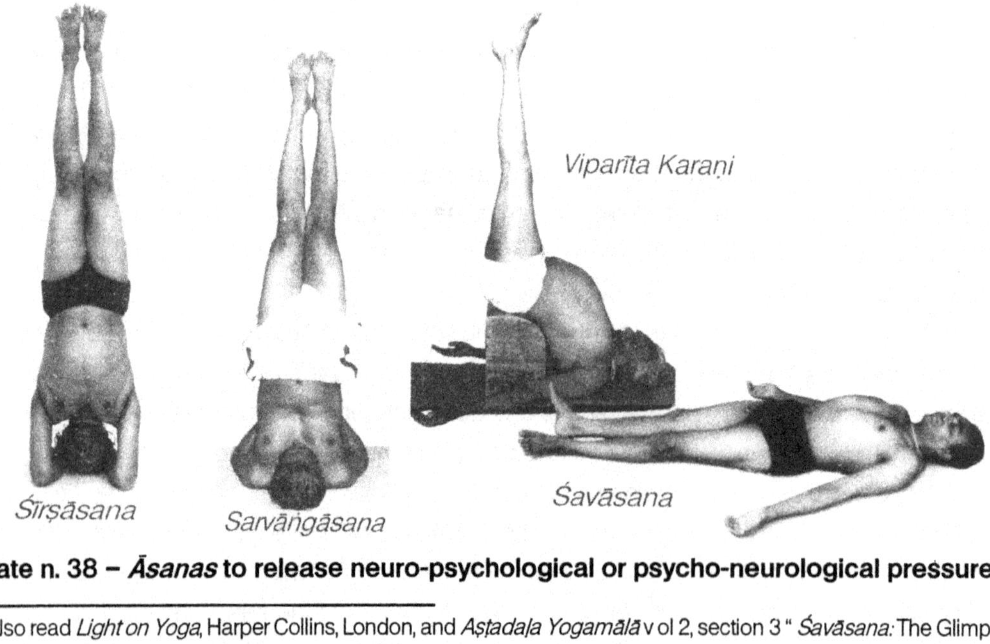

Plate n. 38 – *Āsanas* to release neuro-psychological or psycho-neurological pressure

[1] Also read *Light on Yoga*, Harper Collins, London, and *Aṣṭadaḷa Yogamālā* vol 2, section 3 " *Śavāsana:* The Glimpses of the State between *Jāgradāvasthā* and *Tūryāvasthā*".

Q.- I have quite a few students with multiple sclerosis, and we are working with yoga. That is one thing I am going to tell them, because they are really involved with their nervous system. Are there specific poses that you would give to someone who came to you who was hypertensive?

Yes. You know, when we use the word 'hypertension' the stress is on the brain, hence we have to know how to make the brain 'hypo'. Sometimes we keep weight on the floor of the brain, as tendencies come from this aggressive part of the brain, the frontal brain. Due to the weight, the energy of the frontal brain recedes towards the back of the brain and hence becomes quiet, so the patient cannot think. The brain becomes hypo in certain *āsana* like *Setu Bandha Sarvāṅgāsana, Dwi Pāda Viparīta Daṇḍāsana* and *Halāsana*.

When you find that the patient is hypertensive you can make use of the weight plates on those areas where the tension builds up. The nerves that get inflated due to the tension begin to get deflated and calmness begins to set in.

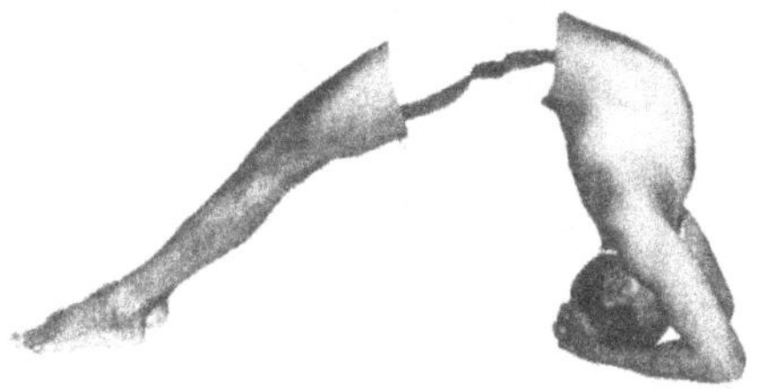

Dwi Pāda Viparīta Daṇḍāsana

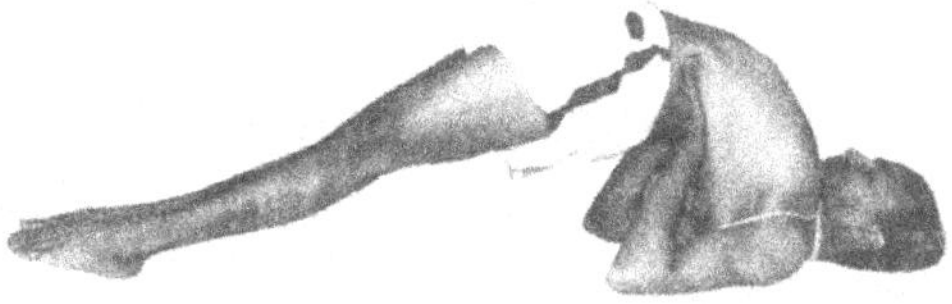

Setu Bandha Sarvaṅgāsana

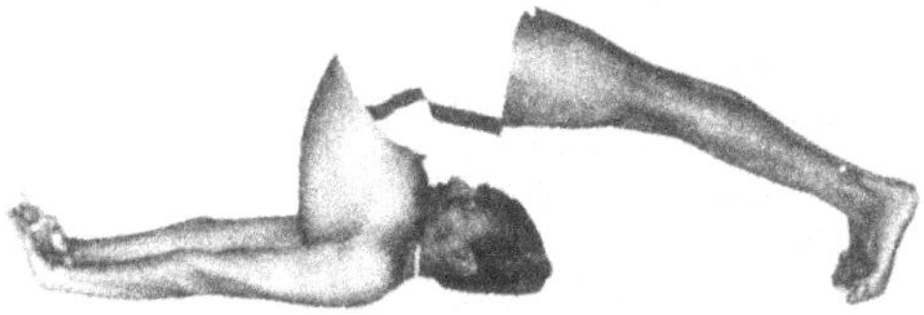

Halāsana

Plate n. 39 – The brain becomes hypo in certain *āsana*

Q.- Does the breath play any important part?

Normally each inhalation is a stressful action whereas each exhalation is a non-stressful action. Normal inhalation is not done by the lungs, but by the brain as well as the entire body. One can easily mark the normal inhalation breath causing the movement in the body. The muscles of the body get puffed up, and while exhaling the release of the compressive movement of the muscles can be seen very clearly. In other words, during the normal breathing the entire body inhales, the entire body exhales; but in yogic or *prāṇāyāmic* breathing the brain and the extremities of the body are made to remain passive and only the lungs are activated. In *prāṇāyāmic* breathing, the role of the thorax, diaphragm, ribs, intercostal muscles, lungs and that of the abdomen differs from normal breathing. The respiratory system is used totally without straining the nervous system.

In normal breathing, the blood is sucked by the brain. By the current of inhalation not only does the brain draw the energy, but also sucks the blood, and in exhalation the brain releases the blood as well as the breath. So such types of so-called normal inhalation and exhalation are nothing but the pumping of the blood in and out from the brain. Because of this kind of inhalation, the stress is built up in the brain. In such normal breaths the brain cells are continuously inflated with inhalations and deflated with exhalations. Therefore, instead of getting energised, the whole body and the brain get dissipated. So the yogis advise to pay attention to normal inhalation and quiet soft exhalation, so that there is no load on the cells of the brain.

- *So paying more attention to a quiet soft exhalation?* -

Yes, so that the stress is taken off once and for all. If the scientists explain the pressure of inhalation and the pressure of exhalation on the brain, then we and the scientists can meet and show the way for ordinary people to relax.

Q.- Another area which is kept very tight is the diaphragm, which is the main breathing organ. How could the layman get in touch with his diaphragm?

It is very interesting, is it not? When you get nervous or frightened, which part do you hold first? *(She points out the bottom of the sternum towards the abdomen and says, "Here.")*

That is why I always use the word that the diaphragm is the medium between the physiological body and the psychological body. Learn to release the diaphragm, then the tension in the brain disappears.

Q.- So how would you tell the students how to release their diaphragm?

When we do *Setu Bandha Sarvāṅgāsana*,[1] observe the movement of the diaphragm, which expands towards the sides. Medical science knows only up and down movements, but the yogi knows not

---

[1] See *Aṣṭadaḷa Yogamālā*, vol. 4, plate n. 23.

only the vertical movement but also the horizontal movement of the diaphragm. The moment we give a lot of attention to the horizontal movement of the diaphragm, then the brain becomes quiet and appears as an object or a thing.

Q.- So would you use props, bolsters and so on?

Yes, for any beginner we have to use props so that the diaphragm does not move up and down but sideways like *Viparīta Daṇḍāsana*, *Setu Bandha Sarvāṅgāsana*, even *Ūrdhva Dhanurāsana* on a rolled stool or drum, so that the diaphragm is kept stretched from the extreme ends of one side of the bottom ribs to the other.

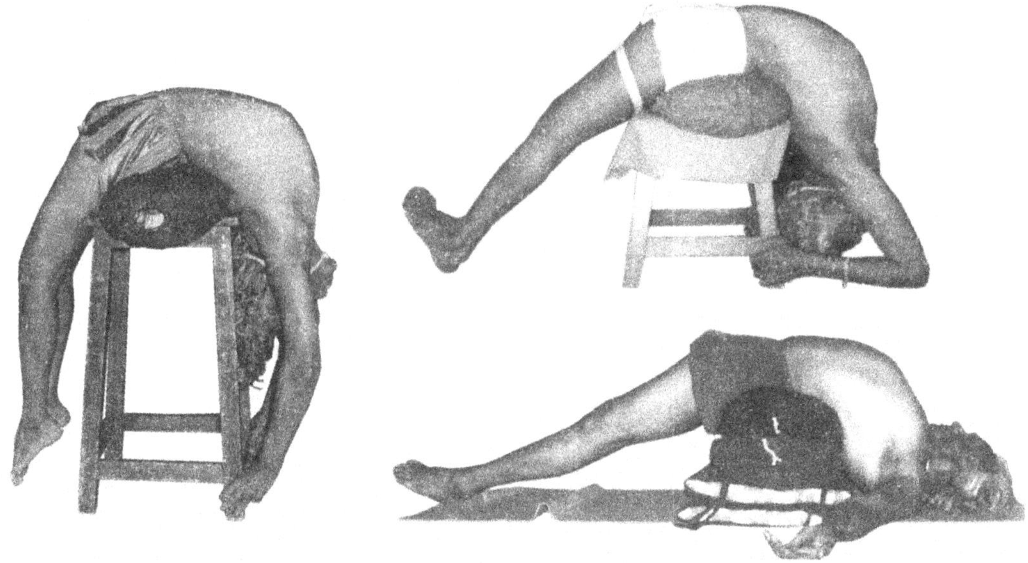

Plate n. 40 – Using props so the diaphragm moves sideways

Q.- And that will keep it naturally softer?

Yes. In all cardiac diseases the first indication is the tightness of the diaphragm muscle, which makes the breathing shallow. Nature sends a warning that this type of breathing is going to be a problem for their heart later. The first warning comes from nature to those who open their mouth to breathe, that their heart is going to be affected soon. It means the diaphragm is hard and tight. The moment one makes the diaphragm elastic, naturally the breathing becomes deep and the strain on the heart is lessened.

There is an inter-connection between the diaphragm and the heart, which I think the doctors have to explain to the common man for his good. One who practises yoga can understand the value of such breathing. The yogi may not be able to explain the inner functioning of such kind of movement of the diaphragm on the heart as clearly as the doctors and the scientists. But he experiences it. I think that the scientists should work with the artists of yoga, and the artists of yoga should work with the scientists, for the benefit of people so that they are convinced.

– *And it is coming!* –

Slowly coming – in time we may find a lot of improvement and mutual understanding between the two.

– *The more information we get and the more myths we can dispel, the more quickly it will happen.* –

Yes, you are right.

Q.- I would like to talk a little bit about yoga and meditation. Perhaps you could define meditation, and tell us how it fits into the system of yoga?

My friend, meditation is yoga, yoga is meditation! Meditation – *dhyāna* – is the penultimate stage in yoga. It is a part and parcel of yoga but not a separate entity.

– *Definition done! (Laughter).* –

Yoga is known as *samādhi*, *samādhi* is known as yoga. The seventh aspect of yoga is *dhyāna*, meditation. Meditation is not a separate subject beyond the yogic principles. Yoga has got eight aspects: *yama, niyama, āsana, prāṇāyāma, pratyāhāra, dhāraṇā, dhyāna* and *samādhi*. If people say, "I will teach you meditation" and "*āsana* are not necessary", was Patañjali then a fool to use that word *āsana* as a third stage and *dhyāna* as a seventh stage? A perfect body is needed for the mind to be free from the contact of the physical body. Patañjali says, do the *āsana*. When the mind is freed from the contact of the body, then it is fit for meditation. Meditation is not for peace of mind, it is meant to humble the pride or ego. *Dhyāna* is for *ahaṁkāra nivṛtti*. *Ahaṁkāra* – the 'I-ness' – is subtler than intelligence. As such, meditation *(dhyāna)* is not so easy as compared with that which is practised these days, without having any ethical or moral character, physical health or dispassionate nature.

Q.- So start from the periphery and work from there?

Yes! All the earlier aspects lay a firm foundation for *dhyāna*, and therefore *dhyāna* and yoga are not different subjects. It is all intermingled in yoga. The definition of *dhyāna* is to bring the complex mind to a state of simplicity, and to live in a state of innocence. That is the quality of meditation. These days *dhyāna* is considered as sitting in any posture with the eyes closed, having no bearing of any discipline on one's mind or on oneself.

– *That dispels the myth that* haṭha yoga *is physical only. Each* āsana *is a complete meditation.* –

Yes!

Q.- I have been listening to you as you have been talking with your teachers, asking them to keep the purity of your work in the *āsana*. Is it possible to keep the purity of your work and still be an individual within your system?

Certainly. There are several ways one can take to reach the railway station, but the end aim is to reach the station, isn't it? Similarly, I say, go anywhere but come back to that point. Many of them forget that they have to come back to their original point.

I am not telling them to imitate me and lose their individuality, I am asking them to maintain the methodology in spite of having freedom of expression.

Q.- Is there the possibility, though, that a teacher, in trying to adhere to the purity, could become very rigid?

No! Rigidity is insensitivity. Purity is sensitivity, not rigidity.

– *Ah! (Laughter).* –

Dhyāna has to follow all the earlier aspects of yoga. One cannot hop on the seventh aspect of yoga at once without earlier preparation of the yogic background. Such hopping may bring distress and disharmony. Hence follow what Patañjali says, then it brings *śreyas* or auspiciousness in the person. It is not a rigid discipline but a progressive discipline that builds purity of purpose in the *sādhaka*.

As far as the teachers are concerned, the art of presentation and expression of the language in teaching has to be simple. That is what I do in the class. I do not want teachers to use words that cannot be understood by the doer. They should use simple words and stop or give a pause in between so that the students understand and grasp what the teachers have said. Before they say further they should wait and see the students' body language and whether they understood that and put that into their efforts. Then the purity in teaching is maintained.

If you have been in the class, you might have noticed that I have built up the void they create; in some I destroyed their wrong expression so that they can relearn; in some I guided so that they move further and, in some who could not go further, I constructed words for them to carry on with confidence. I have used these methods for teachers, to understand and proceed in imparting knowledge.

Yesterday in one class I 'destroyed' a person so that he could relearn. Destroying means destroying their old thoughts and wrong conceptions. The presentation was very bad. Naturally I had to destroy that habit. I have to be strong so that he can learn to forget that habit fast and start in the right method. He had to forget the old habits of using the same words and start anew. You need to clean the slate to write again.

– Get them thinking very quickly. –

No! They do not think quickly. Wrong is wrong! Eradicate that faulty method and give them the constructive way of thinking.

– Yes. (Laughter). –

Q.- Could you give some advice to people who might be sparked to begin a yoga practice?

It is very simple. I say, don't go to the very depth of yoga in the begining itself. Your body is your capital. God has given this body as capital or a bank to start anything. Take care of this divine capital that God has given to you. Look after yourself. See that your joints, your muscles, your nerves, your blood current run rhythmically in the body. Please learn so much. Then I say, the other aspects of yoga will automatically follow.

One should not just say the body is the temple. Make the body a sacred temple for the soul to live in. Make the body purposeful for the intelligence and the heart to do good work.

Q.- Sir, it has been an honour to speak with you, and I thank you very much for being with us.

Thank you. You are all so very kind to me. God bless you all.

ART OF YOGA*

"In yoga you express in each and every tissue the basic art... I have only refined the art."

A dynamic man with formidable eyebrows jutting out over penetrating eyes, B.K.S. Iyengar orchestrated the class, playing upon the physical instruments to release the music of each individual cell. This stern, but by no means humourless, man was living testimony of the effectiveness of his art. Despite a sickly, bedridden childhood he has developed himself into a renowned and revered teacher of haṭha yoga *to over two million followers from all over the globe.*

Yoga has its roots in ancient Indian philosophy and offers its followers a guide to reaching balance, health and harmony in their physical, mental and spiritual existence. While haṭha yoga *emphasises control and rigorous discipline of the body it complements* rāja yoga, *the control of the mind, and together they form the approach towards yoga's goal – union with the Universal Spirit. Mr. Iyengar's refinement of* haṭha yoga *stresses correct body alignment, endurance and the development of strength and flexibility. His way of practising the* āsana *or yoga postures exercises every joint, muscle and nerve and benefits the internal organs.*

Mr. Iyengar lives in Pune, India, where he trains senior students at the Ramāmaṇi Iyengar Memorial Yoga Institute. He made his first teaching visit to Edmonton, Canada, on September 7th and 8th, jointly sponsored by the University of Alberta's Faculty of Physical Education and Recreation and the Iyengar Yoga Association of Edmonton. His pupil, Dr. S.V. Karandikar, gave a comprehensive slide show and lecture on the "physiology of Trikoṇāsana", rather an awesome experience for me, a relative beginner at yoga, seeing all the intricate detailing of muscles and joints involved in just one posture.

The following day Mr. Iyengar instructed a three-hour workshop that left me feeling like I'd just been struck by lighting. Never had I seen a teacher speak or move with such authority – he frightened and inspired. I interviewed Mr. Iyengar after the workshop.

Q.- How long have you been studying yoga?

---

* Interview by Molly Smith, September 1990.

This is my fifty-first year. The basic points were given by my teacher, my brother-in-law, sister's husband. Later I developed myself. I never went to anyone else. I carried on... For an artist the most important things are his own skill, direct perception, analysis and synthesis. One can buy the books and read so that he can understand the art. For a yogi, a student of yoga too, it is direct perception, logical calculation, factual imagination, the skilful application and all the available sacred literature on the subject. All these made me develop the art of yoga.

Q.- Why do you teach?

I had neither decided to teach nor did I claim anywhere that I wanted to be a teacher. People wanted me to teach. It was just a coincidence.

I was an unhealthy child and when I went to my brother-in-law he made me practise certain simple *āsana*. I was a bit forced to come to this line or let me say that destiny made me take up yoga.

I was quick enough to be good in my early days as far as the performance of *āsana* is concerned. Those who saw my performance must have liked (what I consider now) my crude presentation of yoga postures in the 1930's and people forced me to teach. And when they insisted I teach, I had to learn. So I say that it was God's will and I had to learn to do well in order to learn to teach.

I had to learn by looking at people how to bring the grace, the form, the shape and the beauty of the *āsana* in the body not only from outside but from inside as well. The above expressions of feeling had to be expressed without any other instrument than the body. Next year my third book, *The Art of Yoga*, will be published. In that book I may explain in detail what I mean by yoga as art.

So I think, as people demanded that I should teach, I started and along with teaching I discovered the artistic quality of yoga as well as its science and philosophy.

Q.- Do you travel a lot?

Between 1952 and 1976 I travelled alot on invitation by my pupils. I used to go every year but I was away from my country for only three months each year. I would go to Europe, South Africa and America...

I have travelled but travelling was not my aim. Yoga was important for me. Who knows, I am going to curtail my travels and settle to practise for knowing the subtlest parts in the body which might not have surfaced in me. I like to penetrate further so that I reach the core in my *sādhanā*.

- You've never had a desire to live elsewhere? -

Not at all, though many people offered me the opportunities. I say if God had wanted me to live elsewhere, why did He make me take birth in India? In 1976 I said I would not come to the West again. Even now I say, I propose that I should remain in the land of my birth. But as the saying goes, "man proposes and God disposes." So here God is disposing of my proposal. Somebody in England asked me to come and help. I went there and then Australia asked me, then France and now America; so I came because when they ask me, out of compassion and love I go to share the knowledge and benefits of yoga with others. And if I fulfil wishes of one country, I need to do so for other countries too. This is the first time I have taught here but this is my second visit to Canada. The first time I came to see the Niagara Falls. My heart is for my pupils. I have to serve my pupils first. Then I can think of sightseeing and my friends.

In the early days I was teaching only the "cream" of the world, many of the political leaders, musicians, artists and writers. Then in one of the papers that interviewed me they wrote that yoga is "King of exercises" and that yogis always move with kings and queens. So the day I read it, the next day I decided to go to the common man. Now the kings and queens must make an appointment to see me while other people get me easily.

However, I never had any intention of going outside my country to settle. I have seen almost the whole world. I am contented in my own country.

Q.- Why do we do *āsana?*

The body is the instrument available to us to serve the people and serve ourselves too. We cannot exist in the state of bodilessness. Therefore, our duty is to keep the body healthy and clean.

Often we, the human beings, experience the nearness of the mind to the body. If the body suffers, the mind is affected, if the mind suffers, the body is affected. Similarly if the body enjoys, the mind is satisfied. If the mind enjoys, the body is satisfied. All our experiences, enjoyments, enchantments, entertainments, enticement, are through these instruments that are close to each other. The organs of action and senses of perception work as a medium between these two – the body and the mind.

While practising the *āsana* we reverse this process and change the role of these instruments. While practising the *āsana* we not only have to give attention to body but to mind also and take them nearer to the very core of our being. The core of being is nothing but a part of God. This is how you find or reach God. God is nothing but the Ultimate Truth.

The body is an essential instrument for experiencing the world and emancipation as well.

Q.- Where did you learn English?

I learned by talking to people like the way I am talking to you. I had no formal education. But all my books are written in English. *Light on Yoga* took six years to write. *Light on Prāṇāyāma* took fourteen years and *Art on Yoga* has taken three years.

Despite his captivating depth and strength of character I detected a feeling of almost protectiveness in the devotions of Mr. Iyengar's retinue – as if he needed some shielding from a life that could be at times too demanding. He gives much of himself. His choice of words, while witty and funny at moments could also be sometimes mystifying as to meaning. But I believe his following remarks seem to point towards man's struggle for a purity, that is after all intensely private.

Q.- Once in a question and answer session, after a class someone said, 'See how Iyengar attacks people. What magnetism he has to attack people?' Can you comment?

Certainly, I've got magnetism. Tell me who is able to come near me. My magnetism keeps people out. So how do you say I haven't got it? The magnet pulls iron. Similarly, those who are able to face my fire, anger, demanding discipline can come near me. Those who have not got strong will, strong pull or gravitation towards yoga won't come to me.

What anger or fury I have is now less intense. Earlier, I could not tolerate anything going wrong in practice. Now, I am a little better than before. I've quietened a great deal. The fury has lessened in me. But when I teach, it comes back: the fire, the purity in art. While I practise or teach, that time I am not I. I am beyond I. Something moves beyond me. I can't control it at all. I'm out of my body. I am absolutely on a different level. The sense of 'I' goes and sense of purity and divinity enters. Therefore I am beyond my 'I'.

For me, yoga has been a confrontation with myself: my weaknesses and my strengths. No other exercise programme has been as difficult or as rewarding – physically and spiritually. Good fortune indeed was mine to be able to see and hear the unforgettable B.K.S. Iyengar.

Having seen a newspaper picture of himself in his white flowing robes, sitting in full lotus position on the steps, Mr. Iyengar softly remarked:

"This is like a flower, really like a lotus it has come."

INVOKING PATAÑJALI*

Q.- We would like to ask you some questions about the invocation.

What's the problem? If you tell me then I will know it. See, what we are doing is that we are only praying for the blessings of the Father of yoga, Patañjali. We are praying so that he blesses us in our practice. It is completely a universal prayer. According to the story from the *Purāṇa,* Sage Patañjali was the incarnation of Ādiśeṣa, the couch of Lord Viṣṇu. Hence, he is depicted holding a conch in one hand and disc in the other, and half the body in the shape of the cobra and top in human form. Being incarnated in India, the *ṛṣi* thought of this shape.

Q.- Right, that's where the problem is. They (students in the West) don't understand the form.

The invocation to Patañjali, which is in Sanskrit, speaks of neither any cult nor religion. Probably the translation in English could be made easily available so that invocation prayer has no room for suspicions in the minds of the members to think of it as Hindu culture or religion. This conveys only a way of respect and gratitude to him who gave us light on the knowledge of body, mind and speech. The doubts may not arise if you give the translation of it, which is in *Light on Yoga.* Then you can convey that what was said in English is in the original form in Sanskrit.[1]

As we pay respects to our parents for our existence, the yoga practitioner pays respects to Patañjali who showed us ways for physical, mental and spiritual health and harmony.

Q.- Could you elaborate a little bit on the meaning of each of the symbols: the conch, the disc, the cobra, and the human torso?

* Interview by Bonnie Anthony. Published in *Newsletter* of the B.K.S. Iyengar Yoga Association of Southern California, Spring/Summer 1991, pp. 2-4.

[1] The full translation is available in *Light on Yoga Sūtras of Patañjali.*

As the conch can be blown, it represents a kind of alarm if any danger such as evil spirits or diseases interfere, and the disc indicates that one can destroy the evil thoughts, evil spirits or diseases. These are the two important things which have been expressed in texts about Lord Krishna. In *Gītā*, you read them as *śankha*[1] and *cakra*[2] held by Lord Krishna, *śankha* is the blowing of the conch, which keeps out all other sounds so that the pure sound of the conch is heard, and the disc *(cakra)* is to destroy the evil thoughts and actions. That's the significance. The disc is meant for destruction of evil thoughts and actions.

Asī means a sword. On one hand he holds the sword of knowledge to destroy nescience. On the other hand he blesses those who practise yoga.

In another aspect, he folds his palms and salutes the seat of the *antarātman* - the God, symbolically showing that through yoga, one reaches God.

Q.- And then the cobra.

You know the cobra is the one which is holding the Earth. It is the Protector of the universe. In the *Haṭhayoga Pradīpikā*, the first stanza of the third chapter says: "Ananta, the Lord of Serpents, supports the Earth with its mountains and forests, similarly *kuṇḍalinī* - serpent energy - is the main support of all yoga practices", which is again indicated in the form of a snake.

The divine serpent is considered to be thousand-headed and regarded as an emblem of eternity. This divine serpent is considered to be supporting the seven nether worlds below and the seven aerial regions above.[3]

From early civilisation almost all the religions have worshipped the Snake God. Every mythology had some sort of serpent worship. It was a belief that snakes do not die but they shed their skins and emerge as new. This eternity of snakes became symbolic. This ageless quality of the serpent is known as *ananta* - never ending.[4]

---

1 *Bhagavad Gītā* 1/15

2 *Bhagavad Gītā* 11/17.

3 See the author's *Light on the Yoga Sūtra of Patañjali,* under *sūtra* III.27.

4 The Indian serpent Goddess is called Kadru. Babylonians too worshipped the snake with a similar name. Egyptians too called the serpent as the great mother. Akkadians worshipped the Goddess snake and called her Mistress of serpents whereas Babylonians called her heaven-Goddess. Jews have their own version of the myth that the serpent was the first lover of Eve. The serpent was worshipped in Palestine too. The Jews were considered as the 'sons of the great serpent'. Persians had faith that there is a connection between menstrual blood and the serpent's secret of longevity as the continuity of pregnancy. Many gnostic traditions identified the serpent with Jesus. Some Christians considered the serpent as the father of Jesus which overshadowed the bed of the virgin Mary and begot the human form of Saviour.

The snake is a symbol of eternity, fertility and regeneration. It is the symbol of wisdom too. The snake is depicted with good and bad deeds of man. Is it not? All religions say that we have to conquer the emotional upheavals like lust, greed, anger, malice, and so on. The snake is poisonous but its venom is medicinal too. Similarly anger, lust, etc. are poisonous. We have to convert our nature and develop the opposite qualities such as quietness, control or continence, love, contentment and so on. The divine snake indicates how it can be close to God.

The prayers are done by everyone. Hence prayers in various forms got into various religions of the world to be free from evil deeds. When the human weaknesses are conquered you are one with the soul. That's in the meaning of the invocation. It is to uplift us (the yoga practitioners) for liberation from the effects of *avidyā*.

Q.- And then the fourth is the human torso.

Yes. The above half is depicted in human form because he has to explain the background of yoga with its ultimate goal. You must have heard the story of Patañjali's birth. He was like a worm which took human form, and his mother Gauṇika was a virgin, just like Mary. The virgin mother of Patañjali said while praying to the Sun God, "Now, let me give back that knowledge that I learnt under your shade and which I got through so much of penance. As I have not got one student or a son to whom to impart this knowledge which I earned by your grace, I would like to offer it to you." Saying this, she closes her eyes, palms filled with water to offer the water as an oblation to the Sun-God thinking that her experienced knowledge may merge in the universe through that water. Before offering, she just opens her hands and looks and there she sees a worm in her palms, which immediately transforms into tiny human form. This indicates the process of evolution, how one can progress from small creature to human being. It is the growth and expanse of intelligence. This head in the human form is to explain the essence of yoga. That's why we call Patañjali "born of his own will power". This is one side of Patañjali.

Now, here is another invocation about Patañjali by Vyāsa, he says:

Let us prostrate before Lord Ādiśeṣa, who manifested himself on earth as Patañjali to grace the human race with health and harmony.

Let us salute Lord Ādiśeṣa of the myriad serpent heads and mouths carrying noxious poisons, discarding which he came to earth as single-headed Patañjali in order to eradicate ignorance and vanquish sorrow.

Let us pay our obeisance to Him, repository of all knowledge, amidst His attendant retinue.

Let us pray to the Lord whose primordial form shines with pure and white effulgence, pristine in body, a master of yoga who bestows on us his yogic light to enable mankind to rest in the house of the immortal soul.

This, you will find in my new book, which I am writing: *Light on the Yoga Sūtras of Patañjali.* When Vyāsa comments on Patañjali, he invokes this prayer for Patañjali's blessings and I have translated the same into English.

On account of the enormous calibre of Patañjali, these invocations are constructed by the yogis of yore for his blessings in our practices, and these have become sacred to all of us.

TRANSFORMATION OF *PRAKṚTI* TO BE IN PART WITH *PURUṢA**

Q.- In the *Haṭhayoga Pradīpikā*, it is said: "Taming lions, elephants and tigers requires a lot of time and prudence; similarly *prāṇāyāma* should be progressively practised according to the capacity and limits of the practitioner. Otherwise, it will maim him".[1] In that sense, would not your last book, which speaks on the practice of *prāṇāyāma*,[2] represent a danger for the practitioners of yoga?

To subdue a lion is very difficult; similarly, to subdue the breath is also very difficult. You have to wait and watch to seize the opportunity and be in a position to subdue a lion. As long as you have not found its weak point, you will not be able to control it. But if you have a lot of patience and perseverance, you will find an opportune moment to do it.

Not everyone can find a master to learn *prāṇāyāma* correctly. I had many requests regarding teaching it and I finally decided to write a book about it. It took me fourteen years to complete it. The book begins with the basics and the simplest practices, i.e. techniques of normal breathing and how to improve the normal breathing into a *prāṇāyāmic* breathing.

All these questions that are not found in my first book[3] have been explained in detail. Anyway in my *prāṇāyāma* book, I speak, first of all, to the non-initiated. I explain how, step by step, they can master respiration without danger. I have explained each *prāṇāyāma* from its simple form to an advanced version. This can be sensed, if one reads the book carefully. Hence, each practitioner can watch his own capacity. One can introduce each stage of *prāṇāyāma* gradually though it may take one time to learn to do things safely. As I often say, a good book or a good manual is better than a bad teacher.

Actually, what I have done in this book is to remove the fear complexes but also the damage that may arise by wrong introduction.

---

* Interview for Yoga Centre of Victoria, May 1991.

1 *Haṭhayoga Pradipīkā* II.15.

2 *Light on Prāṇāyāma*, 1981, Harper Collins, London

3 *Light on Yoga*, Harper Collins, London.

Q.- What is the goal of practice of yoga postures?

The goal of these postures, which are known as *āsana*, is to keep the neurological body in good shape and at the same time not to allow the mind to be afflicted by the body; freed from all attachments, the mind is able to come in contact with the self. According to tradition, there are innumerable movements to achieve a posture. It is often necessary to introduce intermediate position in order to reach the main *āsana*.

The *āsana* cleanses the whole system. The body is established in each *āsana* in such a way that the mind and breath do not waver. The intelligence is sharpened to look within and penetrated to reach the very core of the being. They are practised and perfected so well in order to make the *prāṇa* move uninterruptedly supplying energy to each nook and corner of the body.

Q.- Do you teach techniques of mastering the mind as you teach the postures?

You cannot learn postures by using only physical force. For instance, you cannot gain elasticity of joints by forcing them. Of course, practice requires a tremendous power of will, and extreme attention frrom the mind has to be brought to feel all movements of the body – external as well as internal. Consequently, in order to master an *āsana*, three conditions should be observed at the same time; strength, will and direction.

In the early stages of practice, the practitioners use a lot of physical force. The organs of perception and the mind do not witness or register every other movement of the body. It takes time to feel the actions and the effect of the actions, whether correct or incorrect, during the practice. In that witnessing process, a state is revealed that is felt as a pause.

The understanding of the body comes from this state, and the body "feels" if the position or inner movements are in harmony. So the position is readjusted in order to reach homogeneity in the flow of the energy. At this stage there is a clear reflection on the *āsana*. At the same time there remains no more disparity or any obstacle between body and mind. Thus the *āsana* becomes contemplative. When this state of contemplation is well established, one has mastered the *āsana*.

At that moment, the effort which is complete, becomes an effortless state. The practitioner forgets his body, his will, his intelligence and becomes "one" within. This is nothing but the shaping of the mind. The mind is made to involve itself in the *āsana*. Hence, the mind too is cultured and mastered.

All *āsana* should be practised in this way, with this intention. But in the beginning, there is no connection between body and mind. The body acts, but the mind cannot perceive it. Body and mind have to be made to interact in each *āsana* in an uninterrupted and attentive manner to achieve a greater harmony between body and mind.

Q.- So, to acquire such a level of understanding, a relationship between body and mind has to be realised. You say this relationship is a result of an uninterrupted awareness. Does classical yoga recognise existence of that awareness?

Patañjali says, in one of the aphorisms[1] that the practice of *āsana* puts an end to the dualities and disparities. The differentiation between body and mind as well as mind and soul ceases. This integration happens because of the new awareness, the discriminative awareness.

Even other scriptures such as *Bhagavad Gītā* explain this state using a different expression.

When the senses come in contact with their objects, the dualities set in such as heat and cold, pain and pleasures. When one is established in yoga *(yogārūḍha)* and gets *samāhita citta*, the pairs of opposites do not affect him.

This way, yoga knows the existence of that kind of awareness. Patañjali and all scriptures speak about it. The problem is that most practitioners don't understand it.

Q.- Does the process of mastering the posture imply a step-by-step progression?

Of course, *āsana* implies step-by-step progression. Each *āsana* has its own hierarchy. Firstly the physical practice is conative. A connection must be established between the organs of action and the senses of perception. In other words *karma* and *jñāna* have to go together. One should be clear about the action and purpose behind that action in *āsana*. This is the second stage where the *āsana* becomes cognitive. We become aware of all the movements and the functions of the body. When the *āsana* is performed with conscious awareness, the mind is drawn along with the body to begin an inner journey.

The third stage is the discernment that comes from the intervening mind. The fourth stage is the reflection on the *āsana*. This stage precedes the state of contemplation. If *āsana* are practised in this way, one reaches the state of contemplation. The tensions of the body, of the mind and of the will vanish.

All these stages are step-by-step progression in the *sādhanā* of *āsana*. The practice of *āsana* builds up positive strength and subdued will power to proceed for *prāṇāyāma sādhanā*.

Q.- What do you mean by the word "subdued"?

---

1 *Yoga Sūtra* II.48

When we act, the tensions and stress are built up in the body, as well as in the organs of action, senses of perception and mind. At that moment breath cannot flow smoothly and easily. It is as though while driving a car you press the accelarator and the brake pedals at the same time. Breath is the accelerator. The fibres of the organs of action and senses of perception become tight and prevent this smooth flow, which causes a detrimental effect on *prāṇāyāma*. In order to succeed in *prāṇāyāma*, the power of the will has to be quiet and serene. The nerves, mind and breath have to be tension-free. This is a taming process. When a lion is tamed, it remains humble. This is called the state of subdued or passive sublimation. The senses, breath and mind, emotions and impulses are channelled and purified.

Q.- The yoga of Patañjali states that there are seven steps of yoga before reaching *samādhi*, which is the eighth step. In your book, you present them as separate but in a certain order. Do you advise practising them in strict order?

Nowhere does Patañjali state that there are seven steps of yoga. There are eight steps, or aspects. He calls them limbs. I call them petals of the flower of yoga. These are *yama, niyama, āsana, prāṇāyāma, pratyāhāra, dhāraṇā, dhyāna* and *samādhi*.

According to Patañjali, all these aspects of yoga should be practised together. The approach of the practitioner should be to adopt all the aspects in certain degrees. It is impractical to adopt all the five principles of *yama* first and then switch over to *niyama*. The *sādhaka* needs to have an all-round approach. He did not mention that one step should follow another except for *prāṇāyāma*. If the practitioner has not yet mastered *āsana*, he should not practise *prāṇāyāma*. This is the only point where the practitioner has to master one step before moving to the *prāṇāyāma* practice. Here too he indicates that since one needs to sit steady for a certain duration, the body, nerves, breath and mind have to support and be made conducive for *prāṇāyāma*. Therefore mastery over body and mind has to be achieved to some extent to proceed towards *prāṇāyāma*.

Samādhi is the eighth aspect of *aṣṭāṅga yoga*. As there are five *yama*, five *niyama* and several *āsana* and *prāṇāyāma*, so also there are eight stages of *samādhi*. These are *savitarkā, nirvitarkā, savicārā, nirvicārā, sānanda, sāsmita, virāma pratyaya* and *dharmamegha*. *Savitarkā* takes us towards analysing, *nirvitarkā* takes us beyond analysis. *Savicārā* takes us towards deliberate reasoning while *nirvicārā* takes us beyond reasoning. So, the first four lead towards awareness in which thinking, analysing, doubting and reasoning cease, resulting in serenity.

Therefore, a state of bliss is experienced in the fifth stage of *samādhi* called *sānanda*. The sixth stage of *samādhi* is experiencing depth of being which is closer to 'I'-consciousness. In the seventh stage, there is complete suspension of movements of the consciousness. That is what is called "a spiritual desert" – *virāma pratyaya.* The practitioner stays on the threshold of awakening but he does not know how to cross this passage. It is a precarious state. It will bind him, taking him after accomplishments or uplift him to take him towards emancipation. This *virāma pratyaya* is an independent state of absorption that is free from all kinds of supports. In this state, emptiness emerges. At that moment, if the active and attentive practitioner maintains the strength of awareness with great faith, he reaches the last stage of *samādhi* known as *dharmamegha samādhi,* where all functions of mind, conscious or unconscious, stop – inhibit themselves completely. And the very self-intelligence emerges and reaches its peak and wisdom flows as a tempestuous river; that is the superconscious state. It is a state of unsurpassed bliss.[1]

Q.- Let us come back to more modest levels. Which kind of condition of disposition has to be acquired before one attempts to practise *jñāna yoga*?

First of all, be clear that there are no categories of yoga. Yoga is one, *karma, jñāna and bhakti* are different aspects in our yogic experience. Finally there is a union between individual and Supreme Soul.

The yoga of Patañjali begins with self-discovery on different levels, understanding the body, organs of action, senses of perception, mind, intelligence, 'I-consciousness' and finally the Self. The practitioner does not always have a correct understanding or perception of all these aspects, visible and invisible, or measurable or immeasurable. To reach understanding, he has to practise *āsana* and *prāṇāyāma.* So, the physical body is perceived and mind enters in to be in contact with the unknown aspects of both the body and mind that can be only understood through direct experience.

Patañjali speaks about studying and observing the evolutionary growth of the tangible, visible body. It is a known fact that the body is made up of five gross elements. The muscles, bones, cellular organs, the organs of action are consisting of the five elements. The practice of *āsana* and *prāṇāyāma* brings the awareness in the practitioner to analyse and balance these five elements. In *savitarkā samādhi* these five elements are realised in a very subtle level but the clear foundation is laid in the practice of *āsana* and *prāṇāyāma.* From this point one proceeds to study the senses of perception and mind. The mind, which gravitates towards the body, begins to gravitate towards the intellect. And the mind, intellect as well as the five subtle elements come together for the sake of cleansing the intellect. Here begins *jñāna* in practice. From these one proceeds to bring the evolutionary growth in intelligence, consciousness and conscience. The *sādhanā* for evolutionary growth of body, organs of action, senses of perception, five gross and subtle elements and mind has a strong

---

[1] For more details, see the author's *Light on the Yoga Sūtras of Patañjali,* I.18 and I.42-51, and table n. 5 in the same book.

bias. Here the path of *karma* is involved. The *sādhanā* for evolutionary growth of *citta*, *mahat* and *mūlaprakṛti* has the element of *bhakti* in it. Finally, self-realisation leads towards the maturity of devotion which culminates and terminates in *dharmamegha samādhi*. Thus, yoga does not only pacify the mind in order to create an emptiness but to discover the very source. One realises that light and energy are not inherent in the mind, but the mind draws it from pure consciousness – the *ātmā*. This drawing or inheriting process can be done only through the body since it is the first outer envelope of the soul.

Therefore, practice of yoga covers not only *karma* but also *jnāna* and *bhakti*. It is a complete path in this sense.

Q.- What exactly is a Self, for a yogi?

The soul is an entity, with its covering sheaths of the body, organs of action, senses of perception, mind, intelligence, "I-ness", consciousness and conscience. Self is latent and exists everywhere. However, due to our ignorance, we identify soul with body, mind and intelligence. When we speak about ourselves, we speak about our body, mind and intelligence. This mis-identification is recognised as 'Self'. The 'Self' expresses this identification whereas it is pure and a separate entity. 'Self' gets tinged on account of the closeness with its sheaths.

The yogi through his yogic practices searches for this untainted Self, realises its presence, witnesses its existence.

The Self or Soul is the seed from which the self sprouts as *jīvātman*, which expresses its closeness to body and not to the soul. This *jīvātman* expresses itself as individual self. The whole process of yoga is to separate or disassociate from all the shackles of body, mind, intelligence and self to perceive the soul, which is in a pure form.

Q.- What happens between stages of physical attitudes and the stage when the beginning of understanding takes place?

To know, to reach the Infinite, the finite is a means. The body has limits and is mortal while the soul is immortal. This mortal body is only a part of nature, built of five elements; earth, water, fire, air and ether. The senses of perception are related to the qualities of these elements.

For Indian philosophers, the mind is the eleventh sense, a "super organ" of perception and conception, which helps other organs and senses to function. By practising *āsana* and *prāṇāyāma*, the organs of action, senses of perception and mind are poised and made silent. The five elements and their functions enter in fusion due to vital energy. Obviously the body gets impregnated with cosmic energy. This is what happens between *annamaya, prāṇamaya, manomaya, vijñānamaya* and *ānandamaya* sheaths.

As long as these finite instruments are not sublimated, the infinite *ātman* will not manifest itself. The clouds in the sky don't allow the rays of sun to reach or touch the earth. When clouds dissipate, there is no more obstacle for the light of the sun to reach the earth. Similarly, when the obstacles such as the elements of body, mind and other evolutes are not dissipated, the Self cannot manifest. Practice of *āsana* and *prāṇāyāma* removes these obstacles. When the obstacles disappear, the light of Self shines more and more. Thus, without going through finite you cannot experience infinite. But having only finite, you cannot "see" infinite.

When the finite is fully mastered, it dissolves in the infinite, the infinite shines itself. But to come to this stage, much effort has to be made. If the effort is not pursued, there will still be clouds between Self and consciousness. Work has to be continued and that is the essence of yoga.

Q.- Do you recognise different levels of consciousness in yoga?

The seed sprouts and grows as a tree. Similarly, the intelligence of the heart rises and becomes intelligence of the head. The seed is *ātman* – the soul. It starts slowly sprouting as *asmitā* – individual self. From this sprout, springs consciousness, which is known as *citta*. *Citta* is something like the stem of the tree. From the stem, branches sprout. These branches are nothing but ego, intelligence, mind, senses of perception and organs of action.

Citta or consciousness is composed of ego, intelligence and mind. This *citta* or consciousness functions at different levels and with practice of yoga undergoes transformation. This transformation takes place in steps since they indicate different states of consciousness.

The *citta* is consciousness according to its characteristic functions at different levels. Obviously the levels are recognised according to these qualities. They are namely; *mūḍa* – dullness, *kṣīpta* – negligence or distraction, *vikṣīpta* – oscillation or agitation, *ekāgra* – one pointedness, *niruddha* – restraint or control. The *citta* disposes, delivers and deliberates thought according to these levels.

However, with the practice of yoga the level of consciousness qualitatively changes from *mūḍa* to *kṣīpta*, from *kṣīpta* to *vikṣīpta*, from *vikṣīpta* to *ekāgra* and from *ekāgra* to *niruddha*. The first five aspects convert the consciousness from *kṣīpta* to *vikṣīpta* and the remaining three aspects convert the consciousness from *vikṣīpta* to *ekāgra*. Lastly, at the highest stage of *samādhi (dharmamegha samādhi)*, the consciousness reaches the level of *niruddha*.

To ascend from one level to the next, the consciousness undergoes a transformation. The levels are not climbed as steps but through transformation. The first five aspects of yoga cleanse and purify the consciousness. Thereafter the consciousness transforms itself from *vyutthāna citta* – generating consciousness – to *divya citta* – pure absolute consciousness. These states of transformation are recognised as *vyutthāna, nirodha, śānta, ekāgra, nirmāṇa, cidra* and *divya citta*.

When you sleep, *ahaṁkāra* does not manifest; the principle of individuality is completely dissolved. Thus nature nourishes the consciousness. It gives an enormous amount of energy to an individual. Man can use it to entertain himself or to search for felicity and liberation. We say that it is necessary to tame nature through yoga. Evolution is when a little seed becomes a tree. From the top to the root the tree is one.

As fruit is in relation to the root, Self is in relation to the body. Techniques of yoga give the opportunity to capture energy from the exterior as well as from the interior and to utilise that energy to accomplish such an evolution.

ALIGNMENT OF BODY AND MIND WITH THE SOUL*

Q.- What is yoga?

Yoga is a subject which deals with the health of the body, clarity of mind and growth of intelligence, to experience the hidden, eternal core of Being, so that one experiences the joy without any colouring. It is a science, it is a philosophy, it is an art which deals with the perfect physical firmness of the body, cultivates the mind to face the mental turmoils and upheavals of the world and guides the *sādhaka* in acquiring the sensibility in the intelligence, so that his thinking is clear, direct and precise, and it is not made to oscillate on account of want of understanding or a lack of clarity within oneself. Yoga helps to develop all these characteristics in an individual. Yoga means to yoke, to unite, to bring together. It also means yoking the body to the mind and uniting the body and mind to the soul.

Q.- You are right now writing a new book about Patañjali's *Yoga Sūtra*. Would you like to clarify how one can find the eight pillars of Patañjali's yoga in your teaching?

Yoga is divided into three compartments in order to understand it. It begins from the base and shows how to reach the ultimate emancipation and freedom from sorrow and pain. Patañjali did not introduce the subject of yoga but codified it for the first time. The very first *sūtra*[1] of Patañjali explains the traditional practices of yoga, assembling together the scattered parts as a codified subject. He conveys this with the word *anuśāsanam*. *Śāsana* means conduct, code of behaviour, *anu* means traditionally followed. Hence, Patañjali says, "I am explaining what yoga is, which has been spoken of traditionally for developing the discipline in ourselves to understand the mutations of the consciousness."

---

* Interview by Carles Bruno, Jordi Marti and Patxi Lizardi, July 1991 in the Library of Ramāmaṇi Iyengar Memorial Yoga Institute, published in the Spanish magazine *Cuerpo Mente*, no. 22, February 1994.

[1] *Atha yogānuśāsanam* (*Y.S.*, I.1).

Hence *yama* and *niyama,* which have been introduced in the field of yoga, are not new terms. They are traditional. The two ethical disciplines exist from time immemorial and are mentioned in scriptures such as *Veda* and *Upaniṣad,* which Patañjali explains in detail for an average intellectual to understand the depth of an ethical life. Secondly, when he refers in the very first *sūtra* the word *anuśāsana* or discipline, or the behavioural pattern to be followed, he means that one has to follow the disciplines said by the earlier sages, which include all types of disciplines – ethical, physical, moral, mental, intellectual and spiritual. As he deals with the eight aspects of yoga, the first two, *yama* and *niyama,* have been from time immemorial for the growth of each individual. These are the pillars on which one has to build up further to evolve towards the sight of the Self. So in order to evolve – physically, mentally, intellectually or spiritually – the other three aspects – *āsana, prāṇāyāma* and *pratyāhāra,* are given as progressive stages of yoga.

The first two are the base - the foundation, which one cannot overlook. The evolution is possible by living in these two principles. *Āsana, prāṇāyāma* and *pratyāhāra* were introduced to build up one's body, mind and soul, from those two pillars, *yama* and *niyama.*

When you are working in the office, you get your salary. When you teach yoga, you make your money for your livelihood. Whatever job one does, the effect of that is in the form of salary or goodwill or may be in any kind. Similarly, when you follow the five aspects of yoga, the goodwill of yoga is the properties or the effects known as *yoga svarūpa.*[1] The last three aspects of yoga are *yoga svarūpa,* which process the consciousness towards developing the highest sensitivity in it. These three are *dhāraṇā, dhyāna* and *samādhi,* which I say are the effect of yoga or the *pariṇāma* – the properties. Though *dhāraṇā, dhyāna* and *samādhi* are explained as separate entities, they are triggered together. Though these are dealt with individually, they are treated as a single unit as psychological distance between each of them is short. Therefore Patañjali later uses the word *saṁyama* or the integration of these three i.e. *dhāraṇā, dhyāna* and *samādhi* into one. The practice of yoga is perceived in the first five aspects and is conceived in the last three.

– But what about siddhis? –

You derive the benefit of each action you do. Similarly, by doing perfect yoga the effects (*siddhi*) of these actions are explained in the third chapter of *Yoga Sūtra* known as *Vibhūti Pāda.* Whether one believes or not is immaterial for the simple reason that one accepts a certain part of the author's treatise because it is pleasing and adaptable and reject what is impossible even to grasp. If you do not accept, then that does not mean that there is no truth in those said facts, which may not be appealing to you. But some people say that they do not believe the *siddhi* or

[1] *Svarūpa* means a natural state. The first five aspects are *sva-prayoga* – self application. In other words, where one has to practically practise them in order to get *svarūpa* – the natural state.

accomplishments, yet practise yoga, then how can they believe some parts and degrade the other parts written by the same author? Patañjali explains the esoteric powers achieved by the *yogi* as powers, which are in fact the fructification of the conquest of body, mind and soul. They come as natural effects because of the conquest of the seemingly unconquerable. The elemental body, senses, mind, vital energy (*prāṇa*), intelligence, I-ness and consciousness are not easily conquerable. One has to work tremendously with total attention to have control on them. When our practice has not reached that level to experience those powers that Patañjali explains, what right have we to reject them? Have we reached that pinnacle of the *sādhanā* to criticise?

When one has not reached that level, one has no right to criticise. When one reaches a certain state, then one says, "I have reached", but when one has not reached at all, one has no right to doubt the author who has written this treatise more than two thousand five hundreds years ago. If you had put this question directly to Lord Patañjali, probably he would have answered easily and directly, as he was a great master. His *sādhanā* was supreme, intense. And if you read carefully the third chapter, he says that some certain developments do come by the practice of yoga. Take yourself or your friends who are here. You have been doing yoga for several years, they too. What were they, what was their mental calibre before yoga and what are their mental calibres today? Are there changes or not?

– *Yes, certainly.* –

Is there any change in you or not?

– *Yes, yes.* –

Are you not humanly better than you were before? Now would you like to do what you were doing then? That itself is a proof that there is some truth in the words of Patañjali because you are experiencing, in your practice and in your daily way of life. As you are progressing in yoga, many of the desires are dropping away and many of the needs are lessened. You may not be very pure; you might not have reached the zenith of purity as Patañjali has reached. Yet, ethically, physically and mentally have you not improved?

– *Yes.* –

So this is a proof of what Patañjali has said. It is a kind of self-examining process to see whether our *sādhanā* is of that calibre. If *sādhanā* is not of that calibre, it should be understood that one is not fit enough to experience them. For instance, Einstein came to the conclusion that $E=mc^2$.

That was his *sūtra* like Patañjali's aphorism. The scientists later worked on this *sūtra* and came to know nuclear energy. Could you imagine, years back, about the atomic bomb and nuclear weapons? Has not the brain developed to have new discoveries and new inventions? So materially when we are becoming accomplished, can't we be spiritually accomplished?

Then why do you distrust a person who has said something about accomplishment 2,500 years ago? The guide for us is the third chapter. Patañjali speaks of diverse wealth, which comes through the *sādhanā* – they are thirty-four to thirty-five properties or powers which a yogi can get. Yet I will request the students of yoga of ten to fifteen years of practice to read and re-read it carefully and find out whether any of you have touched a drop of what he has said in that chapter or not. You might have experienced what he has said, but he has not said that it is made for exhibitionism. His idea was not only to have the impetus on the *sādhaka* but to experience the properties or the wealth or the power which has been dealt with in the third chapter. Even if the experience is of one per cent of what he has explained, then take it as a guide that the *sādhaka* is on the right track of the *sādhanā*. Otherwise, how does one know that the *sādhanā* is on the right track?

So the third chapter is the stepping-stone to know whether you are moving in the right direction or not. From this angle, the third chapter is an essential chapter. If you don't get even, as I've said, one per cent of what he has said, then you have not followed the right *sādhanā* at all. If there is something missing or some fragrance is missing in your *sādhanā*, I don't think that it is right for one to criticise a man of Patañjali's calibre.

Q.- Your book *Light on Yoga* is the international reference book for the practice of *āsana*. Your book *Light on Prāṇāyāma* is the real revelation of the breathing techniques, but still some people consider your yoga as physical yoga. What place do *āsana* and *prāṇāyāma* occupy in your teaching?

My friend, is it ever possible for any individual to demarcate the body, the mind and the soul? If those who criticise me can demarcate body, mind and soul, then I may understand them. But as long as they themselves do not know where the body ends and the mind begins, where the mind ends and the soul begins, they have no right to remark on me when they do not know or practise, or if at all, practise superficially. There is no depth in them. If there is depth, then probably their language may change.

Who are they to say that what I am doing is physical or mental or spiritual? Is it their right or my right to say what I practise? Who is the practitioner? They or I? Have they entered into my heart? Have they entered into my brain to measure my vibrant physical action or mental action to say that this is physical? Now, you read philosophical books, right? The content in them is spiritual, isn't it?

– *Yes.* –

But how is it explained to you? Isn't it explained to you in a physical form? In order to explain, the person has to buy paper, the person has to use a pen, the person has to use the pencil, an inkbottle...

– *Of course.* –

So, are these not physical things then? Without physical means, can they express their spirituality? The painter, when he says, "I'm divinely involved in it", what does he use? The brush, the colour, the paper... Are these physical means or spiritual means? As you put the first question, "What is yoga?", this is the answer. Yoga is the divine marriage of the body and the soul. As the lover embraces the beloved or the beloved embraces the lover, similarly the matter is the beloved and the soul is the lover and they embrace each other in yoga. Through the practice of *āsana*, I as a practitioner embrace matter and as I embrace matter, the matter comes and embraces me. So my practice of *āsana* is nothing but the divine union of my body with the soul and the soul with the body. But if they don't understand, it is not my fault. It is not for me to give answers for each and every question that is raised by the critics. You cannot go on answering all the questions of the people. If there is logic one can answer, if there is no logic one remains silent.

Hence, it is wrong on anyone's part to say, "I'm practising spiritual *sādhanā*. Mr. Iyengar's is physical *sādhanā*". This very statement expresses the egoistic quality of the sayer. After all, the body is the vehicle of the soul. Then why do they need sleep in the night? Why do they need food? Are they not physical states for survival?

– *Absolutely.* –

The body has not been denied or neglected by those who are on the spiritual path. Though it is not the main instrument, at the same time it is neither cajoled nor made to indulge in pleasures. I keep my body healthy, so that my mind may move in my body without any hindrances. My body and mind both freely allow me to have my inner journey to be close to the core. Is it physical if it is making the avenue for my consciousness or the seer to move freely in my body without any abstractions? I do *āsana*, so that I can see my inner universe very well.

I don't think that you or my pupils should get disturbed by such type of criticism. I began hearing this type of criticism since the day I started yoga. Even if you read my *guru*'s book, my *guru* starts answering the same question, "Is it not physical? Why do you need to do *āsana*?". The world moves on through such doubts. Doubting is not wrong. One needs to do the reasoning behind doubts.

People want all the enjoyments of life. Then why should they want the enjoyments of life, if they are spiritual? Even the so-called philosophers want a huge applauding crowd in front of them to provoke their thoughts. If you look at your own body, it is physical; but if you gaze at a candle, it is spiritual. Is that logic? What is the candle? Is it a physical object or spiritual thought? It is a physical object. Somebody says, "Gaze at a candle, so you improve your concentration", and a person like me says, "Gaze at your toe for correction." Which is superior? If there is a defect in your toe, at least you correct your toe. If the flame of the burning candle goes out, your mind also goes out. So where is the spirituality? Is it not a fluctuation? But here, if your toe moves, you are controlling the toe, which is a better thought than gazing at the candle.

Know that the body is the expression of the inner soul. *Āsana* are the expression of the inner soul. If you have read some of the *Yoga Upaniṣad*, it is clearly mentioned that a man who has mastered the *āsana* becomes the master of the three worlds.[1] Why did they say that a man who practises *āsana* conquers the three worlds, if it is just physical? Why then did Patañjali recognise *āsana* as one of the eight aspects? Remaining in the sensual world one should not talk about the spiritual world. So sensually talking and saying that you are spiritually far advanced is cheating one's own self.

Never mind. Even if it is considered as physical, it has given me light. I am happy. If people consider *āsana* as the movements of the body, then I can also say that *āsana* and *prāṇāyāma* help you to remove the veil, the cloud that covers the intelligence. In medical language you talk about cholesterol formation, which blocks the space in the blood vessels as well as blockage in the heart causing narrowness in them. Obviously the heart has to pump strenuously in order to make the blood to flow through.

Similar to cholesterol in blood we have the lack of understanding in our intelligence. The flow of intelligence in the *jnānanāḍī* (senses of perception), is blocked which causes lack of awareness and sensitivity. Practice of *āsana* and *prāṇāyāma* removes the clogging in the intelligence. As the coronary blood vessels get blocked causing heart attack, similarly the intelligence gets blocked causing hindrances in the process of self-realisation. The two key limbs *āsana* and *prāṇāyāma* are meant for the evolution of the aspirant.

As effort is needed to flush the cholesterol formation in the heart and blood, a similar attempt is needed to remove the cover that clouds the intelligence.

Q.- You speak very often in your classes about the consciousness of the self, alignments, body and mind integration, etc... Could you explain what you mean by these expressions?

[1] *Śāṇḍilyopaniṣad*, I.III.14.

Yogis say equanimity *(samatvam)*[1] is yoga. Therefore, for me, aligning my body, senses, energy, intelligence and consciousness is *samatvam*, which is yoga. Is it not very interesting to learn now that a disease such as AIDS is opening the eyes of the scientists of the world more and more? If AIDS had not developed so rampantly, probably medical science would have missed those points referred to in the question.

Medical science now has come to the conclusion that cells have their own intelligence, cells develop their own memory and hence one has to keep each cell healthy. A copious oxygenated supply of blood is required to nourish them to retain the memory. The cell can itself change through the experience of its memory for the better usage in the system. Patañjali said this 2,500 years ago, that the cells of each individual have their own intelligence and hence they have to be kept healthy.

Here, I am not talking about the physical health. I am talking about the inputs and imprints. When the body dies, the cells die, yet the imprints are carried. As the plane has the black box and every detail is noted on it, the cells too register their experiences on consciousness (*citta*), which are carried by them to the next life. Now the science talks about DNA, which Patañjali has spoken of centuries back though he does not use the word DNA. Patañjali does not consider body as a hindrance for self-realisation. On the contrary, he demands a complete transformation of this body for higher purposes and spiritual experiences.

He does not even deny the importance of the health of the body. Disease is the first impediment he speaks of, where the alignment gets missed between the body and the soul.

So unless you give a bath, unless you supply sufficient blood to those areas, how can they be healthy? How can you keep the system away from diseases? Whether the science accepts it or not, yoga as science has said that you have to align your inner and outer bodies, so that they understand each other and run parallel to each other. When they run parallel to each other, communication is established between them and they send messages for you about what to do, what not to do, how much to do and how much not to do. Hence for me alignment is a metaphysical word. If the muscles or vertebrae of the spine are unaligned, one gets a lot of aches and pains. Scoliosis makes the patient suffer because of non-alignment. If one organ fails in its function, the other organ takes the responsibility and wears out gradually, though the body-machine continues to work. Stress is experienced. The non-alignment is the cause of such stress.

Take *Haṭhayoga Pradīpikā*. Do you know the meaning of its name? What *haṭha* means? You have all read that right side is *piṅgalā* (sun), left side is *iḍā* (moon). In other words it means that the right side of the nerves – *piṅgalā* should communicate with the left side of the nerves – *iḍā* of the body, and left side of the nerves of the body have to communicate with the right side of the nervous system of the body. This is what exactly *haṭha* means. So what does it convey to you? It conveys the

[1] *yoga-sthaḥ kuru karmāṇi saṅgaṁ tyaktvā dhanañjaya /*
siddhy-asiddhyoḥ samo bhūtvā samatvaṁ yoga uchyate // B.G., II.48

alignment, does it not? Does is not convey that the right side speaks to the left side, left side speaks to the right side? There should be a healthy understanding between the right and the left, so that they run without any deviation in their systems. This is the alignment of the nervous system, but Patañjali's alignment is to align the consciousness with the cells of the body. In your practice of *āsana* and *prāṇāyāma*, is your intelligence running parallel to your body? I am sure that this is very difficult to understand in the beginning, but later it strikes the practitioner as he goes on practising and absorbing the reactions of actions.

– *Oh, yes! Very difficult!* –

Yes, alignment is difficult. Alignment means delicate, skilful adjustment in action.[1]

Now you are all doing the practice of *yogāsana*. Lift your hands up in *Vīrabhadrāsana I*. You lifted up. Feel the intelligence on the right hand and left hand, which is strong, one is generating more power, whereas the other is not generating power. Right?

– *Yes.* –

Now is there any alignment, though you are lifting your arms, between the right and the left? One is active, one is sensitive. One side of the skin, the cells are sensitive, but are they sensitive or insensitive on the other side?

– *They are different.* –

They are different. Now, I say, try to bring the alignment by watching the feeling of the right with the feeling of the left, or the feeling of the left with the feeling of the right, without any deviation. Can you get it?

Now you have done it.

– *Yes.* –

Is your body stretching or your intelligence stretching inside your arms? What is stretching?

– *Both.* –

---

[1] *buddhi-yukto jahātīha ubhe sukṛta-duṣkṛte /*
tasmād yogāya yujyasva yogaḥ karmasu kauśalam // B.G., II.50

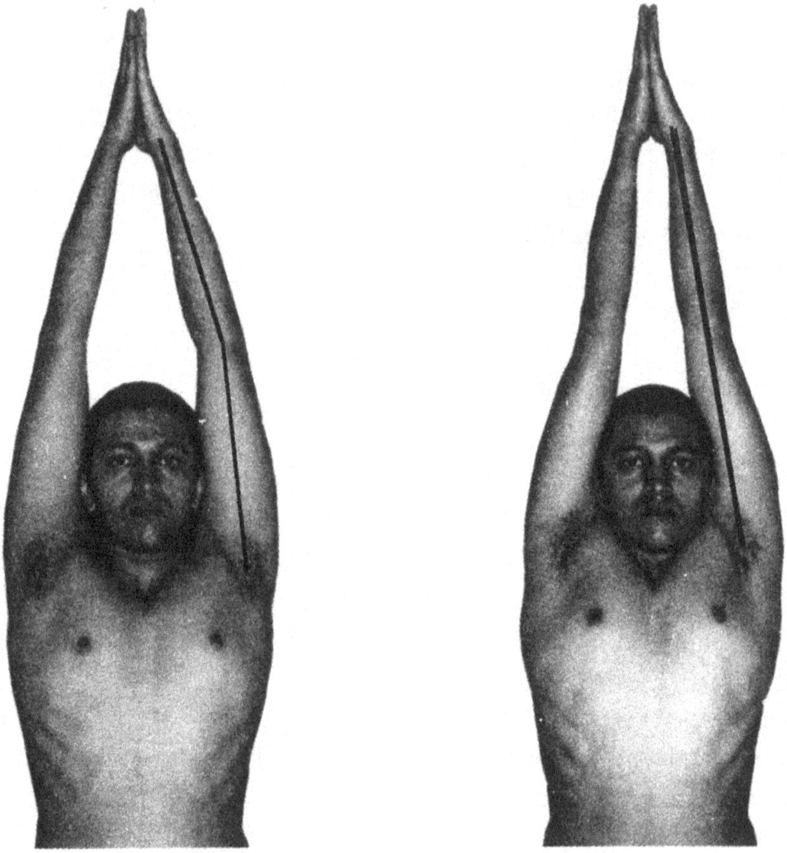

Plate n. 41 – Is your body stretching or your intelligence stretching inside your arms?

You may stretch your arms physically but are you aware of the other areas and other muscles of the arms co-ordinating evenly? Is there equanimity in the stretch? Did your mind go up with the arms? Did your mind reach there? Did your intelligence extend further or not? This way of observation in *sādhanā* touches the frontier, does it not? Repeat again and observe. See whether your intelligence is touching the extreme end of the skin of your fingers equally on both sides or not. There is a difference, is there not? Then you have to work for it, don't you? Why do such inequalities or unevenness remain? It is not inadvertence or a sort of defect in the thinking mind. It is the failure of mind to observe or watch. It is the absent mindedness and unawareness. It means that the mind did not align itself with the body. When you act unconsciously, you say, you were not aware of it. But here, you are conscious. You stretched your arms with conscious attention, yet the disparity in stretching the arms is visible. So the moment you apply intelligence, you get a feedback. You know the disparity causing non-alignment. At that time you cannot allow your mind or intelligence to waver. This is the alignment of body, mind and soul. Patañjali uses the philosophical word *śuddhisāmyatā*.

Now, is that spiritual or physical? Are you moving your soul inside to reach, or just touching the skin? Is just your finger going up or your mind going up?

- Mind. -

This is known as practical experience. Through practical experience, you realise that your practice of *āsana* is not physical. It is a pure alignment of intelligence with the body and the self.

Why do you listen to others when I bring you to have the experience directly? In the practice of *āsana* the mind is greatly involved in action, and so it is the culture of the mind and not the culture of the body. You are using the frontier of the mind – the body as a means for the mind to travel in the body in order to culture it.

Suppose, I like your pen and ask you to give it to me, you present your pen with a smile, saying "With great pleasure", and I take it. But the other side of the coin is that from your heart, you may not want to part with it. Physically you give it but with the unwillingness of your mind. Your action may be on the principles of etiquette, though the mind had a different view. Or you gave it to me, because you do not like it. This way the attitude of mind could be differing from the attitude of the head. Very rarely do both brain and mind go together with action. While practising *āsana* the body, the brain and the mind have to go hand in hand without the tinge of emotions, such as likes, dislikes, attachments, detachments and so forth. Mind, brain and body have to work hand in hand with the heart of the soul. Hope you understand now the meaning of alignment of body, brain, mind and self.

- Very clearly. -

So why do you listen to people who criticise without knowing the subject or with no revelation of experience in themselves?

Now again take your arms up. And retain them. Well, do it. *(We bring the arms up again).*

When you are retaining it, what does the body say? You should drop, right? What do you do then?

When you lift them again, do you lift them with the body or the mind? Do you lift with the mind or with the consciousness?

- First with the mind, afterwards... -

Ah!... afterwards... A little longer, what happens? The *prāṇa* (energy) moves and *prajñā* (awareness) engulfs. This is consciousness. Then where is the mind or where is the will?

- *The mind begins to disappear, and another one appears.* -

Yes! There is another. What is that "another"? That is the known (*citta*) moving towards the knower – the *Self.* This evolutionary study from body to the Self in doing *āsana* is the spiritual way in the path of *āsana*. Now, bring the arms down.

That is how one has to learn to get and understand the spiritual insight (*vedānta*)[1] in the *āsana*. The Self-realisation is not only individual but practical also. Those who talk about the *āsana* have no right to talk unless they as practitioners experience the spiritual background (*ātma-jnāna* or *puruṣa-jnāna*).

I said earlier that one has no right to criticise the powers that Patañjali speaks of, because one has not reached that)level to give an opinion on his experiences. Similarly, those people who make such remarks should examine themselves as to what is lacking in them before making statements on others.

Many say, "I'm doing *dhyāna yoga*". When I say, "I am doing *dhyāna yoga*", is it a spiritual experience or an egoistic expression? Tell me. "I am doing *dhyāna yoga*, and not physical yoga." What does it show? They want to say that they are slightly higher than you and me. So is it not the expression of *ahaṁkāra?* I thank God, when they are telling me every now and then that I am a physical yogi. The more they say that, I become humble. If I said, "I'm doing *dhyāna yoga*", people would have said, "Ah, he is great because he is doing *dhyāna yoga*", probably, my pride would have gone up. On the contrary, they are doing good to my practice by providing food for reflection. I'm happy that the more they criticise, the more I get humble and spiritual advancement in me is possible. This feeling of mine is so very subtle that it is hard for others to understand. If I criticise you, I indicate that I am greater than you, which means that my ego has horns.

The *dhyāna* and building of ego both cannot go together. *Dhyāna* and ego cannot exist together as *dhyāna* acts as an instrument to subdue the ego or *ahaṁkāra*.

I will give you another example. You know about the adrenal glands. Adrenal glands are defensive glands. Their functional aim is "flow with or fight". You are a practitioner of yoga and I also am a practitioner of yoga. Both are practitioners but you know that I am your teacher or I am a step ahead to you. Then don't you become nervous? You run away from me. But if you face me and give a good fight, you are no more afraid of me. The defensive adrenals instead of flying prepare to fight. Adrenals have defensive and offensive characters. If its secretion increases it gives you courage to

---

[1] See *Aṣṭadaḷa Yogamālā*, vol. 2 – "From *Moha* to *Mokṣa*".

face and fight the situation and if it decreases, you may run away and not face the situation.

When some criticise me, I don't run away. I face their criticism, because my genuine practice is my answer to their criticism. You have no answer so you become nervous. The *sādhanā* has to be of that level to face them. I don't say that I am doing *dhyāna yoga*. My *dhyāna* is there in everything that I do. You have several moods in your *sādhanā*; I have only a meditative mood in my *sādhanā*. To say that the *dhyāna* yoga practice is superior, is nothing but psychological egoism. If I say that *dhyāna* is in my profound practice of *āsana* or *prāṇāyāma*, then you may also brand me as a spiritual egoist, but note that this is an essential quality. Psychological ego can be shaken because it is built up on inexperience, whereas the spiritual ego is based on the profound experience.

Each one has a personal point of view, but as we cannot demarcate body, mind and soul, no one has the right to say that this is physical, this is mental, this is spiritual. Even Patañjali or the commentators have not used such words as physical, mental and spiritual. However, they have used the words *bahiraṅga sādhanā* and *antaraṅga sādhanā*. I have added one more term as *antarātmā sādhanā*, which you also find in *Light on Yoga*. These are the common terminologies used by one and all.

When the word *bahiraṅga sādhanā* is used, it means that you are using the external means in your *sādhanā* to reach the internal gate of the outer sheath. Or, you can say that your external efforts and discipline are a kind of threshold to enter into one's own being. And when the word *antaraṅga sādhanā* is used, it means not only that you are using the external vehicles of the soul, but also the internal vehicles of the soul. That is along with the body, *karmendriya*, *jñānendriya*, mind, intelligence, I-ness and consciousness are used in your efforts. *Antarātma sādhanā* is without any aid of those vehicles of *bahiraṅga* or *antaraṅga*. You deal directly with the soul. Patañjali has not divided by using the words physical, mental, spiritual, but he has used the words *antaraṅga* and *bahiraṅga* in the second and third chapter. And do you know where this demarcation has been shown, for whom he has shown? Those who are advanced. He says that even the internal appears external to the innermost. He says that for those who have reached *samādhi* through *dhāraṇā* and *dhyāna*, their vehicles are so co-operative and supportive and hence they are in an integrated state. We all know the eight aspects of yoga. But Patañjali adds one more aspect to it. When the last three *dhāraṇā*, *dhyāna* and *samādhi* are eventually mastered, they culminate into the state where the practitioner is in an integrated state.[1] He has clearly mentioned it according to the quality of the intellectual growth of an individual and according to the growth of the intellectual sensitivity of the person that has developed through the practice of yoga. As the level of *sādhanā* is relative, the standard of intelligence too is relative and hence the level of progress changes. But Patañjali has not defined *bahiraṅga sādhanā* as physical yoga.

---

1 *trayamekatra saṁyamaḥ* – *Yoga Sūtra* III.4

The commentator says that up to *pratyāhāra*, it is *bahiraṅga*, since you have used the external means in order to penetrate the inner gates of the soul. From *pratyāhāra* onwards it is *antaraṅga sādhanā*, since the journey towards soul is from the internal vehicles – the *buddhi*, *ahaṁkāra* and *citta*. Note the difference of the language people speak and what Patañjali and Vyāsa say. The external vehicles are the means in order to penetrate the inner up to *pratyāhāra*. That is why the word *bahiraṅga* is used. You see, *bahir* means external, *aṅga* means aspect.

Using the external organs such as the body, the senses of perception, organs of action, mind, to penetrate the inner is *bahiraṅga*. In *dhāraṇā*, the *antarāṅga*, the internal means such as intelligence, discriminative power of the intelligence are used. The discriminative power of the intelligence is dealt with in *dhāraṇā*. *Dhāraṇā* is not mind control. It is the control of the very intelligence. The mind has no power of discrimination. When the discriminative power of the intelligence is brought to the surface, *dhāraṇā* begins. That is why it is called internal yoga, because the intelligence is utilised. At a higher stage even the intelligence also becomes an external means or external cover to the seer. So it becomes external to the person who uses the very core of the being for *sādhanā*.

When one does everything with the core, then there is no intelligence, there is no mind, but only *antarātman*, who is hidden inside. From then on, the *sādhanā* is done directly from the core and not with the help of its vehicles.[1] Beyond that I cannot go, it is impossible to question, because all three are involved in the growth of a person.

Now, when there is an orchestra, how many musicians are there in an orchestra?

– *Many.* –

There is also solo music, there is also chamber music, is there not? Varieties of music are there. But when hundreds and hundreds of people are playing, why don't you say, it is all physical, this man is scratching something, that man is beating something? Is not playing the violin or beating a drum physical? But you call the music divine. When hundreds of people are playing hundreds of instruments in hundreds of different ways, you call it spiritual. Here while doing *āsana* you are moving your legs this way, your hands that way, so you term it as physical. Now can you see that no one knows how to integrate? Why don't you see that one moves one body in hundreds of ways, in an orchestrated manner? Is it not integrated? Actually it is an orchestra. The solo player is inside. So if you can damn the musicians saying that orchestral music is physical, then you have the right to damn me.

The body, mind, senses, intelligence, all these aspects are like an orchestra for the soul. The various movements, adjustments, alignments, stability etc. are different sounds or vibrations,

1 *Tadapi bahiraṅgaṁ nirbījasya* – *Yoga Sūtra* III.8

which can be produced in various *āsana*, so that you can listen to the sounds. The sound of *Vīrabhadrāsana* is not the same sound as *Hanumānāsana*. In *Trikoṇāsana*, the sound of the legs, the vibration of the legs is different from that of *Hanumānāsana*. So what type of vibration do you get in this *āsana?* What type of vibration do you get in that *āsana?* You have to watch.

I listen to this inner vibrated sound of *āuṁ*. *Japa* of *āuṁ* has become very popular in your country. Having the *japamālā* (the chain of beads used to count the chanting) in your hand, you people are asked to repeat the sacred syllable *āuṁ*. Is not the movement of the beads physical? Is not the chain of beads a prop used for counting? They keep on saying, *āuṁ - āuṁ - āuṁ* and the word goes topsy-turvy "māu-māu-māu" – (Māo-Māo-Māo) – the name of the world's famous man – Mao of China. The vibrations of the body, mind, senses, intelligence, I-consciousness are at least orchestrated in the practice of *āsana*. While practising I listen to the sacred, mysterious inner sound while you do not listen to the sound within. This is the difference between your practice and my practice. Your TM becomes MT (empty!). For me, the inner meditative orchestra becomes totally complete.

There is a very good story in the *Rāmāyaṇa*. The author of *Rāmāyaṇa* was Vālmiki. He was a robber. He was absolutely uncultured and illiterate. One day Sage Nārada was passing through the forest and he saw this man coming to rob him. The robber thought, "Now I have got my food, the sage is coming, so my wife and children can be fed", so he wanted to stab the sage. Sage Nārada realised his intention and said, "Just wait, you can kill me, I don't mind, I'm your prey, but before you kill me, go and ask your wife whether she has got any share in your action of killing and murdering. Go and ask whether she can share your sins. Ask your children whether they are ready to share your sins". He said, "But how can I believe that you are going to be here? You will run away". Nārada said, "You can tie me. You can do anything, but please ask her. I give my word. I will not leave this place". So he went and told his wife that he had found a prey today and the prey was asking him this question: "Do you share the sin, when I'm killing the people, the *hiṁsā* of what I'm doing, the violence I'm doing? Do you share, as you are my wife?" She answered, "You have to protect me because you have married me. Why should I share your sins? Your job is to look after me because I'm your wife. I'm not a part of your sins". He asked his children and the reply was the same. He was surprised and shocked by this answer. Then he went back and told everything to the sage Nārada. The sage said, "Now you have understood that your wife and children are not willing to share your actions or the reactions of your actions". Then suddenly the robber realised his mistake and he asked, "What have I to do?" The sage gave the *mantra* of Rāma and said: "You say the name of Rāma and Rāma will come to you to protect you". He could not pronounce the word. Whatever way he tried, he could not get the word. So Nārada reversed the word and said, "Say *Marā-Marā-Marā-Marā*." Then the words of the *mantra* become Rāma-Rāma-Rāma. The robber sat there, closed his eyes and started repeating the word *Marā-Marā-Marā*. He did not realise when the word *Marā* became 'Rāma'. So *Marā* was given by Nārada to Vālmiki who got cleansed in his heart and head and became enlightened. Later, he wrote the epic *Rāmāyaṇa* about how Rāma appeared on this earth as an incarnation of Lord Viṣṇu. He became a great scholar.

Those who speak of spiritual life, who say, "I am doing the *mantrajapa*," are they doing the *mantra* as it should be uttered? If not, it is as good as not doing it. The *japa* or the continual recitation of *mantra* has to be very clear. That is why Patañjali says, *tat japaḥ tada artha bhāvanam*[1] (I.28). Sage Nārada realised the potential spirituality in Vālmiki. Therefore he could give the *mantra Marā-Marā*, which became meaningful and emotionally touched the heart of Vālmiki. That is why he could write the *Rāmāyāṇa* later. If there is no inner urge then there cannot be any transformation. As *marā mantra* changed into Rāma in Vālmiki, the change to TM may turn into MT bringing emptiness. Even the *mantra Harihi Om! Harihi Om!* may end up with *Hari home*, Hurry Home and Hurry Home.

– *(Laughter)* –

Therefore, what I say is that you should not be confused. No practitioner of yoga should get disturbed by the words of others, because the words are very often used with pride. When the words come with experience, then they are for the growth of the individual. The human nature is to criticise. We should not become victims of it. We should accept if it is constructive for our betterment. You are not a neophyte or a beginner that you do not understand that they are misguiding you. Now when you are practising for so many years you know that the change has come. As the changes came subjectively and directly, that is enough proof for you to continue.

Q.- About this accuracy, it is always surprising the knowledge that you manifest in your teaching, the depth of the inner connections of the body, the correspondence between the nerves, muscles, bones, cartilages and tendons in the living body. Where did you get so much information, which is not available in the books? How do you know so much about the human body?

It's a very difficult question to answer. See, if you had asked me about fifty years ago, I would have said that I'm moving my limbs and I do know nothing beyond that. But fifty years I churned my body as you churn more and more to get butter out of the milk. I churned my body to a great extent and I am still churning, and that has given me the depth of knowledge. That knowledge is experienced knowledge, and as it is experienced knowledge, the words are few but the depth is more. So I say

---

[1] The *mantra āuṁ* is to be repeated constantly, with feeling, realising its full significance.

that it came to me with my *sādhanā*. You all use the word intuition. I say intuition, because I have developed the knowledge after doing for more than fifty years or because something clicked inside. I was tutored from within to learn all these things. I got tutored from my own body, from my own cells, from my own intelligence to know this depth. Hence I'm tutored from within and that gave me the depth.

I was *muḍha*. I did like a *tapasvin* and perhaps this is the result of it.

Q.- Props are used in your way of teaching. What are they for and how did you create them?

The challenges from the suffering people on me were very very great. Lots of people, who had incurable diseases, wanted some solace, some relief. The diseased people used to come with the hope of cure. So it was a challenge and a chance for me to improvise the methods. Often I have to put a lot of effort in order to bring progress. I used to utilise my hand, knees, legs, back as a support to help them. I had to think of ways and means to see that yoga gives them some benefit.

Though the support and help was not an easy job, the patients used to ask me how they should practice on their own. On account of their queries, ideas started coming to my mind, to create props as self-help so that they could make use of them to continue practice independently. I began experimenting and I succeeded in finding supporting instruments to perform *āsana* independently. But unfortunately many are using them as a luxury which I feel is not fair.

I discovered it for the simple reason that when *Haṭhayoga Pradīpikā* says that yoga is meant for children, youngsters, old people, ripe old people, weak people, diseased people, I took these last three: *ativṛddha* (very old), *vyādhita* (diseased), *durbala* (weak) person.[1] How to deal with such disabled or physically challenged people, how to make these three categories of people do yoga, was a big question. You are healthy, I can make you to do *Sālamba Śīrṣāsana* anywhere. But a person whose arm is amputated, what have I to do to make him do *Sālamba Śīrṣāsana*? I traced the ways and brought joy to them. When *Haṭhayoga Pradīpikā* says that yoga could be practised irrespective of age, irrespective of diseases, irrespective of weaknesses, that gave me an idea that I should think that if a person cannot do *Sālamba Śīrṣāsana*, how can I make him? What is the way to make him do it?

That is how I converted the available commodities in the market, things which we use daily in our houses such as chairs, bricks, bed, and sofa into props, which you all see. As they can be used for any household purposes, they can also be used for yoga, not as a special yogic instrument.

---

[1] *Haṭhayoga Pradīpikā*, I.64.

I did not invent them as special instruments as people could not have afforded them. I picked up those things we use for common purposes. Those which could be used for common purposes, I used them also for this extraordinary purpose, and that's how I went on finding various props.

I feel in my heart of hearts that if I had not discovered all these props, probably the struggle would have been more to learn this art. In one way it lessens the struggle and gives right direction to do the *āsana*. If you do on a chair for example, *Sālamba Sarvāṅgāsana* or *Dwi Pāda Viparīta Daṇḍāsana* from the edge of the chair, you can understand which part you are touching, which part

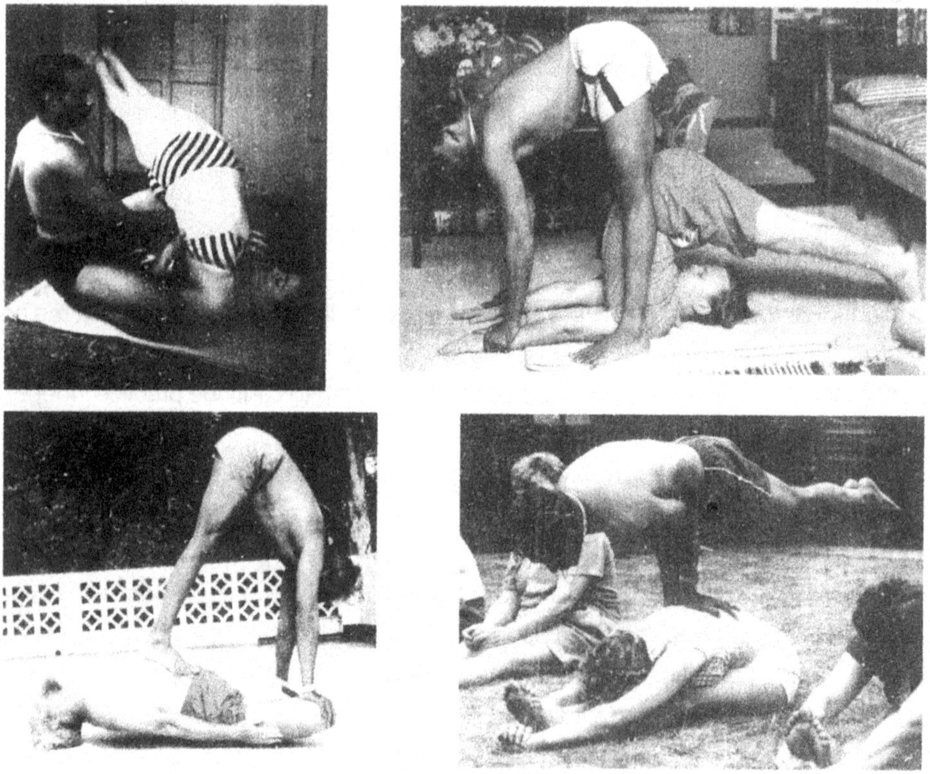

Plate n. 42 – Using my body as a prop to help

you are not touching, how much you are lifting or curving, where the life is and where it is not, which part of the spine is above or below. You get enough time to feel and think with the help of the props, whereas when you do all these independently you cannot watch because you are afraid that if you try to do something you may lose balance. So in order to have the correct sensitivity and have the grasp of the positions in *āsana*, or even in *prāṇāyāma*, we use props to reach accuracy soon. For that I created them.

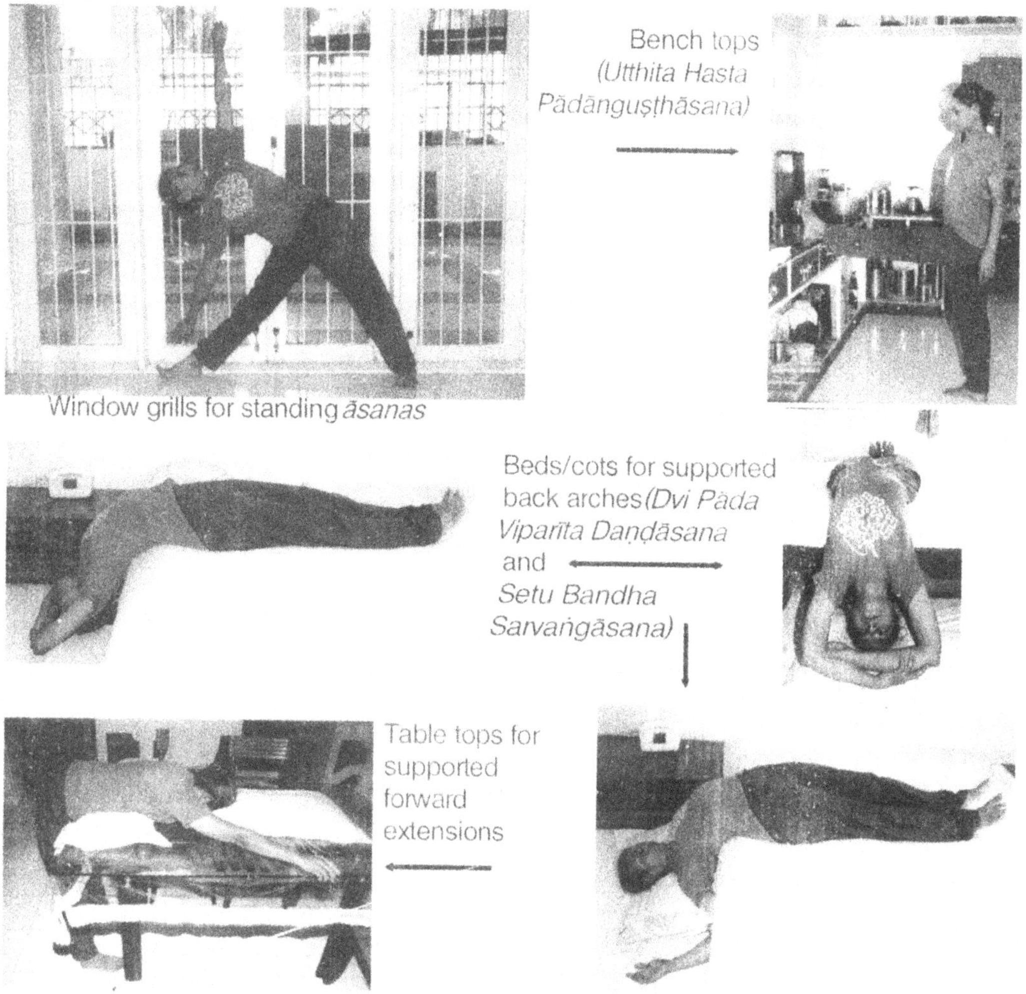

Plate n. 43 – Using household commodities as props

Take this bandage cloth, which you all use. It was an experiment with J. Krishnamurti. All his lectures were based on alert passivity, which he used to say is very, very difficult. Having done *Ṣaṇmukhī mudrā*,[1] I had the experiences of alertive passivity in the brain. This is how I started helping patients suffering from insomnia first. Now a days the handkerchiefs are very small. In earlier days people were using neckties, long ones. Now it has gone out of fashion. I used neckties, because they were longer than the handkerchiefs. Then one day I told Krishnamurti, "Sir, you often talk about alert passivity which is difficult, but with this necktie the alert passivity will come in no time, since it is an easy method". So one day I tied him and he also experienced the value of this.

---

[1] See plate n. 15

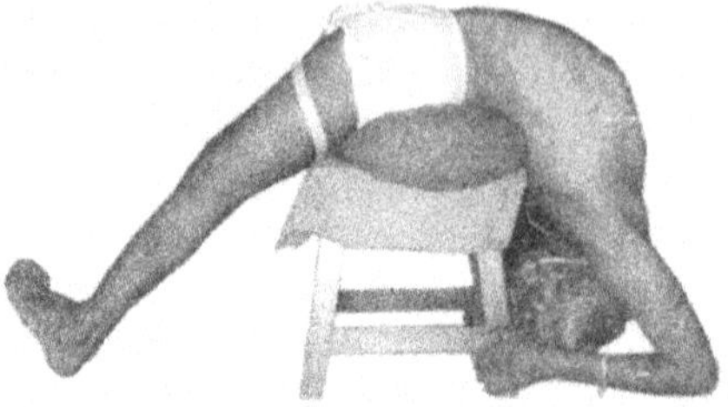

Dwi Pāda Viparīta Daṇḍāsana (stool)

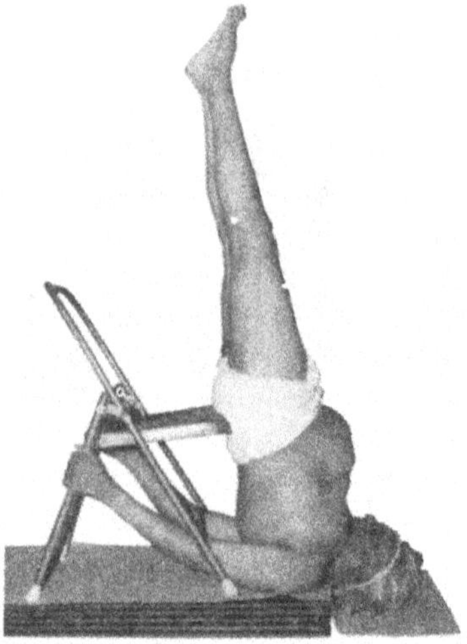

Sarvaṅgāsana (chair)

Plate n. 44 – *Sālamba Sarvāṅgāsana* (chair), *Dwi Pāda Viparīta Daṇḍāsana* (stool)

Then I started using it for patients suffering with blood pressure, glaucoma of the eyes, displaced retina and so on. Such people cannot work, they cannot see, but they could rest their eyes. Through the resting of the eyes, the nerves rest and brain would become silent. Though I experimented with Krishnamurti as per his explanations, in the back of my mind my idea was how to save him from the pressure in *Sālamba Śīrṣāsana*. How not to allow the eyes to become red or capillaries to break in *Sālamba Śīrṣāsana*.[1] That is how I started the bandage cloth, but today you are using it for everything, and it has become a blind spot. But I don't use it. Have you seen me using it? Tell me. I am the inventor, but the inventor is not using it at all, and nobody thinks why I'm not using it. When the need comes, then I use it, but when there is no need, why should I use it? When you use it without any reason it makes you dull and does not lead to passive alertness.

Though I am the creator of these props if you asked me, "What is the good, what is the bad?" I can tell you that if you use them constructively they do more good, but if you use them for the lazy type of yogic practices, then you are definitely on *tāmasic* lines. The *tāmasic* and lazy practice may give a state of beingness but it cannot be witnessed since there is no light. The *sāttvic* practice gives the state of beingness, which is witnessed. You use the props as a need to get the understanding and sensitivity.

No doubt, props are good, you can increase the time of stay in the *āsana*. As the duration of stay in these *āsana* gets prolonged, use it as a powerhouse to increase the intellectual sensitivity in your system. Then I say the props are great friends and great boons. But if you completely depend

[1] See plate n. 45

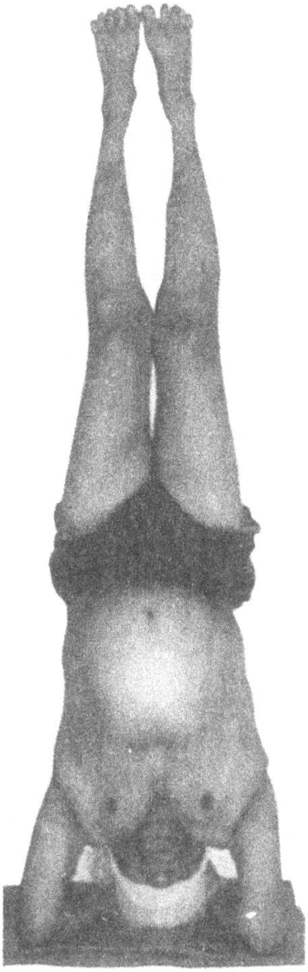

Plate n. 45 – **_Śīrṣāsana_ with a bandage**

on them as resting *āsana*, it makes you dull and inactive. Then it is a curse. Yoga is freedom. Here instead of freedom you are in bondage. The same props can be the cause of freedom as well as bondage. It depends upon how and why you use them as well as for what reason.

Q.- Let us change the subject. We know that the Indian cricket team practises your yoga. What is the place of yoga in sport?

When you know that lots of people in sports are coming to learn, that means something is missing in their needs. It tells that something is wanting in their methodologies and the word used before, i.e. alignment, is very, very important for sportsmen. Because they use their energy in the shortest period in order to win or get fame or medals, whatever it may be. Yoga may not build up muscles but it builds up endurance. Endurance in the sinews, which are the feeders for the muscles. The sinews, the tendons, we call them *snāyu,* maybe you do not know that word and I will try to explain that to you. Now, these are the biceps, this is the muscle, but the sinew is here. Sinew is the tendon joining the muscles to the bones. The sinews build up muscles. The energy in sinews is more. If these sinews can supply energy, then the person is strong. But if they cannot supply, then the speed wanes. If the muscles are not close to the bones they lose the power. Yoga helps in storing, strengthening or rejuvenating the sinews and makes them store energy to use when needed.

In sports certain parts of the body are activated and certain parts are dragged. The players are not aware of their bodies. They concentrate on the game, therefore the body is dragged. Just now when you lifted your hands you noticed that one hand went up very fast, being alert and active; the other hand moved slowly. So when we are educating, what do we say? Use both the arms with equipoise, equistretch, and equiunderstanding. Because you use each and every part of the body differently, may be spindles, cells, fibres, sinews, or even muscles, right and left, so education of equistretch is needed. Hence yoga teaches you to use these parts accurately and precisely without showing any deviation between the right side and the left side. For the players this gives not only speed but also control. In any game or sports they cannot give the same speed evenly on both parts of the body, and that is why yoga helps all other exercises. A sportsman might be a good runner but he does not realise how he can improve his performance by properly training the legs.

Sport makes the joints stiff because lactic acid gets collected in the joints, so the fatigue comes to them due to the acidity in the joints. Due to maximum stretching, maximum flexing and proper relaxing in yoga, the formation of the acid dissolves in the joints. Therefore, the muscles and the joints do not develop fatigue, which is a great advantage to athletes as well as sportsmen.

On account of this, I have said long back that yoga makes a sportsman a better sportsman, as we say yoga makes a man a better man. If yoga makes a man a better man, a religious man a better religious man, then yoga also has to make a sportsman a better sportsman. You cannot deny that. *Āsana* helps them a lot because of the proper alignment of the bones and joints, a good circulation, flexibility and quickness.

The way we teach strengthens the cartilages of the knee, therefore the injuries in the knees are avoided. We strengthen them, educate them, bring their attention to see and interpenetrate the actions. While doing *āsana* the action is felt inside the body, whereas in other activities, it is felt outside. So integration between the outer body and inner body comes on its own in yoga.

In *āsana*, the integration of the joints with the muscles, muscles with the joints, then with the nerves, nerves with the bones, is felt. The Integration takes place on its own if the *āsana* is done accurately. Even if you view from the physical angle, the practice of *āsana* is a foundation for all other exercises because the total system of the body is attended at the same time. Whereas in other fields of exercises they cannot pay that attention of interpenetration.

Therefore, I say that yoga is good for the sports people, that's why they are coming. They say, "I'm very good on the right side, I'm not good at all on the left side"... Some say, "My heel is strong, my ankle is not strong; my thighs are strong, my calf muscle is not strong". They have their own problems. Now I ask, though yoga is a spiritual subject, remember what Lord Christ has said: if a man comes and asks you for bread don't give him stone. An athlete comes to yoga for physical fitness. If we give them the sense of well being in order to fulfil their wants and their demands in sports, then that does not mean that yoga is at a physical level. Yoga is for all. It can yield benefits according to the needs of each individual. Hence, yoga is essential for them in order to perform better, develop skills, avoid injuries, increase endurance as well as stamina, maintain emotional stability and to recover from fatigue as well.

Q.- After many years of being ignored by the Indian authorities and after a complete international acknowledgement, the Indian authorities recognised officially your merit when they bestowed on you the *Padmaśrī* award, one of the biggest civil recognitions. What do you feel being recognised by the authorities of your country?

(Laughing) We won independence forty-five years ago, in 1947. With all the good growth in the field of art after independence, yoga was not at all recognised as an Indian cultural and spiritual heritage, though outsiders consider it as one of the heritages of India. I don't know how the government opened their eyes. No doubt it is a matter of great satisfaction. I am not saying that I've been boosted by this award, because I've received several awards and honours, from various parts of the globe. One happiness is that at last after forty-five years, the Government of India has awarded me for my work in the field of yoga. That means the subject of yoga is honoured and has at last come on the national map of India with this award, that's all I can say. *(Laughing).*

Q.- We heard in India that western people can practise yoga techniques but it is very difficult for them to live in yoga totally. What is the maximum that any western yoga practitioner can achieve by following your teaching?

Don't you need food, don't you need sleep? You need food, you need sleep, whether you are a Westerner or an Easterner. Can you forego that? As long as you are eating food, you need some work to digest it, do you not? Yoga is as essential as food and its digestion. If you don't eat food at all, then I can say yoga is not at all needed. If your body-machine works without forming any toxins in the system or does not need to throw the carbon dioxide out and take oxygen in, then yoga is not needed at all. With all the advertisements about nourishments and nice food, particularly in the West, I don't think that the majority of the people are eating nourishing food. Yes or no?

- No. We eat whatever is available. -

You just run after whatever is available. Ready-made foods are available. How do you know that that commercial food is really nourishing food? You don't know, right? So that means they are forming toxins in the system. You want to save time because you have to work at the office, you have to make a little money, so naturally what do you do? You eat whatever is available in the market, so that you can prepare food in a few seconds, such as instant coffee, instant food, tinned food. You should know, as you are intellectually and technically advanced, you should know that this kind of life style is a disease monger. The body is a machine, which needs attention. If your car is not running, you give it for servicing. Even the car needs lubrication. Is it not the duty of each individual, whether in the East or the West, to lubricate one's body every now and then so that the machine can function without any problem? Let us not get away with the feeling that we have no time to do yoga. The health consciousness has grown more in the West than in the East with all such ready-made products of food that you are eating. Still you feel that you need something to keep yourself fit. As Westeners you can use your available time for yogic practices to keep the inner body fit, while all other methods keep the outer body fit.

I use the word inner body. If you take a bath, your skin is cleansed, but does it clean the blood, does it clean the joints? If you want to clean a gutter, you have to call the fireman, do you not? Similarly, in order to clean the inner gutter you need a fireman who is in you. You have to give a bath to the inner organs, not by external water but by your own blood, which is running in your system. The blood is hot. You take hot bath. The blood circulates and creates warmth in the joints, and as I said before, it removes the toxins formed in the joints. As it removes the toxins, is it not worth doing it, to live in it? The whole world is facing and fighting diseases such as AIDS and cancer. Such diseases are afflicting humanity all over the world. Hence, let us work to keep these afflictions out of yogic discipline. Yoga being an internal cleanser, let us devote our time to do it and keep free from diseases.

By the by, do we brand cancer as American cancer or as Indian cancer? Cancer is cancer.

- *Cancer is one.* -

In the same way body is body; mind is mind. You have emotional problems; we have emotional problems. You have physical diseases; we have physical diseases. You want to sharpen the intelligence and we too need to sharpen the intelligence. All want life's realisation. Then what is the difference between Easterners and Westerners? In yoga you are using your own will power to cleanse your inner system – body, mind, intelligence and consciousness. You are not depending on external means for your health. Yoga is economically cheaper. Remember that word, yoga, is economically cheaper. You have to pay the teacher, but in the long run you are not continuing your practice with the teacher. You learn by yourself, and then maintain health and stability both in body and mind. Even the emotions are economised. There will not be worries and anxieties. The anger and desires are all lessened. Problems are the same for you and me, so yogic practices fix the brain, fix the cells. Here, fixing means disciplining.

If you do *Sālamba Śīrṣāsana* you give proper blood supply to the brain, if you do *Setubandha Sarvāṅgāsana* you give blood supply to the kidneys, if you do *Sālamba Sarvāṅgāsana*[1] you supply blood to the chest, if you do back bends you draw the blood to the entire spinal muscles. Again each and every *āsana* has its own characteristics to give help to the areas such as mind and intelligence that even the present medical science has not penetrated. So you have to remove the doubt from your head about whether yoga fits in or not with you being a Westerner.

You all suffer from physical problems and emotional problems. Practice of yoga brings cleanliness in the nerves. So the nerves can scan the load of the speedy western life. Life is speedy there; therefore there is strain. As there is strain, toxins form in the system. So please do not use such words as East or West, but ask, as human being, as a man, how yoga could fit into a way of living which is highly artificial today? Yoga is the natural means to maintain health. Any age group can adopt it. Can you buy health in the market? How long can you buy medicines to buy health? Is it a real health? Yoga gives positive health. It gives physical, emotional and intellectual health, whereas the present medicines help to keep life going. Hence I say yoga is the only home-made medicine to keep oneself healthy and happy. You know, if the house is clean, tidy, you love it. If it is dark and dusty, would you like to stay?

– No. –

So what is the house for your core of being? The body is the house of your core of being. Is it not the duty of each person to see that the house in which the being dwells is kept tidy, airy and healthy? Yoga is the only subject which keeps the abode of the soul, the temple of the soul, the house of the soul, healthy, whether you are in the East or the West, North or South.

That inner sanctity which comes in *āsana* does not vanish. Sanctity means holiness, purity. The clean body is the holiness of the body. The soul dwells in the holy place. Yoga is for each and everybody, without distinction of place or class, without division.

Now, whether one is an Easterner or a Westerner, he has to follow the ethical and moral disciplines of yoga. Spirituality and morality go together. Therefore, Patañjali while speaking about *yama* and *niyama* says that they being universal law have to be followed by one and all. No religion has omitted moral principles. No human being can deny the importance of moral health. As far as the esoterics of yoga are concerned, it totally depends upon the individual to see how to bring the spiritual progress in oneself. No one is denied Self-realisation or God-realisation. No one is denied devotion and knowledge. So the question is not at all where you are born on the earth. The question is of your total approach and involvement. Be devoted, know the subject and practise thoroughly.

---

[1] See plate n. 30

Q.- May we request you to give some advice for the yoga practitioners of the West?

See, again you are using the word West! *(Laughter).* Don't use the word "West". Yoga, as I said, is a cleansing process. You have a house. You buy a house. Why do you paint it every two or three years? Tell me.

– *Because it will be more beautiful and better protected.* –

So the building is protected. You've paid so much attention, every three years you get your house painted outside and inside so that it shines, it may not crack, it may not leak, it may stand for several years. So also practise yoga, to keep not only your body but also your mind, senses, intelligence and emotions clean, untainted, spotless and pure so that the soul shines from within.

– *Thank you very, very much.* –

EXCHANGE OF IDEAS BETWEEN MR. IYENGAR AND SWAMI RADHA*

Swami Radha: What is the procedure in order to practise *haṭha yoga*?

Mr. Iyengar: *Haṭha yoga* starts from the body and goes directly disclosing, from the body to the breath, from the breath to the mind, from the mind to intelligence, from the intelligence to the self and from the self towards the soul one after the other.

Swami Radha: It is similar to when we look at a picture. At first we may not be able to see everything at once, so we begin by looking at one area and then at another. Finally, we can see the whole picture.

Mr. Iyengar: Yes, then we experience in totality with complete alertness. For example, the body for me is the gross soul. So how can the envelope be separated from the content?

Swami Radha: Right. Duality is the creation of the mind.

Mr. Iyengar: No one can demarcate where the body ends and the mind begins, where the mind ends and the soul begins. These terms are all for the sake of convenience, when it is explained that one is the gross body, one is the subtle body, and one is the causal body. We express it as *sthūla, sūkṣma* and *kāraṇa śarīra*. Patañjali explains using this in different terminologies. He calls it *viśeṣa, aviśeṣa, liṅgamātra* and *aliṅga*.[1] The soul is encased in them. The body can be perceived, therefore it is distinguishable. The mind, I-consciousness are nondistinguishable therefore have to be conceived; whereas intelligence is differentiable from the soul. Therefore as our existence is expressed from gross to subtle, for the sake of convenience we express it as body, mind and soul.

---

* Victoria Yoga Centre, June 1992.

[1] See the author's *Light on the Yoga Sūtras of Patañjali, sūtra* II.19, and *Aṣṭadaḷa Yogamālā*, vol. 2, p. 202.

Swami Radha: For the sake of communication...

Yes, purely for the sake of communication. The body is expressed as having five sheaths of the body. We have the anatomical body called *annamaya kośa*, the physiological body - *prāṇamaya kośa*, the mental body - *manomaya kośa*, the intellectual body - *vijñānamaya kośa*, and the abode of the soul - *ānandamaya kośa*. *Ānanda* here means eternal bliss and not mere happiness or enjoyment. There is no *ānanda* for the mind; only pleasure of enjoyment. *Ānanda* is for the soul, which is the eternal unmixed and untainted, which never fades. That *ānanda* is pure *ānanda*.

The practice of *āsana* is not merely doing or being in *āsana*. Each *āsana* is done in such a way that you communicate the body to mind and mind to soul. Sometimes the body is the subject and self is the object and sometimes the self is the subject and the body is the object. While teaching my approach is different as I have to transfer my experience through expression to the pupil. Hence I have to teach and bring the understanding in my pupils so that they do not experience duality or demarcation.

For me, each cell is a self. The body is a God-given gift. The cells of the body might be dying every moment but if the cells die new cells arrive. Then who brings new life into the cells? The new life comes in cells because they are connected to the Self. The energy of *ātman* - *ātmaśakti* - flows in those cells. In order to fully understand what health means one has to understand this *ātmaśakti*. This is my way of teaching, and that is how I work. The cells are new, second to second. They are born, they die; and if we don't do the *sādhanā* for even one day, we don't make use of the cells fully. We are then creating artificial or induced death in the cells. Why should we not create natural death in the cells by making use of them before they die? Why not leave good *saṁskāra*, good imprints on them? Let the cell die with good and auspicious *saṁskāra*. Here come the *āsana* and *prāṇāyāma* to rescue the cells. Through the practice of *āsana* and *prāṇāyāma* each cell is made full use of. This way, we live totally in the cells, we live totally in our body, mind and self without difference in body, mind and self.

The river of energy *(prāṇa)* and the river of consciousness *(citta)* have to flow together in the river of tranquillity - *praśānta nāḍī*. These are my words. *(Laughs)*. Patañjali puts the same idea in different way while the content remains the same. He says that the restraint of rising impressions brings about an undisturbed flow of tranquillity (*Y.S.*, III.10). Again, Patañjali at another place says, "By the practice of yoga the impurities of the body and mind are destroyed". Tell me, how can this happen? He uses the word *aśuddhi kṣaya*. He further emphasises that even if you reach the state of *samādhi*,[1] the *sādhanā* has to be continued daily, otherwise the tranquil state becomes very shaky. There are nine types of obstacles that come in the way of progress, and the

---

[1] *Samādhi* is the state in which the aspirant is one with the object of meditation, the Supreme Soul pervading the Universe, where there is a feeling of unutterable joy and peace.

last one is *anavasthitatva* – inability to maintain the achieved progress. After reaching the state of *samādhi*, the practitioner may take pride in his success and achievement which may cause instability thinking that practice is not necessary after reaching the state of *samādhi*. This brings about a downfall in the *yogi*. Therefore, one must remember that if one stops the *sādhanā*, the downfall is certain.

I am sure that today we have lost a great deal by neglecting the concerns of the body which becomes *atapas*. If we get just a glimpse of higher states such as *samādhi*, it does not mean that we have to neglect or forget the earlier aspects, which have taken us to these higher states. The *anavasthitatva* happens because of our callousness and negligence. Communion between body, consciousness and self gets lost. The fragrance of the flower is only there if the plant is healthy. The quality of the fruit depends upon the health of the tree. The spiritual end of a small plant is in the tasty fruit. So, in order to maintain that fragrance, that flavour, we have to maintain and sustain our practice of yoga regularly. If there is no fragrance or flavour, what is the use of that life? I may be able to talk philosophically but what is my inner condition! Does it not remain in a conflict? How do I feel inside? How does my consciousness react? A talk or lecture on philosophy is something that comes from the brain. It is easy to advise *(upadeśa)* without a practical base. It is difficult to be in *upāsanā*. *Upadeśa* is merely an advice whereas *upāsanā* is an actual practice with dedication.

Here, I would like to mention that *upāsanā* is of two types – egoistic *upāsanā* and devotional *upāsanā*. Both need dedication. If one is egoistic dedicational practice, the other is divine dedicated practice. One who does *upāsanā* with devotion, his advice comes from the heart and he does not demarcate between the body, mind and soul.

Swami Radha: Under the name of spirituality one cannot neglect the body .....

Yes! We are not supposed to neglect or deny it. The body is not something separated from our mind and soul. The practice of yoga is meant to live spiritually using the various sheaths of the soul divinely and at the same time to die with a natural majestic death. And if we don't practise, if we don't care for the cells, we kill the cells artificially before they die naturally, and life fades away without our making use of it.

It is unethical for a person who is doing his *sādhanā* to miss it even for a single day. If I do not do my *sādhanā* today, I am definitely unethical within myself. If you take the stories of Vaśiṣtha and Viśvāmitra, the celebrated Vedic sages, two of the seven great *ṛṣi*,[1] showed no negligence

[1] The *Saptarṣi* or Seven Hermits appear anew in each age of Manu; the *Saptarṣi* of the present age, Marīci, Aṅgiras, Atri, Pulyastya, Vasiṣṭha, Pulaha and Kratu, are the mental sons of Brahma. The *Saptarṣi* of the current age are placed as the seven stars of the Great Bear constellation.

to their bodies. Their health was in the highest state; at the same time they knew that the body is a vehicle, which is essential to carry on the *sādhanā, tapas* or *upāsanā*. Even Patañjali warns that one should not end up as *videhin* or *prakṛtilayin*.[1] According to the *Kaṭhopaniṣad*, the body is the chariot, which must not be neglected. A charioteer requires a good chariot. But today what has happened? The charioteer is there, but there is no chariot! Both the chariot (body) and the charioteer (Self) have to go together. A musician can express through an instrument. A yogi has nothing through which to express except his own instrument – the body. So whether it is the yogi as an artist, the yogi as a scientist, the yogi as a philosopher, he always expresses through his body, senses and intelligence.

Swami Sivananda: Didn't you have some disability when you were seventeen or eighteen?

I suffered from tuberculosis in my childhood. At that time there was no streptomycin, or penicillin or any medicine as such. In fact, there was no treatment. So I said to myself, "If one has to die, what difference does it make anyway. It is all the same whether I live or die. At least let me die peacefully, that is all I asked. If my health does not improve, at least I will be able to say that I die doing yoga. Beyond that, nothing mattered. Death has to come, does it not? That is certain. So let it come in a noble way." That is all I thought – and I have not left my *sādhanā*. Even now I am a very rigorous and vigorous practitioner.

Swami Radha: Oh, I can see that! *(Laughter).*

People say that one cannot see the infinite through the finite. But show me one man who has seen the infinite without finite means. Each and every person has used finite means to reach the infinite. When the finite submerges in the infinite, everything is infinite. We are beings in which the finite also becomes a part of the infinite. So that is why I am practising yoga hours together even today.

Swami Radha: The practice rejuvenates you?

Yes, of course it is tremendously rejuvenating. Apart from that it is for me an inner discipline. It is a *tapas* for me, so that the mind gravitates towards the soul.

---

[1] *Videhin* and *prakṛtilayin*. See the author's *Light on the Yoga Sūtras of Patañjali*, I.19 Harper Collins, London.

Student: Did you say you did ten hours of practice a day?

Yes, when I was young I practised hours together. Then it was a forced discipline, as I had to struggle to master this art! Now it is a natural discipline. I can't call it a discipline any more, because it has become an inner passion. In the past, who knows, I might have turned my back on it having TB. So my motive was, "Let me conquer, let me conquer." And to be frank with you, even today, when the doctors examine my ribs, they say that my ribs are as tender as a boy of twenty years. They say, "You must have suffered from TB," and tell me that according to their findings, these ribs cannot carry this body at all. Yet I am carrying it.....

Swami Radha: Yes, you do very well! *(Laughter).* For me, coming from the West...

But I appreciated you, because you were very sincere, honest in your ethics, telling people to be ethical!

Swami Radha: Build character first.

Because ethics is one wing and spirituality is the other wing. The bird can fly only with two wings, not with one wing. So one wing of the human being is ethics, the other wing is the spiritual life. If they go together, the seeker can definitely fly and reach the spiritual height of the Everest. Not otherwise.

Swami Radha: And discipline......

Yes! Discipline is a part of morality. My discipline is not mere strictness as you hear from people. When I am conducting classes, sometimes I am very strong and demanding. Some pupils do ask me, "Why are you so demanding?" I answer, "I am demanding because I do not want to withhold knowledge from you but transmit so that I can die in peace."

Knowing the art, if I do not teach what I have experienced, I will be questioned there in the heaven and not here on the earth. If I had a limited understanding of this art, it would have been a different thing. The innocence can be pardoned, ignorance is bliss sometimes. But unfortunately, God has made me to know so much in this art, that if I can't share it with the pupils or the diseased ones, it would be unethical on my part. As a yoga student, when I know that I can help diseased persons and others, I should do so. Otherwise I will die with unhappiness.

Now see that girl. *(Mr. Iyengar points to a student with a "bamboo" or fused spine, who has been developing flexibility in her back through his guidance).* I helped her and she is improving. I would have been very unhappy and my conscience would have pricked if I had not helped her. Why should I not help when I knew that it could be corrected and worked out? I took the risk to work her hard with strictness and it has helped her.

Swami Radha: But the secret is also your motivation.

That is there.

Swami Radha: That is why you can take the risk.

I have tremendous confidence also.

Swami Radha: Motivation.

Not only motivation but also faith and confidence.

Swami Radha: Yes! How long have you known Gurudev Shivananda – my *guru*?

Oh, since 1937. *(Laughs).*

Swami Radha: Ah, just when you started your practice.

No, after three and half years of practice.

Swami Radha: How did you meet him?

Well, we were always corresponding, because I was having lots of problems when I started practising. I used to approach not only my *guru*, but all yogis, whoever they were. I said, "I am having this trouble, I am having that problem with my practice. Can you help me?" But the guidance I received was not sufficient. They would say, "Rest if so and so problems are happening." The answers were negative rather than constructive. So I used to question them, "Why do you say don't do it? Have you done it, have you suffered with the same problem? If you have suffered, then tell me what was the remedy." I used to write to them and say, "Come what may, I am not going to stop my practice unless I know why the problem happens." This way I fought with them throughout! I said, "Give me the right guidance but don't say don't do it; tell me instead, by doing it what are the things that will happen? How did you experience these things?" That is how the dialogue used to go *(Laughs)*..... Later, in 1950, I met Swami Shivananda in Pune and showed him an album with my *āsana* practices. He looked with keen interest and said to me, "You are Matsyendranāth!"

Swami Radha: Why did he call you that?

Because he looked at my *āsana* in the album and said, "This I can do. This my pupils can do – oh, this one!" Only the advanced *āsana* impressed him so much and he called me Matsyendranāth.

Swami Radha: What does that name mean?

Matsyendranāth was the founder of *haṭha yoga*. Let me tell you the story. Pārvati, Shiva's consort, wanted to know from Him about yoga. So, Lord Shiva said "I will explain it to you, but we must go where no human beings exist." As both of them were moving, Lord Shiva saw a beautiful lake and said, "Let us sit here, because the weather is very good, and the lake is calm, with no movement at all." Lord Shiva started explaining to Pārvati about this art of yoga. There was a fish in the water, which listened to their dialogue so intently that it did not disturb the water at all. After some time, when the discussion came to an end, Lord Shiva saw something moving. He said, "What is this? When we looked, there were no movements at all. And now there is a movement." And he looked into the water and saw the fish. He blessed the fish, and the fish got transformed into a human form called Matsyendranāth, the King of the Fishes. *Matsya* means fish.

So Swami Shivananda used to call me by that name, and tell me I was the modern day Matsyendranāth. In fact, he insisted that I should join his *āśrama*. He said to me that he would give me *sannyāsa*.[1] I point-blank refused and said, "I want to be a married man. If I want to take *sannyāsa* (a *swāmi*), I will come. I'm not interested at present in becoming a *sannyāsi*."

---

[1] *Sannyāsa* = renunciation of all worldly possessions and earthly affections.
Sannyāsi = a renunciate, *Swāmi* = the title with which the renunciate monks are called.

Swami Radha : Why did you want to become a married man?

Because the common people had this notion that only *swāmijīs* can do yoga, only *sannyāsīs* can do yoga. It was the belief that yoga is done only by renunciates.

Swami Radha : Oh, I didn't know that....

Yes, I am speaking of the 1930's, when yoga was unknown even in India. So people thought that either a *sannyāsi* or those who are a bit mad or fanatic, practise yoga. At that time we had to struggle to establish yoga. Even today, many think that those who are dejected or rejected by society do yoga. Or those who must have been completely disappointed in their lives and lost interest in everything take to yoga.

If I had become a *swāmi*, then people would have said, "Of course he can do it because he has nothing else to do. But living in the turmoil of day to day, can he practise yoga?" I proved that one could practise living in this turmoil. I can live in the world and practise. Also I can practise living in *āśrama* where the Ganges is running. I practise in the city, in the world, meeting all the ups and downs in life. So when Swāmiji asked me about *sannyās*, I said, "No, I will do it facing the ups and downs in the life. I don't want that security, the quiet life." So I refused to take *sannyās*. And now I am a *sannyāsi*, because my wife is gone. So God has given me *sannyās* without even asking for it!

Student : Weren't you worried your attention would be between two things, your home and yoga?

No, I chose to prove whether a man in turmoil could do yoga. If I had been a *sannyāsi*, everyone would have said, "What is there? What problems has he got in life? So he can practise." But I live amongst the people and my practice is still on top. Not one has done the way I practised. That is why I say to those who come to me, "Show your practice. If you do better than me, I respect you and love to become a *śiṣya* again. I prefer to see the practical aspect, so that I can gauge and compare my standard of *sādhanā* with those practices."

Swami Radha: No, wait a minute! You had . . . . . .

That will power!

Swami Radha: You had to make money to feed your family, you had to give time to your wife, and you had to give time to your children.

Yes, and I still had to practise.

Swami Radha: Right. How many hours did you sleep? Four?

You ask my children and they will tell you. Did I not maintain the whole family? Did I not look after everything? Did I stop my practice for even one day, you can ask them that too! *(Laughs).* I maintained everything. That is why I said I am a responsible person. I can explain this to any one who is married and practising yoga.

Geeta Iyengar (Mr. Iyengar's daughter, one of the main teachers at the Institute): That is very important, because there are some people who call themselves spiritual, and who are married and neglect the whole family. I mean financially also. The family is not properly looked after, and you find the family members suffering in such a house. But this didn't happen in my father's case. It has happened in many a case, when the man has left to become a *swāmi* or a *sannyāsi*; the whole family has been left to suffer, without money, without food.

Mr. Iyengar: Even as Gurudev Swāmi Śivānanda says that we should have the blessings of the *gurus*, why should I not have the blessings of my children?

Swami Radha: So you don't feel you have missed anything?

No. Neither I have not missed anything nor attention on my children. Why should my children say, "On account of my father, see my fate?" They can say this now, for I have given them all.

Geeta Iyengar: But this has not happened to other families, with the man going off to become a *sannyāsi* and the family suffering on the other side.

Swami Radha: Yes, I have met one in Shivananda Āśrama in 1958, when I returned for four months. There was a young man teaching us *haṭha yoga* and he told us that his father had been a yogi, and had left his mother, himself and two other children, to the mercy of the rest of the family. And then one day, when the young man was twenty-one or so, his father told him, "Come, I want you to witness something so you will understand what I have been doing". The father said that he was now going to consciously enter *mahāsamādhi* – the final stage of *samādhi*, or divine union, where the life force is withdrawn, because he had no more desires. The young man sat there watching his father seated in the meditation posture. Time passed, and more time, and more time, until finally the son touched him to tell him, "Well, this is enough now, why should I sit here and watch you?" The body fell over. His father was dead. And now he, the son, having witnessed this, was so impressed, even though he had gone through so much suffering as a child, that he left his wife and two little daughters and went to pursue yoga. I think that this was the reason his father had wanted his son to witness the *mahāsamādhi*. I asked him, "How much time do you spend to look after yourself? That time you can also give it to your family!" There was also some discrepancy.

That is why my life is a balanced life, because I have seen everything in life. *(Laughs).*

Swami Radha: I have not been able to understand how you can achieve the Highest at the cost and tears of someone else.

Yes. Then that is not liberation. That is not proper at all! And the episode that you narrated just now is not making any sense to me. The one who said that he is going to *mahāsamādhi* found dead. And tell me, what kind of attachment was that when he called his son to witness his achievement? So, I do not call it liberation. One need not invite the public to see one going into *mahāsamādhi*.

Swami Radha: Right! *(to the other students in the group)* I'm glad that you hear that! I met another Indian somewhere around Rishikesh, who said to me, "I am a full-blown *brahmacāri* (celibate)!" I asked him what he meant. Well, with the help of his *guru* they had purchased a little village girl of fifteen or sixteen. He described it as

simiiar as being in a room where food is being stored. If you eat all the food until you almost burst, you don't want any food, you don't even want to see it anymore. And here the same principle was applied to sexual indulgence – if you have had all the sexual pleasures, you have had enough. I said, "But the body digests the food and you get hungry again. The sexual desire will also return again. You are not logical – and what happens to the girl? Now she will not be able to marry. If she becomes pregnant what happens?" "Oh, she can put the baby in the hills, and wild beasts will eat it." Do you call that spiritual?

Students: No, no.

Swami Radha : Oh no, no, no. She can drown herself in the Ganges, because nobody will want her, or she can become a prostitute.

We have spoken earlier of ideals. We have to have ideals as teachers. If we have no ideals, we should not even speak on the subject of yoga.

Now this controversy has been going on between my pupils and myself recently. Your ideas about ethical life in America are quite different from those of ours. Your way of living and our way of living are quite different. I never say that the West should be like India. In India marriages only take place with family consent. The bride and groom do not meet before the marriage. In your country there is contractual living together, which is part of your ethics. I'm not objecting to that at all. I do agree because according to your ideas the man has to understand the woman, the woman has to understand the man, so after two or three years they should marry. Up to this point it is fine. But how is this possible that, in the daytime they are students, in the night they are sharers of the bed. I said, "That is not ethics. You cannot do that or you must marry." You see what is going now? I said, "No, I will not encourage such things in my life."

Student: That's just what *Matājī* says!

Swami Radha: *(Laughing)* I don't care how old you are, you cannot stay in the *āśram* in the same room if you are not married.

You are absolutely right. This is the only way we can teach. In the olden days, even in the western countries, they were behaving like that. There was some code of conduct. But all of a sudden it has taken a change, it has become a pleasure: everything is a pleasure – then yoga is a pleasure. Then why call it yoga? There is a word *bhoga* for pleasure. Yoga is an auspicious thing. Even if you want to have *bhoga*, I say, "Marry and enjoy!"

Swami Radha: There it is, the same.

I am not saying, "Don't marry at all." I am not a fool to say, "Don't marry," because as my daughter said, if you are wanting it in your head, it is better to be mentally pure, too.

Swami Radha: Yes, I often have given you as an example to me. "But look, Mr. Iyengar is married." I said, "I have heard Mr. Iyengar has been a widower for a number of years. So if he only married for the sake of sexual pleasure, I'm sure he would have found a second or third wife. But he didn't."

That is true. I always give many examples to my Indian students who go to America. I say, "In the West, if you have got an art, it does not matter whether you are ugly or handsome." You know, there were lots of people who fell in love when I went to England for the first time in 1954, I was in the prime of my youth. Yet even today I fold hands (*namaste*). I have spoken to *swāmijīs* who travel in the West, and asked, "Why do you kiss women? It is not good for you to do that as *swāmi*." They say, "No, we consider everyone as children." But my question to them is, "how do you know the way in which a person will respond?" Secondly, how even *swāmijīs* consider themselves pure? They need to ask their conscience.

Swami Radha: Right, I agree. I get my own viewpoints very well confirmed, thank you for that! I have to struggle sometimes with it.

But even now I am struggling still with all these people! It is difficult to convince people since they get carried away with such behaviour. They think that they are blessed by such *swāmijīs*. Some foreigners come and say, "Just see the magnetism of this other leader, and how many people he can attract!" I say, "Don't you know I have the magnetism which keeps you far away from me? *(General laughter)*. You cannot come near me! Why are you afraid of me the moment you come near? Why are the people afraid of me if I just walk by them? That is my magnetism. *(Laughs).* When I teach in the class I attract their attention more towards the subject of yoga. I teach the subject in such a way that they attentively listen and practice. For me the subject is more important than me as a person. I make them do intensely and bring their minds on to the subject, so that they forget the surrounding colleagues and make them watch their own inner mind.

Swami Radha : Do you treat women differently than men?

Why should I, tell me! If the soul has gender, then I may have to tell differently. If there is a feminine soul and a masculine soul, then I will say what the difference is. Whether you are a woman or a man, the emotional feelings are the same. Are not they? So I do not treat differently as I do not feel them differently.

Swami Radha: I do think that a man has more physical strength and a woman has a little more endurance.

Yes, I do agree with that. It is a different matter. But coming to the subject of yoga, *sādhanā* is important and not the *sādhaka.*

Swami Radha : But that is all. Right?

Yes! But, that is all. It should not make much difference as far as the subject yoga is concerned.

Swami Radha: Years ago I asked Swami Venkateśānanda who he considered to be the finest *haṭha yoga* teacher, and he said, "Well, I think Iyengar is the best." So I got a copy of your book *Light on Yoga* and as I held it in my hands for a while, I felt a great sense of peace. I often go with a feeling like this, so I said to myself, "I will open the book at random, and in the first three lines on the top of the right hand side of the page I open the book and there was something which confirms my feelings." After I had this sign, I put the book on the list for our students, even before I had read it completely. I based my decision on my own impression, and read it afterwards.

As I said before, I think that in the West you are the only person who has insisted on ethics. Even the Indians don't see this attitude, which hurts me tremendously. Ethics is the base of yogic practices.

Swami Radha : I am presently writing a book on yoga from the psychological viewpoint. In your book you had a small paragraph in the introduction: "We must see that we live in the world with many other creatures." That sentence gave me, finally, the clue. I have always been interested in symbolism, I would sit by my lily pool and watch the goldfish, and reflect on what it means to be a fish in the water. I searched for information on all the various animals and other life forms for which the *āsana* are named, even when I felt I knew the meaning from my own practice.

I came across many delightful legends and stories, such as the conversations of the king Milinda and the Sage Nagāsena about the tortoise, one of the animal names used in *haṭha yoga*. Nagāsena tells the king about the five special qualities symbolised by the tortoise. For example, when there is danger and temptation, the aspirant should dive to the bottom of deep meditation and hide himself until the temptation is over. He should protect himself by drawing in his senses as the tortoise draws in its limbs for protection. These symbolic stories are easily understood by Westerners, so I have searched for anything I could find.

I also used the same technique I used in the *kuṇḍalinī* book *(Kuṇḍalinī : Yoga for the West)* of asking people to write on a paper to clarify their thoughts. What does the fish mean to you? What does the tortoise mean to you? What does it mean to stand on your head?

During the last three weeks I was at the *āśram* in Rishikesh, Gurudev Shivananda said, "Now that you have seen some of the *āsana*, show me six of them." I showed him what I had been practising, and he said, "Now, what is the psychological meaning?" I was stunned. I hadn't even heard about this. So I started to think about it, and said, "If I can twist my body in so many ways, my mind can certainly twist in as many ways." So one thing followed another, and he said, "Now, what would be the mystical aspect?" I didn't even know where to look! So I went to the *swami* who was teaching *haṭha yoga*, and he said, "What are you talking about?" I went to another one who said, "I am only devotional, I don't do *haṭha yoga* anymore." So I went back to Gurudev and I said, "You have to give me one example so I know where to search." And he gave me the example of the mystical meaning of standing on the head, and that put the whole thing together: learning to become my own opponent, and looking at things from the opposite

end; but also the insight of what is termed "nectar and ambrosia". Now I help people to discover the psychological message: "If you can't do the *āsana*, what is the reason? Are you stiff-necked?"

First of all, as the practitioner of yoga we should know that though the *āsana* is performed by the body, its boundary is not the body but beyond it. The body is merely an instrument for the practice of *āsana*.

Suppose you are doing *Ūrdhva Hastāsana*, you stretch your arms and fingers. When you stretch your arms mechanically as physical action, you do not witness the arms totally or all the fingers or the disturbance that takes place in the legs. You just lift your arms over the head and get carried away. Your legs do not remain steady, your mind does not reach the stretched arms. When you become totally aware of the arms, the intelligence too has to reach there as it is the connecting link between you and your arms. When you stretch, the intelligence also has to take the shape of the arms. Suppose you have stretched your fingers, you stretch them only longitudinally. When I stretch, I see whether my awareness is touching the inner and outer edges of the fingers evenly. I see whether with my extension and expansion of the fingers on the back, the front and sides, I become aware of my fingers totally. This way, I not only send a psychological message but also a mystical or spiritual message to the entire body while doing *Ūrdhva Hastāsana*.

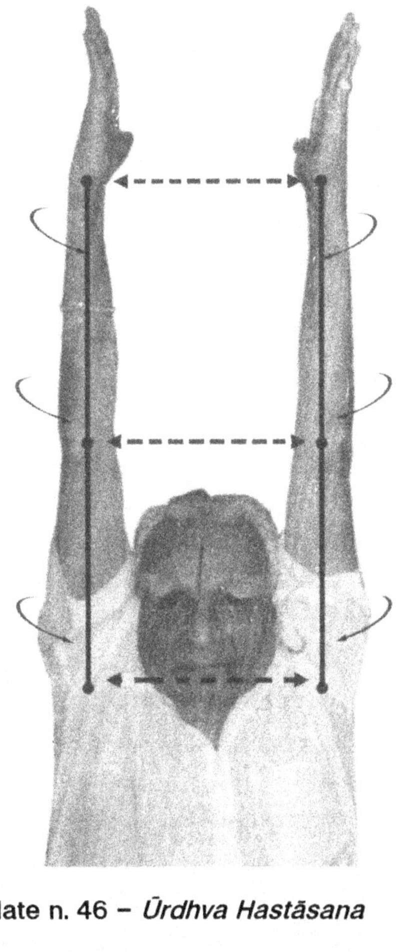

Plate n. 46 – *Ūrdhva Hastāsana*

While doing the *āsana* we need to build up consciously an intellectual layer, which has to run parallel to the physical body. I see while stretching my arms whether the layer of the skin, arm, is surrounded by intelligence or not and touch the arms with intelligence. While doing *āsana* I create eyes everywhere to witness my movements, actions, adjustments and feel my presence everywhere. Then do you consider this awareness physical or beyond it? We know the feel of touch. In yogic practice we develop the feel of touch from outside in. For example, in *Ūrdhva Hastāsana*, I touch my arms everywhere evenly not only from outside but inside as well.

Similarly, when I am teaching the *āsana* I say, "The feeling in upper arm, the feeling in lower arm, the feeling in the inner and outer arm should be the same." At the same time, I see that they keep the feel of touch evenly in the legs also. We have eight directions: North, East, West and South as well as Northeast, Northwest, Southeast and Southwest. We also have top and bottom. So in our body, we have ten directions as God has created. When we do each *āsana* we have to penetrate all these ten directions, then a unity is built up within. Then your body, mind and intelligence penetrate everywhere evenly.

Swami Radha: I'm glad we have that on tape! *(Laughter)*

This is how the *āsana* have to be done. I tell my students in the classes, "People say to concentrate on a lamp, to gaze at it, and call that spiritual practice. I say, Look at your toe. Why do you make your right toe longer and big and your left toe small?" This way I build up intelligence in them. But intelligence does not come by looking at a lamp. It may strain the eyes without bringing positive results. There is a torch of intelligence within you. Each *āsana* has to be done in such a way that the torch of intelligence within is switched on, and use that light while performing the *āsana*. Just by standing on head the mystical aspects do not come. When you rest on the crown of your head, do you know what the crown of the head is? Often while doing *Śīrṣāsana* resting on the head, people are aware only of the front part of the head and the balance of the body and not of the crown of the head and therefore the intellectual awareness touches the frontal body while the back of the body remains in the state of insensitivity. The fear of losing the balance blocks the intelligence. Therefore, one loses the logic of resting the crown of the head to run parallel to the arches of the feet. Now, I should explain to you that the middle of the arch is the crown of the foot. If a line is drawn from the centre of the head to the centre of the foot, these two points should be in a single thread from the head to the arches of the feet. This single connecting thread from the head to the arches of the feet is the intelligence. The two heads – the crown of the head and the middle of the arches of the feet – are like the South pole and the North pole. They have to be evenly balanced in *Śīrṣāsana*. This is the spiritual or mystical root of *Śīrṣāsana*. By this alignment the consciousness cannot waver and it takes the shape of *Śīrṣāsana*. Many people, when they do *Śīrṣāsana*, don't know where their right leg is, where their left leg is, whether the head is straight or tilted, whether their feet have gone backwards or forwards.

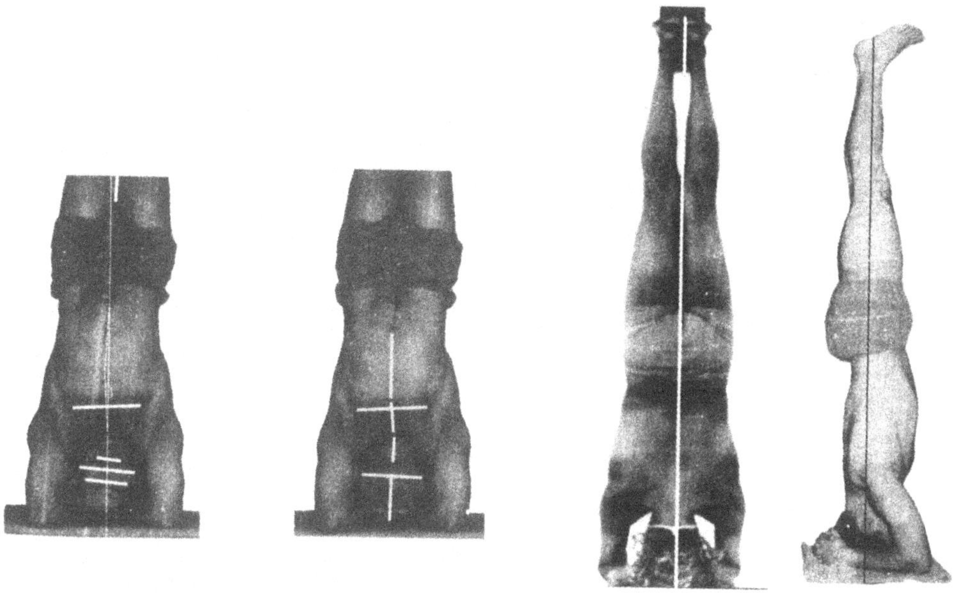

Plate n. 47 – *Śīrṣāsana* non aligned and aligned

If one performs and removes these wavering movements of the body and mind, then it covers the five sheaths of body, senses, mind, intelligence, consciousness and the *puruṣa* (Self).

Swami Radha: No, they only find out, "I can stand on my head for three minutes, or half an hour." That is what is important to them – competition. "I can stand longer than you can." Do you sometimes read the reports about the results of new scientific experiments?

I don't have time to read. I consider myself lucky if I find half an hour in a day to read. Even after the hard work in running the classes my mind still goes on working, "What can I do to help that student? " I am essentially a practical man who believes in practice rather than a 'theoretical' man.

Swami Radha : I am asking you this because many people feel that the ancient teachings are contradicted by the new scientific findings. Yet if one takes the time to study, one discovers that it is just a reinterpretation, and not necessarily a contradiction at all.

For example, when we talk of nuclear energy, now the theory has a chance to change towards growth. We speak of oxygen going into the lungs. I ask, "What is *prāṇa?"* The atom has now been broken into several particles – neutrons, protons, and electrons. All of them are in our system. All of this nuclear energy is contained in the gross atmospheric air. How is that energy consumed into our system? That is what is known as *prāṇa*, which the early yogis explained to us through the techniques of *prāṇāyāma* so we could understand. To a very great extent we can bring the teachings and modern science together.

Certainly, scientific discoveries have substantiated the ancient wisdom of the yogis and sages and I am sure a day will come to see that old wisdom appearing in new formats.

Swami Radha : But then you must have read about these things! *(Laughs).* Otherwise you couldn't explain that right now.

I do read, but not as one must. But I often think when I am teaching. I don't say that I never read at all, but the opportunity is very rare.

Take the case of *prāṇāyāma* again. You know how a magnet attracts iron filings. Now, we all agree that if we develop a good respiratory system by *prāṇāyāma*, our blood contents are normal or better than normal, which changes the chemical properties of the system. Unfortunately, no proper explanations are given for this. This is where I want the scientific members to discover the reason for change by making use of yoga practitioners like me to investigate.

Just as the magnet has the power to clasp the iron filings, in the *prāṇāyāmic* breathing there is a great receptivity in all the fibres of our lungs. In regular deep breathing there is tension since one just sucks and fills the air into the system. In *prāṇāyāmic* breathing there is no tension. As there is no tension, the fibres go into a receptive state. As they are receptive, the energy that is drawn in goes in all the avenues, right up to the tip of the bronchial. This energy is like the iron filings. Like the magnets hold on to the iron filings, all the cells act as magnets which absorb energy and hold it. Regular deep breathing cannot do this; the energy is discharged immediately. Medical science has still to discover what I am saying. Today they may not even think about that, but in some years' time they may say, "Yes, this is the effect of *prāṇāyāma*." No one who is doing research at present can tell the difference between *prāṇāyāmic* breathing and deep breathing. I say it is the nuclear energy, not oxygen alone that is absorbed through *prāṇāyāma*. And that changes the chemical quality of the blood.

Let's take another example – bone cancer. Blood transfusions are given to the patients, yet they do not know why the bone marrow is not manufacturing enough blood. Why do people get bone cancer? The supply of blood to the bones is not sufficient, which brings about the cancer.

Suppose the muscles and the bones are woven together in all our presentations in the *āsana;* then how can bone cancer occur? The muscle is feeding the bone marrow and the bone marrow not only feeds the muscles but also the bones. This way there is an interchange taking place and bone cancer cannot occur. The transfusions are not necessary.

Yet this type of study is not being done at all. Instead the only thing being studied is: "What is the blood pressure when they are in *Sālamba Śīrṣāsana,* and when they come down from *Sālamba Śīrṣāsana?"* It is just a kindergarten test going on. Who wants to know this? When the doctors study some of my students, they find that after *Sālamba Śīrṣāsana* their blood pressure comes down. In other systems of practice the blood pressure does not lower but on the contrary it shoots up. So instead of studying to find out what is the difference in the way my students and others are performing the *āsana;* when the results are different or opposite, they say that the *āsana* doesn't lower the blood pressure. This is what science has to find out: why there are changes here, and no changes there? Is it on account of the differences in the performance of the *āsana* or what?

Some years ago I sent one of my students to help diabetic patients in one of the hospitals in Mumbai. I gave the list of *āsana* and told him, "Don't tell the patients anything, just make them do the *āsana*." And now they are so improved that they have no food restrictions at all except the amount of calories per day. They can even eat sugar if they want to, provided they do not exceed the correct number of calories. Science must find out why some people have been given so many restrictions on how they should live, and others in the same conditions have not been given any restrictions but asked to practise yoga instead, and its effect is the same.

"Let the cell do its job fully and satisfactorily before it dies!" This is what the practice of *āsana* teaches us. I have told the doctors very often but they don't understand. They can't even think!

Swami Radha : But then why is it that some of the yogis that I have met in the Himalayas did not get well in spite of their practice of *āsana*?

The reason is that they don't know how to perform and how to attend to the various parts simultaneously and how to interpenetrate. These things are not observed and followed in their practices.

Swami Radha : You think that is the clue.

That is the only clue. For example, if a person is having liver trouble, and you ask him to reach the liver in *Śīrṣāsana*, he cannot, whereas I can work exactly on the liver alone in that *āsana*. I have worked on my own in that way. Now, how do you work the liver? You know how to work the biceps and how to work the triceps. But how do you work the liver? It should expand, it should contract, it should rinse and it should have lateral movements. There are certain adjustments through which you pressurise or depressurise the organic body. We must learn to think organically. Then we can penetrate directly into the organs themselves.

Swami Radha : What is the influence of the mind on the liver?

What can we say? Unless the mind goes there, how can we influence it? So many people do *Śīrṣāsana*; are they aware of their feet? Are they aware how the bottom of the foot is working? They do not penetrate their intelligence at all in any areas when they do *Sālamba Śīrṣāsana*. They stand on their heads without the sense of the feeling. If you ask me, I can tell you what is happening in each and every area of the body when I do *Śīrṣāsana*. A great deal of inner attention is required. It means the mind has to play the major role in activating not only the liver but all the other organs. If not attended one feels heavy and dull in mind.

Student : So in interpenetration, the cells of the muscles, bones and blood all exchange?

Exchange – yes, it is known as the feedback system in the modern terminology. This was known to us in the olden days. You see! The whole body, what we call the physical body or *annamaya kośa*, is penetrated by mind and energy – *manas* and *prāṇa*. So the liver for instance is not only of muscles but it is a vital organ. We can enrich it with *prāṇa* by acting on it properly by extending, contracting, etc. The action cannot happen unless the mind goes there. When we act applying the mind, then the avenue of blood circulation too changes. So do not think that *āsana* is pertaining to only *annamaya kośa*, but there is a great inter-connection between *annamaya kośa*, *manomaya kośa* and *prāṇamaya kośa*.

Swami Radha : When I have met people who do not have this conviction, I have been as honest as I can that *haṭha yoga āsana* can really take care of healing. What I have done is give people a purpose for living. I ask them, "You want your life to be spared, but if you keep on living in the same old way, there is no reason why your life should be spared. In order to live, you must give something back to life, and have a different respect for the gift of life. Do something selflessly." Sometimes I have said, "You tell me you have a garage full of tools. Take the kids off the streets and show them how to do something!"

Yes, constructively using their life! I learnt yoga to gain health but God had his plans and made me take yoga to fellow human beings for the betterment of society, and many of my pupils follow the same.

Swami Radha : Yes, and anyone who could accept that is still alive.

Yes, I know, because when the cells are cultured gradually the mind also becomes healthy. This helps one to approach health from inside and creates zeal in them to help others.

Swami Radha : So you are saying that the diseased part can be approached and developed from opposite ends.

Yes, yes. We have to work and face the diseased part sometimes with friendliness and compassion or with compassion and admonition. Neglecting the afflicted part is not the right approach.

Swami Radha: All right, I understand. Are you developing more *āsana*?

I keep developing this art for the simple reason that if we neglect our *sādhanā*, then the veil covers from inside and shakes the very being. Hence, the practice of *āsana* and *prāṇāyāma* is a must when one has begun. If you take your lamp and cover it with a blanket, the light is restricted in that area. If I don't do the *āsana*, I feel my intelligence getting restricted. It cannot have clarity or go out into the vastness. The intelligence needs to expand. When I refer to intelligence I mean the constant flow of conscious awareness. I cannot stop my practice, because if I don't practise, then I will have to live on yesterday's memory to explain to you. But if I am practising I can give you what I am feeling today, and not of yesterday. The practice awakens the memory and gives a new look to it. Then one needs not look back to the past. Memory belongs to the past whereas today's feel or experience is present, therefore communication would be fresh.

Swami Radha : When you said more practice...

It is not merely more practice, it is the interpenetration of mind and intelligence to steady the inner depth of this mortal body as the inner body is a very mysterious body.

Swami Radha : Another level, no?

There is no other level. There is only one form, one level, you know. There is no physical level, no mental level, and no emotional level; for me everything is one. I have not demarcated the levels. I say instead, "How much can I interpenetrate? Can my intelligence still interpenetrate more than it is interpenetrating now?" I use the word 'interpenetrate', remember that. In my *āsana* practice, my body penetrates externally and my intelligence penetrates internally. I test these two penetrations to remain one from end to end. This is why I want to keep on practising with further intensity so that *prakṛti* reveals itself more and more. Intensity should increase. In the early days, I practised to get maturity and wisdom. Having acquired them, now there is no doubt now. I am practising to study where it would lead me. With this maturity and wisdom, all trials and errors have come to an end and I practise watching for new wisdom and light.

Actually, I practise for the sake of practice alone. The other type of my practice is to find out ways and means for the sake of those who come to us with their problems and seek solutions. I question myself to find ways so that I can help them and bring relief to their problems. I have to re-create their defects in my body, in my mind, to know how to help them in order to relieve their problems.

Swami Radha : But you do not identify with it?

Why should I? If I identify myself with the defects of others, I am lost. First I imitate to identify their weaknesses. I imagine the problem in me and then work on myself to find a solution. Due to my deep discriminative force, I find the answer. In a way I imitate their problems and work with my intelligence and see what changes occur, which gives me clues to handle.

Swami Radha : When you identify with someone else, don't you lose your own identity?

No. I do not lose my identity. As an actor plays different roles, I presume and act. Imitative identity is quite different from factual identity. I act as the father acts and observe as a witness. Here, identifying does not mean I become someone else.

Swami Radha : *(Laughs)* All right, now I understand how you use the word.

I am a witness. I am identifying as a witness.

Swami Radha : *(Laughs)* Good. Many people identify to the point where they cannot help. I knew that wasn't what you meant.

No. I have to identify for myself exactly what is happening. One needs to identify the defects. So I identify and become a witness and an actor at the same time. I am observing and I am acting. *(Chuckles)* So this is another type of practice.

First I always experiment on myself before I tell others. I don't experiment on others. That would be very unfair. If I don't experiment on my own body, and I say to you, "Try this", it is only an inference, not an experience. I have to be sure that what I say works exactly. If it works with me, I know it will have a greater impact on someone, because my body is very sensitive. This is what I mean by practice. But there are no layers in my practice. I never create layers. The moment I create layers I am creating compartments.

Swami Sivananda : You two are so alike. Everybody who has met you told us that the two of you must meet, because you are so similar.

Swami Radha : Well, we did. *(Laughter)* Yes, I understood what you said. But sometimes we need to use such terms for clear communication.

Student : Do you ever work specifically with medical problems?

Yes, on Tuesdays and Wednesdays we take only medical problems. Some genetic problems, children, adults, everybody!

In one of my classes in Mumbai there was a boy who had a bamboo spine or ankylosis of spine and was completely curved. All the doctors had seen him and could do nothing. I worked on him, and now he has improved to such a degree that if you see pictures of him when he started you cannot recognise him. After two years of training with me he went to his doctor who had been treating him for twenty years, and the doctor said, "Where is your brother who had that stoop?" He could not recognise his own patient! My student replied, "I am the same man" and his doctor said, "No, no! How can you become so straight now? This is impossible!"

In my classes I have students with all kinds of problems. Even cancerous students who have been operated on come to the classes, because they have absolutely no energy at all. How much energy I am giving them! My practice has helped with problems in my own case. If you see me working in the classes, I should have varicose veins all over my body.

Swami Radha : Why should you?

Because the people I teach in my classes weigh from 200 to 300 pounds, yet I just throw them like birds, while teaching the *āsana*.[1] *(Laughter)*. It is not a joke! So much strain to lift, so naturally there is a lot of pressure, yet no varicose veins are visible due to my practice.

Sometimes students grip my legs so hard you can see the blood coming out of their grip. In my life I have had to face all these things. Sometimes if I am teaching and I am too strong, women would pinch me with their long trimmed nails, which are poisonous. I show them the marks and say, "Is this the way to treat me? I do it for your good!"

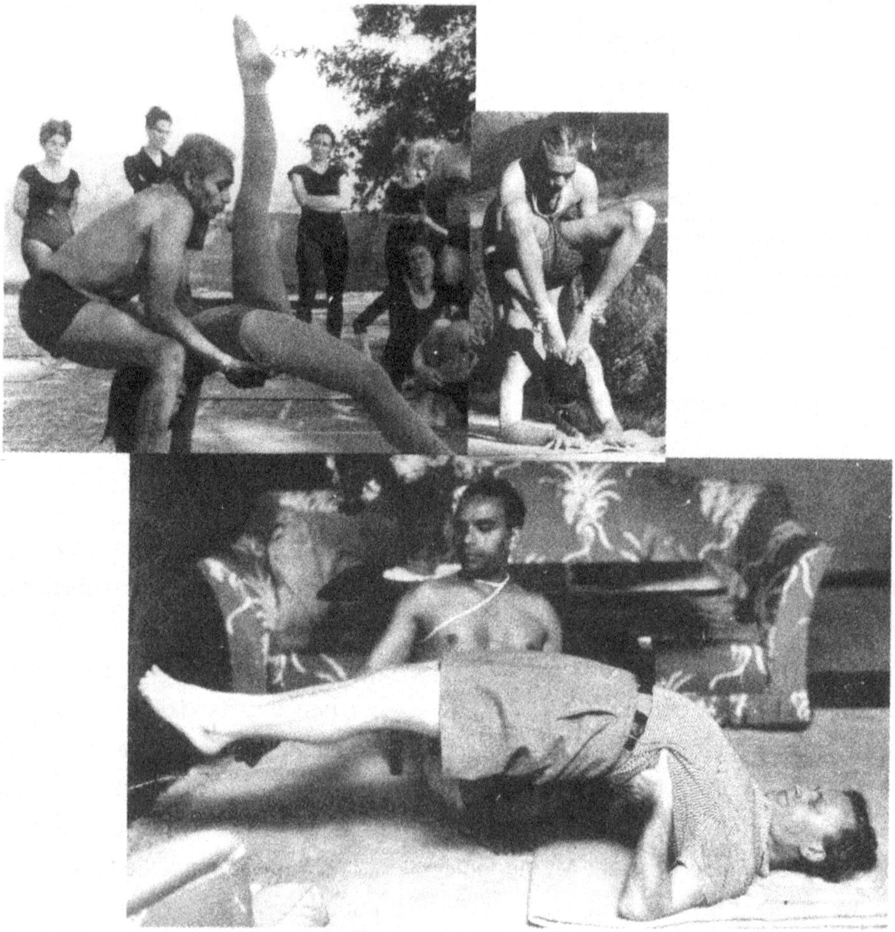

Pl. n. 48 – Lifting the students whilst teaching the *āsana*

Guruji while teaching in the group class used to help all the students whether women, men, heavy, hefty, aged, young, diseased, disabled to do *Viparīta Chakrāsana* and even he used to lift heavy weight people like a flower so that they do not feel their own weight.

Swami Radha : Do they do this because of their fear and anxiety?

There may be a fear. They do not know how to get the balance. Members in the class are many. As I have to move to help all, I cannot patiently wait. Secondly, if I do not handle to the degree that is needed, it becomes ineffective. My way of teaching is special and unique. I pay not only the personal attention but also I see that whatever action, movement and work is expected in that particular *āsana* to be effective, I work to get that effect. Therefore I use my body as a prop for them. To remove this strain on me I do *Śīrṣāsana* and *Sarvāṅgāsana* every day without fail. This is why I have no broken capillaries, no varicose veins. Otherwise I would surely have them by now.

Swami Radha : Do you have any failures, people you can't help?

I am not God. I may fail for the first time, but I use that knowledge as a progressive knowledge. Then, when someone comes with the same identical problems, I give relief where I failed for the first time.

Student : Why are the failures? Are they beyond help, or won't they help themselves?

It is difficult for me to make any general statement. People who have got some troubles will have a negative approach to life throughout. To make them positive takes a long time. Some expect quick results and get disappointed. Some do with fear, or due to the pressure of family members remain non-co-operative. So I do not consider this as a failure. They have no willingness or patience or tolerance to continue.

You see that some cases seem beyond help; it is not true. There are quite a few ascending diseases. In some the basic health itself remains problematic. Some are born with diseases. In such patients if there is a positive approach and willingness, then even if there is not a complete cure they can arrest the disease from ascending. People want to swallow the pills but are not ready to put positive and subjective efforts to improve.

Swami Sivananda : It is the mind, not the body.

You cannot demarcate the body and mind. A patient as a sufferer will not be able to demarcate at all because he or she is in agony.

The fear of nervousness complicates it a little bit more. The mind expresses its fear through the body. You cannot tell the patient that you are treating the mind since the patient is in pain. The negative approach is not expressed only by the mind but by the body also. Hence naturally, we can't just treat the mind alone. We treat the person as a whole. Before we treat the disease, we have to treat the person, which is very difficult. It is not like psychoanalysis where the psychologists ask you what you have suffered from and all. We have to hit the mind directly through the body while teaching. I don't allow anyone to repeat the same complaints over and over again. I tell them that I have heard enough! I start saying, "Now, just do", and I start! *(Laughs).*

Swami Radha : I am speechless...

Yoga can do wonders, definitely! Provided you know each and every fibre of your body – in each *āsana*, how it works. It is tremendous reflection in action. It does not mean quietly sitting in the *āsana*. You have to dynamise inside. Our practice has to be dynamic and reflective. Then only we know how yoga works on our body, mind and intelligence. Later we can decide what to give and what not to give to the pupils and the patients.

Haṭha yoga is a completely revolutionary subject. It revolutionises the practitioner. Probably God made me practise with divine dedication and study hard and made me an instrument for removing the prejudices about this art.

Swami Sivananda : What prejudice?

The prejudice that *haṭha yoga* is only physical and that it has nothing to do with spiritual life. People have equated the practice of *āsana* with physical practice, I have shown the path how to reach through the body, the mind and the soul.[1]

I never go to any seminars or never hold any seminars. I never advertised or indulged in propaganda. Yet I say that I have a good number of sincere followers today and that is enough for me. You will see that all my pupils become very sincere. They are integrated, sincere and whatever little they know, they teach honestly. That is what I have given them. I am happy that I have created a very good purpose in my students. Whether they reach God or not is immaterial; the seed sown in them is very, very good, and so I am very happy. No pupil of mine hides in the art of teaching. That is how I have given. So there is no dissatisfaction for me! *(Laughs).*

---

[1] *Aṣṭadaḷa Yogamālā* vol. 2.

Swami Radha : When people came back from their training here, I asked them, "How was he?" They replied, "He's tough!" I said, "Then he is a good teacher."
One of my students said, "I don't know if I could have taken all this if I had not been to the *āśram*." I understand, because my students tell me that I'm tough. Yoga is very demanding – I demand a lot from people, otherwise it's not worth it.

Yes! I too say to people, "I never invite anyone. When you have come on your own, you have to just obey. There are two ways left to the students. Either they have to learn with me or they have to get out!" There is no middle path for me or for them at all. That is the problem with me. I am merciless to the mind and merciful to the body and soul! *(Great laugh).* That is why people say, "He loses his temper, he gets very angry, he hits!" I say, "Yes, I do so in order to tame the mind."

Student : Mr. Iyengar, you said you are going to stop your classes in 1983?

I am not stopping the classes. I said that I am going to stop the three-week intensive courses, because people exploit these courses, saying, "I have been to the intensive, now I can teach." I have told them from now on that they can come to the general classes or even the beginners' classes, in order to see that they are unfit to be even in the beginners' classes. That is how I want to teach them so that the pride vanishes and humbleness comes. That is the only way to teach humility, there is no other way. *(Chuckles)*

The local people from Pune in the morning classes today also said, "*Gurujī* is very tough!" I said, "Where am I tough? I am laughing and talking, where is the toughness? When I can do it, why can't you?" So I follow them, I make them do yoga with me, so that I can ignite inspiration in them. I never sit on a platform with special dress of a Guru. I wear my yoga dress. If I am there I am there totally so I create interest. I tell them, "No *guru* is coming next to you to do yoga. I am the only one who does practice next to the pupils." Twenty times I may show each *āsana* to twenty people, standing next to them, so that they can learn and can compare to find out what they are lacking. I say, "See my alignment, see your alignment. Where is your head and where is mine? How is your hand and how is mine? Where is my leg, where is my chest? How much have I lifted? So when I can do it, why can't you learn?" But I don't say, "Do it this way. It's all right for today. Tomorrow you will get more." Tomorrow will never come, who knows? I may not be here tomorrow, so why should I wait for tomorrow? *(Laughs).* So I pour out encouragement, which appears tough.

Swami Radha : Yes, you have strong principles indeed! Do you make any discrimination in regard to realisation between men and women? Indians have sometimes said to me, "You can't do this because you have to be born a man."

No, no! Soul has no difference. It is the mind which differentiates. So do not heed what you hear, as it is not true.

Swami Radha : Why would they say that?

The idea must have spread at a latter period. In the earlier period great women had far more wisdom than men, and they also were the teachers for many, many men, which we cannot forget. The present modern way of talking is quite different. They say that the man has the aggressive power, the will power, and the women are poor in will power. But this is all imaginary, you know. For the honest person, it makes no difference in Self-realisation whether one is a woman or a man.

Moreover whether man or woman, child or old, the principles of *karma* do not differ. Nobody is excused from wrongdoing and everyone has the rights to derive the fruits of right and wrong doings. Yoga is an open path to all to cleanse the body, mind, senses, intelligence, I-ness and consciousness.

Those who differentiate man and woman in the field of art, science and philosophy, for me are ignorant.

SEED OF PRACTICAL YOGA SOWN IN AMERICA*

Q.- Gurujī, tell us about your previous visits to the United States. What were your impressions?

When I first came to the United States in 1956, I came at the invitation of the Harkness Foundation. The heiress of this foundation, Mrs. Harkness, had developed a pit in the stomach and Yehudi Menuhin, who was a friend of hers, recommended my name and she invited me to help her. The inverted poses that I gave her did help and she recovered from her illness. At that time I gave two performances, one in Washington D.C. and one in New York.

However the first experience in the U.S. hurt me because I suffered discrimination because of my colour in the airport of New York. That was a considerable shock for me in a country that spoke of freedom. And at that time, it was next to an impossibility to imprint yoga on the Americans. Their approach on life was different in those days. As they were totally material-minded, I had to teach them only on basic physical levels. They seemed only fond of eating. I had a hard time regarding food as I was a vegetarian and no one knew of vegetarian food. I received many invitations to visit the United States after that, but I felt it was not worth visiting America. I decided to wait to see the life style change to visit America.

Then in 1972, Prof. Palmer from Ann Arbor was invited by the Delhi University as a guest lecturer for a month. As Prof. Palmer and his wife were visiting India, they, being friends of Yehudi Menuhin, enquired of India and of Yoga. They heard of me from Menuhin, and Mary the wife of Prof. Palmer, being a practitioner of yoga, requested her husband to allow her to stay in Pune for three weeks' training under me, while he was lecturing in Delhi. Though she told me that she was teaching yoga at the Ann Arbor 'Y', she was not satisfied with what she had been teaching. After visiting Pune, she realised the value of yoga and got impressed so much with my work that she extended an invitation to me to visit America and teach in Ann Arbor in 1973. I came and still saw some roughness in them, similar to what I saw in 1956.

---

* Interview by Laurie Blakeney, Rose Richardson, Sue Salaniuk and Toni Fuhrman, on 9th July 1992. Published in *Yoga '93*, American Yoga Convention, Ann Arbor, Michigan, 1993.

Some members did not like my way of teaching as they thought that I should not command and demand but to be like a lamb. However, when I returned to Ann Arbor in 1976 I was very impressed that people were practising with love, zeal and interest. But even then, because of my experiences in 1956, I wondered if the Americans would stick with it as they were influenced by their wealth and comfort. I had my doubts whether the seed I had planted there would grow. Today, I can say with pride that the Americans have made it a subject of their own. I am very impressed with their progress and discipline. Also health consciousness in general has improved, especially among the young people. In 1956, I saw them always eating on the beach but as time went on, they must have realised the value of life and started searching for natural means to maintain their health, and.they realised that yoga could do this.

After 1976, yoga grew very rapidly in the United States. I never dreamed that thousands would start practising yoga in my lifetime. Even though it took twenty years, I am very happy that the seed, which was planted in 1956, has sprouted at last. In fact, it has grown into a huge tree that not only it engulfed the United States but Canada and other surrounding places as well. It is to the credit of the Americans that yoga has become popular in other areas of the world. I am grateful to the Americans for having proved to be broad-minded towards oriental art, science and philosophy. This Eastern science, this Eastern philosophy has been embraced by Americans. My twenty years' attention and guidance has paid dividends in America at last.

Q.- Do you foresee any changes in how you will guide Americans in the future?

I have a feeling that after this convention the way of life here may change. Through the interest you all showed to become submerged in yoga God graced me tremendous energy to do this yogic service for all. Now the youngsters need a boost to carry on this work. People say, nothing grows under a banyan tree, they think that I am like a banyan tree in yoga. Hence I am handing over the sapling of yoga to the younger generation for it to grow. So I feel that I should be in the background and allow my young pupils to take the foreground, improving and carrying on from where I have left. One thing is certain, I am always ready to come and help whenever I am asked and the initiative should come from you as my pupils. I'll continue to guide and advise but I want youngsters to take the responsibility and grow well.

Secondly, I foresee that my method of yoga practices is sure to become a household product in your country due to the tremendous zeal of today's teachers and students. Now teachers have to learn how to break through and expand to convey the depth of the physical and mental qualities hidden in yoga. Though many students are mild practitioners, the new teachers have to inspire them to develop the intensity. Because of their limitations, they cannot become intense in the subject. Those who want to become intense like to take a high jump quickly in yoga, but such students are in danger of soon dropping out. The mild practitioner though knows that the subject is very difficult and sticks to the practice more than the person who likes to jump very fast. But, whatever development the student has, the teacher has to know his or her physical and mental capacity and work to expand those persons to extend to maximum capacity according to their capabilities. The teachers must learn to bring such students along so that they gradually become more intense. One group has the will to sustain but not the intensity. The other group has the intensity but cannot sustain. The teachers must provide the guidance. This is where I want my teachers to concentrate. Once this problem is attended to, yoga will spread in your country healthily. Otherwise, it will be like all smoke and no fire.

Q.- Can a person's maximum capacity expand?

Maximum for me means to learn to cross the road of the known stretch. It is to try a little more than what is possible so that one learns to cross towards the unknown mind from the known. Yes it is possible, provided the guidance is given. Some people believe they are born with a potential, which they cannot expand. But that is just a mental block. The teachers have to know how to break their mental blocks and give the potential to move further. Here is where my teachers have to cultivate and understand to guide further. The teachers have to restart to see the root cause of weaknesses and failures in them as well as their students.

Today, I told my students a very good story about a student I had. I saw the kneecap had almost moved away towards the outer side of the leg from its centre position. The student was in agony, I immediately ran from the other end of the institute and adjusted the knee at once to its origional position and the party was relieved of pain. I told the story in my humorous way and said, "When you don't like a person, what do you do? You move your lips to the sides. If you like a person you come close to him. The same is true with your kneecap. As you see your knee is not in contact, it means you don't love it. So you are hating your own knee!" We have to see where the block is and from the intelligence of the body the improvement has to come and not from the head alone. We need to see both from the brain and the brawn to release the blocks which exist in the students, consciously or unconsciously.

Yoga is an evolutionary subject. After the optimum level of evolution takes place, then involution begins in yoga. This is known as *pratyāhāra*, the fifth petal of yoga in *āsana*. The practice of the varieties of *āsana* and *prāṇāyāma* are meant to evolve the consciousness to reach its optimum level. After reaching the optimum level, then it is a question of connecting to the source from where it sprouts to reach the optimum level. The question becomes how do you connect to reach the optimum level? That is the involutionary method, but know that the inward journey too is an evolutionary method. The circle is completed from the zenith state of evolution to the zenith state of involution where one reaches the source, the very soul. Here, one experiences an auspicious state, from where there is no return towards *prakṛti*. It is beyond the state of wandering and one-pointed attention, hence the question of stagnation does not arise at all.

While practising the *āsana*, when the life energy spreads harmoniously throughout the entire body, religiousness sets in. At that time you are a religious person because there is no time and no thoughts of the present or the past. At the same time, there is no quality of *rajas*, *tamas* or *sattva* because you have reached beyond time and quality. This state has to be built up to remain continuously in the process during practice so that the intelligence develops the auspiciousness in each and every part of the body. When you have evolved to this level, involution begins. You go inward more and more. Your optimum evolution takes you to that involution method and that becomes meditation. In meditation there is a single mind, a pure mind, and you are in a serene state.

Memory is important in the practice of yoga provided it is used correctly. It is a friend in the practice of the *āsana* provided you retain that memory and work on it for evolution and not merely for repetition. The practice should bring a fresh and new experience. You should use the memory as you use a needle to remove a thorn. Similarly, the pure and cleansed memory does not allow the wrong action to take place. You should use memory as a needle for the intelligence to grow. The memory has to lead you to proceed further. And if progress does not come, you must rely at least on the earlier memory to maintain stability, so you don't lose the potential for evolution.

This is how the teachers have to build the students to cross over limitations of their mind. It is the extension and expansion of mind that is to be considered as the capacity to stretch to the maximum level. The same mental blocks and limitations will return if you do not use your intelligence to flow in the body. Teachers get blocked in their teaching in the same way they get blocked in their practice also.

Q.- And could you discuss the difference between a supple body and a stiff one?

The suppleness and stiffness of the body are relative expressions. However, one prefers to have free movements in the joints and muscles. The restricted movements may affect blood circulation bringing some body afflictions.

Many people see the photographs of *āsana* and think that the supple body alone can perform such *āsana*. But one should know that often the supple body too cannot give any feedback to the brain or mind as the body lacks sensitivity. Though supple bodies do not experience pain, these tax the nerves causing fatigue, restlessness and headache or heaviness. They run out of energy. Instead of receiving the energy, the cells get squeezed and this may introduce hoards of diseases. A supple body does not trigger the intelligence to think what is wrong and what is right in performing an *āsana*. On the contrary, a rigid body has resistance, action and counter-action, which triggers the intelligence to study the *āsana* in the right perspective. There is no action, counter-action or resistance from the supple body to give clues to intellectual thinking and emotional stability. They get the *āsana* easily without inner resistance or response. If one is pregnant and there is no response, then the fear surfaces that the child is still with no life. Similarly, the *āsana* done without resistance is an *āsana* without life, like a stillborn child.

So even if the body is supple, the mind should resist and make itself hard for the body to perform the *āsana* with difficulty.

Q.- When would you say the internal experience is not so refined in a supple person?

Each action should have a reaction. There is a physical intelligence and a mental intelligence in each individual. If the physical intelligence does not respond to the mental intelligence, then the physical intelligence is immature and unrefined. You might call it a lose body but there is no intelligence. Here I use the word intelligence with specific meaning. Suppose you remember a poem word by word without knowing its meaning, does it make any sense to you? The moment you begin to know the depth of the poem's meaning, you begin to appreciate the poem. This appreciation is interaction. You begin to reflect on the poem and this reflection reflects with new thoughts on you.

Similarly, while doing or being in *āsana* there has to be the interaction between the body and mind as well as mind and intelligence. The body may act but the mind has to react. The intelligence has to reflect on the interaction between the body and mind. Intelligence has to demand the feed back from the body and mind. Otherwise, the body does on its own accord without giving any message to the mind or intelligence.

This does not open the gates of intelligence to interpenetrate or outerpenetrate the fullness of the *āsana*.

Q.- So you actually call that a disease of the nervous system, because the connection between the mind and nerves are not there?

I do not call it a disease, but want of understanding due to the lack of communication between body, mind and nerves. As the nervous system is the medium between the physical and intellectual bodies, there should be a thorough response and vibration in the fibres, tendons and nerves each time you move. If you stretch your finger, the response has to come immediately. If it doesn't come then it is as good as a dead body. An *āsana* with no sensation, as in the case of polio or paralysis, is like a paralysed body. It can be considered a disease, as consciousness does not move there.

Q.- How does yoga help with an individual's personal problems? What about particular dispositions that certain people seem to have, for example a person who seems disposed towards dejection? Is that disposition something they are born with or is it self-induced?

We are born with some of these things and some are due to circumstances.

Some problems develop from self-indulgence *(ādhyātmika)*. The person says, "I am very intelligent and healthy, so whatever I do, it doesn't matter. I can withstand anything because I've got my health." These are the proud people. Afterwards they become victims of their self-inflicted problems. They invite problems with this attitude and then get dejected when their defence mechanism fails. Problems may occur because of someone's way of living or by habit formation *(ādhibhautika)*. The elements of a person's system can also be polluted due to their manner of living, their behaviour. A third source of problems is genetic or hereditary *(ādhidaivika)*.

According to Patañjali, all these can be fought through the eight aspects of yoga in one's practice. They can be minimised or conquered. The subject of yoga is like a mirror wherein you can peep in to find out your own positive as well as negative attitudes and *āsana* practice neutralises both these attitudes.

Q.- What about teaching on the emotional level? Would you address this?

If the intelligence of the head is the seat of consciousness, heart is the seat of the sub-conscious intelligence. Emotionally disturbed people convert the conscious mind/brain into a sub-conscious state of mind. The subconscious mind, always in the trunk, is latent in the heart. Subconscious mind disturbs the person more than the brain.

The brain remains disturbed, perturbed and confused, affecting the mind. The Occidentals think that the mind is only in the brain. It is only the conscious mind in the brain, which comes as the precipitate of subconscious and unconscious mind from the core of the heart. The heart is the province of emotions. Therefore one has to open the knots of the heart. Here, we recommend supported backbends such as *Viparīta Daṇḍāsana*, chair *Kapotāsana*, bench *Setu Bandha Sarvāṅgāsana* to make the dormant or passive subconscious mind become active. People who are emotionally disturbed remain disconnected from themselves. Therefore they are made to come in to contact with the body while doing yoga. We ask them to keep the eyes wide open so that the conscious brain is active too. These backbends make the mind become an extrovert whereas in forwardbends like *Paśchimottānāsana* one gets further introverted and dull. When one does *Dwi Pāda Viparīta Daṇḍāsana*, the passive or negative brain comes to an active and positive state. The subconscious is made conscious by moving the head back more and more. In *Setu Bandha Sarvāṅgāsana* or *Dwi Pāda Viparīta Daṇḍāsana* normally the brain becomes quiet, but the subconscious mind becomes conscious. So these psychological transformations that take place through yogic practice have to be noticed by the practitioners and teachers to help those who suffer from dejection.

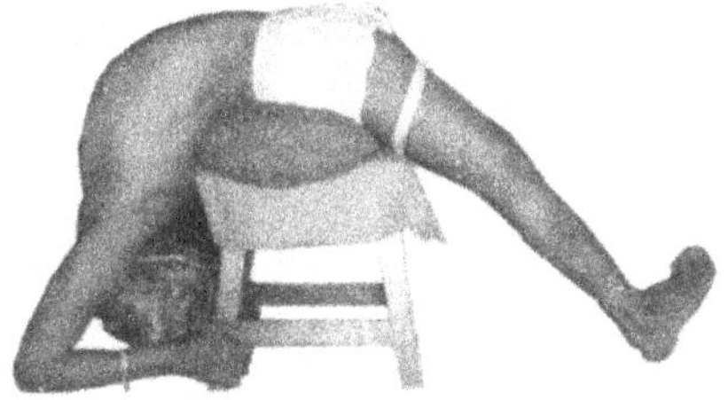

Dwi Pāda Viparīta Daṇḍāsana (supported)

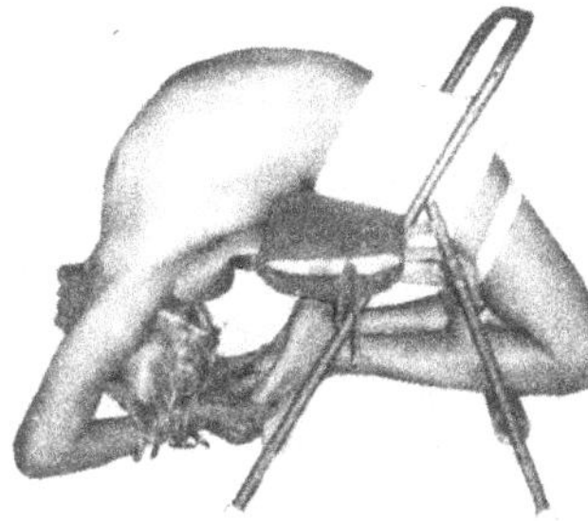

Kapotāsana (supported)

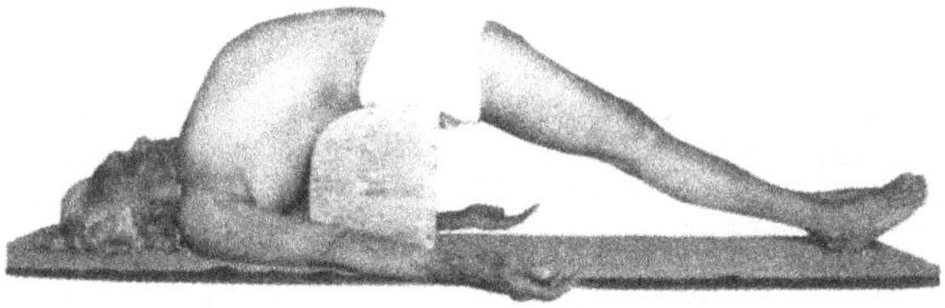

Setu Bandha Sarvaṅgāsana (supported)

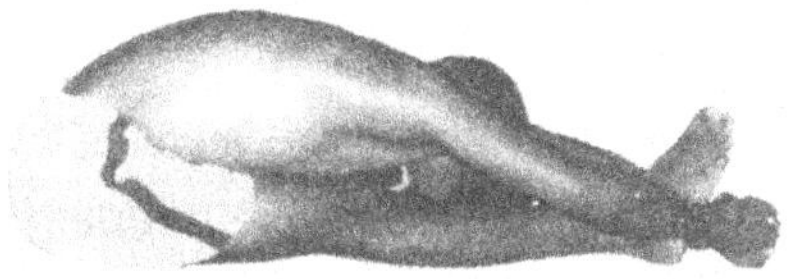

Paschimottānāsana

Plate n. 49 – *Āsana* to bring psychological transformation

Emotional problems take place in those persons who are introverts because they always go inwards. They haven't learned to evolve or bring out the consciousness to surface. Their depression increases in meditation as their thoughts recede and make them further empty. I have just received a letter from England. It reads, "I started attending classes with one of your teachers two years ago but I was keen to experiment with other methods. One of these was Transcendental Meditation. During one of the teacher's meditation weekends I went completely mad with paranoia, confusion, etc. and was admitted to a psychiatric hospital. I was very ill indeed. Fortunately I made a swift recovery and returned to normal life within three weeks. Must admit though, I have become somewhat wary of yoga. On my return to sound mental health I also made a return to my *āsana* practice as I felt that was safe. I have much more faith in it than in Western medicine and continue daily to the present. I have recently been reading some of the *Upaniṣads* and the following question arises. If the divine is within and cannot be realised by intellectual study, then what is the role of texts such as these, the *Yoga Sūtra*, the *Bhagavad Gītā* in the practice of yoga?"

I have answered this question which has come from a dubious mind, "All *Upaniṣads* have said train your body, mind and small self, so that they develop clarity, purity and divinity for the divine, which is within, to shine out with glory. Read them carefully and you feel you get the answer. But you jump to conclusions and this jumping is your intellectual enemy. Learn to take intelligence into your yogic practice. The study of books will guide you later."

Q.- So the study of books is not supposed to be an intellectual exercise?

For me, no not at all. You just gather ideas, which act as a tonic to the intelligence, and if it is used for storing knowledge, then it is not correct. It is a load on the intelligence. Therefore, the gathered ideas cannot be put into practice and that is the problem. The divine cannot be realised by intellectual studies. Taking intelligence to practice is self-culture. That is growth.

Q.- Can you talk about teaching meditation?

Actually, to be honest, meditation cannot be taught by anybody, it comes on its own. What I am teaching takes you towards dynamic meditation. The river flows, the river does not stagnate. So if the mind is stagnant in the lake of the body, what happens to that mind? It gets stale like the stagnated water. So we have to electrify the mind. In order to electrify the mind we do the *āsana*. The *āsana* electrify the mind. This electrification of the intelligence is *dhyāna* for me.

Meditation is the seventh aspect of yoga. What is happening in the world is that people are trying to by-pass the earlier aspects of yoga. So problems increase.

Q.- Gurujī, you often speak of the religiosity of the subject of yoga. Would you expand on this?

All self-cultured growth is a religious growth. Yoga is a universal religion because it does not belong to any one community. When Patañjali speaks of the *yama* and *niyama* – ethical precepts, he has used the word *sārvabhaumaḥ*, which means universal. So yoga is fully a universal culture and a universal religion. A universal religion attracts people from all walks of life and also from different cultures. It is amicable to any community for good health, for good mind, for good thoughts, for good actions and a good feel. I have said very often that *dharma*, wrongly interpreted as religion, is that which upholds, sustains and supports the humanity. In a gross sense, you can call it religion. It is universal because there is no barrier in its *sādhanā*. Do not mistake religion, because there is no correct word in English. We call it *dharma*. Yoga has spread as a universal approach, a universal culture. A cultured person is the one who has cultivated righteousness in physical, moral, mental and spiritual health and lives in virtuosity, then such a person is called a religious person. This is acclaimed universally. Yoga brings, as one goes into the depth of it, the purity of action and thought, which is the religiosity of practice. It may take a long time to experience this, but it is there. So all the self-culturing systems are meant for the growth of the individual to realise the Self. After experiencing the divinity one wishes to maintain that divinity; and that is the religiosity of practice.

Patañjali explains yoga as *citta vṛtti nirodha*, which means to restrain the thought waves. The 17th *sūtra* of the first chapter[1] tells you what happens when you restrain the thought waves. You analyse accurately eradicating the doubts and you enjoy bliss. You differentiate between the bliss which is not permanent and that which is permanent. But often you reach a plateau, not knowing which way to go, you are caught. Then you need to recharge yourself and practise with intense attention to go beyond the plateau which is like a hurdle. If you're so muddled and sick, it's clear that you have to get well. Since you don't know what to do, Patañjali tells us in the 20th *sūtra* of the first chapter[2] that you must then double your practices. Growth does not come when we do not observe our blind spots. If you catch these blind spots or empty spots, then you are eternally intelligent. There is no room for failure. When you have experience you build up faith and with that strong faith, find out if you can still proceed further. God bless you in this path.

---

[1] *Vitarkavicārānandāsmitārūpānugamāt saṁprajñātaḥ* : I.17
Practice and detachment develop four types of *samādhi*: self-analysis, synthesis, bliss, and the experience of the pure being.

[2] *śraddhāvīryasmṛtisamādhiprajñāpūrvaka itareṣām* : I.20
Practice must be pursued with trust, confidence, vigour, keen memory and power of absorption to break this spiritual complacency.

CAN AEROBICS REPLACE A PURPOSEFUL YOGIC LIFE?*

Q.- Aerobics is practised under the care of medicos and dieticians. It resembles *prāṇāyāma*. It is sought for overcoming physical disorders, to gain quickly stamina, strength and to combat stress and tension. They involve inhalation, retention, and exhalation. How do you compare the two?

I am really glad the people have taken to aerobics. Some exercise is better than watching murder and violence on TV day in and day out with all the *masāla* (spices).

Comparison is odious. Aerobics is controversial. I am a dedicated yoga exponent. I introduced yoga. It's catching. Friends and foes call me a "Patañjali fanatic" *(Smiles)*. Yes! I am proud. I have the knowledge and better understanding of yoga.

I have confessed, I am a very very latecomer to *prāṇāyāma*. My *guru* didn't brook the idea, my inadequate lungpower was the snag. I overcame it.

Prāṇāyāma and aerobics have three common actions, inhalation, retention and exhalation, the triad. Aerobics is an exercise. *Prāṇāyāma* is not an exercise. Do not compare *prāṇāyāma* with deep breathing.

I am ardently for *prāṇāyāma*. Yet I make it as a post mortem. I say, *prāṇāyāma* is harmful, damaging, if not done properly. Wrong practice and wrong technique cause hiccough, asthma, headaches, pains, hysteria and neurosis.

I am brutally frank in analysing aerobics. I consider it harmful, even if it is practised methodically.

Prāṇāyāma has four actions: the first three are inhalation, exhalation and retention. I regard the fourth dimension, called *kevala prāṇāyāma* or *kevala kumbhaka*, as supreme.

The fourth dimension is non-deliberate and a natural one. The inbreath energy is drawn in by the physiological cells, the medium between physical and intellectual body. In this phase, the *prāṇa* is held automatically by the respiratory system and heart muscles flushing out the

---

* Interview with M.S.S. Gupte, *The Times of India*, 19th November 1992, 5th June and 30th August 1993. Partially reported by the B.K.S. Iyengar Yoga Association of Australasia Inc., *Newsletter*, Feb.-March 1993.

coating of the heart valves. For me, in medical parlance, it approximates to micro-ventilation.

Prāṇa means energy – physical, mental, intellectual, sexual, spiritual or cosmic. All vibrating energy is the manifestation of *prāṇa*.

Aerobics is an exercise, which excites one with movements, unlike *āsana* or *prāṇāyāma*, which have less motion and more action. Yoga is not motion-oriented but action-oriented. In aerobics, the breath is made to move in and out by force. On the peripheral level, the doers feel that forceful breathing exhilarates the heart muscles, helps them to expand in speed – blood rushing – gushing through the main vessels, aerates and drains the cholesterol deposits. It helps boost the power of pumping out blood.

But at what cost? At the cost of irritation. In aerobics, the heart muscles get irritated due to choking and suffocation. Mentally and physically, dejection sets in. Persons doing it feel like giving up the effort, because it is all forced motion. It irritates the sensitive segments of lungs and heart. Heart is the hub of life. *Prāṇāyāma* is the hub of spiritual evolution.

Hence while teaching *prāṇāyāma* we see that the students feel lightness, quietness, exhilaration and smoothness. Actually, the irritation of nerves and the exhaustion of aerobic breathing is substituted by stimulation and rejuvenation in *prāṇāyāma*.

Aerobics done to taped music is harmful and counter productive. Medical experts feel continued movements of any type cause wear and tear of joints and muscles around. Unconscious or inadvertent movements trigger monotony and fatigue. The initial glow in aerobics is soon lost in the tedium of unconscious effort.

Q.- Work ethic is a new opiate in Japan, South Korea and neighbouring countries. Any comments?

I know Japan has emerged as a giant. South Korea, ravaged by war – the geographical split, division of hearts and minds – is making a fantastic bid to compete with super powers like U.S.

People have gone the full circle – sedatives, sleeping pills, tranquillisers, alcohol, sex and drugs. Now it is work ethic.

Our philosophers, sages and seers advised: "Plunge in work". Work is supreme worship; it is a prayer. It's the backbone of existence to challenge all your power.

In their wisdom they cautioned, *Ati sarvatra varjayet* (avoid all excesses).

Killing work, beyond human endurance, is a new escape. Japan is thinking of compensating work-deaths – people working twenty to twenty-two hours a day round the clock, weeks on end! It's harakiri (suicide).

Where are we drifting? The new pollution has taken over the individual – the community.

Even the children are not spared the strain-stress-speed – the bane of modern life-styles. In an era of satellite communications, the communication gap in and between individual and community is widening – no time to spare, to communicate to and with husband-wife-children.

Where's the time to hark back and talk and listen to your own body and mind?

Q.- Any solution?

The quest for inner peace and contentment through yoga is the solution. Two principal aspects, out of the eight aspects of yoga, are *yogāsana* and *prāṇāyāma*. The panacea to combat three S's – stress, strain, speed is in three W's: Word, Work, and Wisdom that comes of understanding the self and the world.

Q.- Does modern man need yoga? What with myriad exercises to keep fit, nutrition diet, foods vitamins, wonder drugs, physiotherapy and medical care?

A Himalayan yogi or a Tibetan lama may need less yoga but a modern man needs it more. Yoga is needed for more healing and strong lungpower, whether one is a man, a woman or a child.

There is environmental pollution, air pollution with all kinds of toxic gases released in the air by factories and plants. In Japan I heard that children might have to wear masks to enter some areas.

We have not spared ourselves with water pollution, the divine drink for health. How many can afford mineral water!

So the Himalayan yogi or saint needs less of yoga: you and I need it more. Man is drying out the mother Earth and she is working overtime to filter and absorb the obnoxious effluents.

Man's No. 2 foe is self-pollution, our modern life styles, insatiable urge for sensual and sexual pleasure and heavy doses of violence, murder, divorce on the T.V. screen and the print media.

We build up assiduously an "insecurity" net around us, in the rat race of speed, strain and stress. Modern man needs to be calm and retain poise. Only yoga can give the calmness and poise and save us from environmental and self-pollution.

Q.- What is *prāṇāyāma?*

It is regulation of inbreath – inhalation, outbreath – exhalation and retention of breath, which is known as *pūraka, rechaka* and *kumbhaka* respectively for proper distribution of *prāṇic* energy or vital force in the human body.

Q.- What is meditation?

Bringing the complex mind to a state of simplicity and serenity is meditation. Meditation happens when one becomes completely integrated. Sitting in a corner and closing the eyes may not be necessarily meditation. *Japa*[1] is not meditation but a path towards meditation. Relaxation is not meditation. Meditation is an experiencing state of singleness of the mind. It has no expression. Meditation is to subdue ego – *ahaṁkāra*.

Q.- Can yoga fit in for all?

Yoga fits for all and of all ages at any point of time. I taught headstand to the Queen of Belgium when she was eighty-four. Also I taught J. Krishnamurthy in his seventies, when he was having severe prostate trouble. Cardiac patients and the handicapped can also do yoga with props or under correct guidance. So, yoga is for all, the young, the old or the disabled, if you get proper guidance in practice.

Q.- Is yoga a physical culture?

I fought critics for six decades who dubbed yoga "physical". Yoga is culturing the mind with eight limbed discipline: *yama, niyama, āsana, prāṇāyāma, pratyāhāra, dhāraṇā, dhyāna* and *samādhi*. It is a collective integrated package, you can't take one and discard others. The synthesis of body, mind and soul has to be achieved through constant practice – *sādhanā*. Firmness of body and peace of mind can be achieved by yoga.

Speed, stress and strain of modern life send the human system out of gear. The human body is the finest machine created by God. Millions of cells are produced every second and die out also as swiftly. They give strength, fitness and mental calm. The cells have their own intelligence. The orchestra of bones, muscles, tissues, nerves, blood vessels, limbs, organs, the circulatory,

[1] Repetition of the sacred *mantra* or the name of God according to specific rules. Patañjali talks about the repetition of *āuṁ* (*Y.S.*, I.28).

respiratory, digestive and glandular systems are tuned to a veritable dance and kept going by *prāṇa* with consciousness. So in one sense, I say yoga begins with the cult of the body and leads towards the culture of the consciousness.

Q.- What's the secret of your teaching? How are you a different yoga teacher?

How do I know that my teaching is different from others? I teach from my experience. While teaching, the intelligence of my head and the heart blend together, hence I am intellectually and emotionally involved. My teaching is rooted in that experience. I am a doer teacher, not an armchair one. I read books for wider exposure but I don't lift ideas from books to pass them on to my students. I don't deviate from Patañjali who is my invisible, first and foremost *guru*. My other *guru* is my *sādhanā*, my practice. I practise and rub my experience with the words of Patañjali, that's why I can teach with authority and experience. Practice gives me wisdom and conviction.

Q.- Are any of your performances public?

I gave many solo demonstrations. Mind you, I take no drugs or steroids for stamina or endurance. They can test me. And I do it all at my seventy-five. It's grace of yogic *sādhanā* and God.

Some American doctors, after testing me, told my pupils that I have the lungs of a twenty-five year old Olympian. I don't know.

Q.- What about yoga for children?

By all means, but with a different technique minus "meditation". I am deadset against those who are set to teach meditation to children.

Children have speed. They dislike monotony and love variety and newness in everything they want to try. The child's mind is the present, it does not go into the past or into the future.

Adults need meditation due to the emotional turmoils. If you ask children to meditate, they go to sleep immediately. They can be very active, and they become very passive in a split second. They get bored if your teaching is slow or noncreative.

Q.- How do you deal with children who are hyperactive, overactive, naughty, rebellious? Do you calm them with meditation?

No, not at all. They too don't need meditation. I correct their behaviour teaching them *āsana* only. There is a method through which you can divert their energy towards a positive way through *āsana*. You can calm down their nerves and brain through *āsana*. You can call *āsana* dynamic meditation.

Q.- Is yoga for all the classes or the masses? It looks that the dice is loaded in favour of the rich who can afford a diet of rather *sāttvic* food etc. rather than the poor.

Yoga is for the masses.

The affluent and the rich abuse food. They need to restrict diet. The poor find it difficult to get two square meals a day. That's why I don't make a fetish of food and diet.

Food by deliberate choice and thinking from head is a poison. Let the stomach and the tastebuds decide it, not your head.

When hungry you salivate and the human body will change from acidic to alkaline gear or vice versa depending upon the food in the platter.

When hungry, a loaf of bread and a cup of tea will provide all the nutrition if the person does not make it a habit to take it all the time. The poor man cannot be padded with restrictions.

But whether the person is rich or poor, the churning of blood has to take place. This will depend upon the acceleration of the circulatory and respiratory systems, which lighten the burden on the digestive system. They help assimilation and elimination.

The poor need to go for strengthening the immune or defensive system for prevention of disease. What is nourishing for the rich may be their undoing but the poor man will derive at least the minimum nutrition from what little he can afford if he practises yoga. Stress and strain make little difference whether you are rich or poor.

VIP's and the rich shuttling between five star hotels and ultramodem hospitals at home and abroad can afford health disorders. Not the masses.

Q.- You are seventy-six but fighting fit, fit as fiddle. What's the secret?

I have no secrets or sweet hearts. The secret of secrets is the sacred yoga. When I went to Australia early this year, the newspapers wrote that I am old with a young body. My blood pressure is 125/85 and for the last so many years I weigh between seventy-two and seventy-four kg.

Q.- Any ambition target, miles to go?

Nothing! Having taught Queen Elizabeth of Belgium the headstand (*Śīrṣāsana*) and yoga to J. Krishnamurthy for twenty years during his desperate prostate trouble, teaching the meticulous maestro Yehudi Menuhin, speaking to the Pope on yoga privately, and receiving the *Padma*[1] award has given me an abiding sense of achievement in my single minded endeavour. Nothing can rob me of my contentment *(samādhāna)*. I consider *Light on the Yoga Sūtras of Patañjali*, forewored by Yehudi Menuhin and recently published by Harper Collins in London, as my crowning glory.

Moreover, introducing yoga to common people, men-women, young-old, children-sportsmen has given me satisfaction. What else is required?

Q.- What of death?

(Smiles) Birth and death are beyond the will of human being. These two do not ask our permission. It's not my domain. Who am I to think on it! One arrives and departs when the time comes. You know, according to our scriptures, death is *prakṛti* (nature) while life is *vikṛti*, as Kālidāsa says in *Raghuvanṡ*. When one is alive, the mind remains at the level of complexity. There is a mixture of sadness and happiness. The afflictions and emotions affect the mind. One needs to live the life in such a way so that one is not caught in the web of this complexity, then death, which is natural, may come smoothly.

Q.- Death and dying are two different things? Ken Wilber says: Every form of meditation is in essence a rehearsal of death. Zen says, if you die before you die, then when you die, you won't die. And Bob Hope said that he was not afraid of death, but the dying bothered him?

We go to bed each night. Nothing is known in sleep. We wake up in the morning fresh. By this are we not experiencing death and life each day? Yes, in the West the "dying" for the old and aged is like "dating" for the youth. I read it somewhere. I am neither concerned about death nor dying. But I would say this much, "Suppose I had paralysis rendering me fully non functional at all levels, I

[1] The author here is refering to the *Padmashri* award, one of the highest civil awards that India gives to its citizens. He was awarded the *Padmashri* in 1991, and has since been awarded the still higher *Padmabhushan* in 2002.

would consider it as death, though living." Yoga does not allow me to waste time on death and I have learnt to live holistically for every moment. Therefore, I won't say, "Die before you die". Rather I would say, "Live before you die so that the death is also a lively celebration."

Q.- What have you to be aware of having gained what you say a "glorious sense of achievement"?

I recall *American President*, and Harry Truman's wisdom in the film. Power, money and woman can bring downfall of the mighty. Woman does not bother me. I had full marital bliss from my wife Ramāmaṇi. I have five daughters and a son. *Yama* and *niyama* of Patañjali have protected me throughout.

Money, I earned through "sweat". I don't have too much of it to spoil me. I can recall I could hardly afford one meal a day. People called me "raving mad" when I picked up odd size stones and weights, using them for obtaining alignments and freedom in my practice which you call as props now. But I have to be wary if I have power of a sort and perfection in this field of yoga. I do not allow my ego to inflate me, my wisdom subdues my ego *(ahaṁkāra)*, I like to live like a modest average householder. My pride in yoga as an art is another kettle of tea, not the ego.

Q.- What's your immediate concern?

I do not want Patañjali's classical yoga to be polluted. What others do for the sake of money, fame or popularity is not my concern. Yoga should be left pure. A Sanskrit saying goes: *Na bhīto maraṇāt asti kevalam duṣitam yaśaḥ*. My only fear is the zenith of yoga being polluted.

Q.- Your last wish?

I believe in rebirth. I don't like to die as yoga *bhraṣṭa* and fall from the grace of yoga, come what may. Nor do I yearn to be born in a rich household, as *Bhagavad Gītā* says, *Śucīṇām śrīmatām gehe*.[1] I wish to be reborn in a poor humble family dedicated to yoga. For these reasons I keep on my practice without fail.

---

[1] See *Bhagavad Gītā*, VI.41 and 42

Q.- Yoga as a science, philosophy and practice is a sacred legacy of the Orient. What has the West done to enrich it?

I have no hesitation saying that yoga thrived in the lap of the West. We neglected it. The Westeners played in a big way in popularising it. We in the East only talked philosophically and hypocritically about it. We tried to keep it as a secret and individualistic. Westerners with an intellectual bent have the drive and enriched it while we lacked dedication.

The essence of yoga is spiritual discipline, the triumvirate of body, mind and soul working in harmony.

Q.- If you were younger?

If I were younger and mature, I feel I would have done a lot more to propagate yoga and reach out to every home and person.

Q.- Any comment on yoga therapeutics?

Yoga has proved very effective. It deals with live bodies and minds not pursuing the lifeless anatomy and confines of narrow physiological and pathological approach.

The deeper you go into the mind and beyond it, may solve many more riddles of human life and help control physical disorder and ill health.

Q.- How much of sleep?

Even four to five hours is good if you practise yoga thoroughly and systematically.

Q.- What's the barometer of health in maddening tests of blood and other things?

Simple! Your skin. It controls heat and cold for maintaining the balance, it should be velvety smooth like that of the newborn. You might find the texture of my skin smoother than that of a healthy young woman.

Q.- One parting question! Is anybody interested in yoga when there are film stars around?

I am not a film star but a yoga star![1]

Q.- Do you feel that often the animal leads an instinctively "unconditioned life" unlike we humans?

That rings true. But it is not true. In my latest book *Light on the Yoga Sūtras of Patañjali*, I happened to touch this aspect. Have you noticed on the television screen dealing with wild life and nature, the herds of beautiful lean gazelles haunted by marauding predators? But their courtship, procreation, breeding and enjoyment from the rich bounty of nature in no way inhibits them. Don't they know that the inevitable end for them, their spouses or offspring will be in the lion's maw? Why do they keep on running in their shining glistening coat?

The answer is that possibly by instinct they have learnt to live "for the moment". Man as an evolved being has to learn to do this consciously and the eight limbs of Patañjali's yoga will convert their present complex life into simplicity advancing towards serenity.

Q.- It's said Harper Collins released recently your latest title *Light on the Yoga Sūtras of Patañjali* with a foreword by Yehudi Menuhin?

Yes! I am talking about the same book.

– Your latest child! The crowning glory... –

I am quite happy. At seventy-five, I have no ambition. I have always considered myself as a layman in yoga, and as a layman I have done a good job, which I call now as the crowning glory of my life.

Q.- How long did you work on the book?

---

1 In reference to the designation on the 29th July 1988 by the Ministry of Federal Star Registration, Washington D.C., U.S.A., of the star of the Northern Hemisphere, Monoceros RA6h30m46sd + 1º29', with the name "Yogacharya B.K.S. Iyengar".

On *Light on Yoga* and *Light on Prāṇāyāma*, I worked for a few decades. On the *Yoga Sūtra* I worked for fifteen years - worked under tremendous pressure. Harper and Collins breathed down my neck.

I was both agitated and excited, having chosen to write on Lord Patañjali's aphorisms. They are terse and sharp like formulae - profound and a veritable treasure of ancient wisdom.

Since my teens, I rubbed Patañjali's words from the aphorisms – with my work. I was often perplexed and confused. It is only my *sādhanā*, my practice that gave me the clue and insight. Being a "doer" well fortified in my practice helped me to unfold the wisdom in the *Patañjali Yoga Sūtra* and I could write with a greater conviction than others. I tried to import clarity, make yoga practical for seekers – no theorising. I leave the academic cobwebs to pundits. But at the same time, I leave my work for the critics to judge impassionately, impassively and impartially.

Q.- Any idea how it was received in yoga circles?

Some people phoned me to say that they are delighted with contents as well as pricewise, it was appropriate.

Q.- You have a good following abroad?

I think that over one and a half million foreigners practise Iyengar Yoga. In U.S., U.K., Canada and at other places, I believe there are more than 500 Iyengar associations, clubs and circles.

Q.- Yoga is still not a part of the curriculum for physical training programmes. What do you think?

That should have been done years back. Politicians and Ministers and their spouses seek my guidance. They want to practise it in private. It baffles me why they are adverse to its inclusion in the courses. Former R.S. Member and Nagpur Krida Mandal president, Advocate S.W. Dhabe told me that it would be made compulsory in schools. Why does the government drag its feet? The answer is unknown.

Q.- Is there a move to introduce yoga at the Olympics?

I have no idea. It turned out at Barcelona Olympics (Spain), that according to the media, many competitors did personal yoga practices. It was reported that a pressman was asked to wait as Dr Samaranch, Olympic Committee President, happened to be doing his personal yoga practice.

A large number of people are practising yoga from different countries, therefore, there should be no problem in recognising *yogāsana* as a demonstrative sport. Yoga is spiritual besides being a health culture.

Q.- Olympic performance calling for physical endurance has become synonymous with potent drugs and steroids?

Sports and such heats aim at creativity and an effort to bring out the best among the participants. Steroids and the intake of other drugs knock out the basis of ethical practices in this endeavour. Medals are a token of encouraging motivation, not the end-all.

Q.- Many have said that you have given many solo demonstrations of *yogāsanas* – often under gruelling conditions. Is it so?

Yes, I have given demonstrations on uneven flooring, unsteady stage and slippery carpets. I have also performed under -10° (Celsius) during my recent visit to Seoul. My critics say that the pictures of demonstrations are "photogenic" or are the result of a "camera trick."

IS *AṢṬĀṄGA YOGA* INTERLINKED, INTERWOVEN AND INTERCONNECTED?

Q.- It is often mentioned that yoga is of eight limbs. But you insist that the eight limbs of Patañjali's yoga must not be considered as steps or stages or limbs, but as complementary and supplementary to each other. Can you elaborate whether these are parts or limbs of yoga and how they cannot be dissociated from each other?

Well, in order to understand yoga, Patañjali explains yoga as a whole with various facets along with *yama, niyama, āsana, prāṇāyāma, pratyāhāra, dhāraṇā, dhyāna* and *samādhi* as *yogāṅga. Aṅga* means way, manner, mode, a limb or a member. It means a division or the part of the whole. These eight facets of yoga are not only complementary but supplementary to one another.

As both the complementary and the supplementary aspects have close connections with each other, it raises the *sādhaka* to reach the highest point of emancipation and brings freedom from sorrows, afflictions and defects in the way of living.

All these eight facets of yoga put together are called *yogāṅga* (yoga family members). To understand and to weave these eight facets or aspects or *yogāṅga* as an integrated whole becomes the need to actually begin yoga as a whole and not as parts.

Let me bring to your attention what Patañjali explains in III.51. He says that *doṣabīja* – the seed of defective thinking and action – is the cause for disintegration in man and how the practice of yoga frees one by burning out the seed of bondage in him. It is worth studying to understand what this *doṣabīja* means.

Doṣabīja is the instinctive seed of sorrows and defects in the behavioural pattern of the human mind which acts as the cause of imperfection in mankind all over the world. The latent defects of behavioural patterns are: violence, skilful lying, covetousness, sensuality and greed or possessiveness. According to Patañjali, these instinctive defects manifest in thought, word and deed, and should be controlled by discerning right thought, right word and right deed.

---

* Interview by senior students in the library of the Ramāmaṇi Iyengar Memorial Yoga Institute, Pune, December 1992.

Studying and knowing the working pattern of the human mind, Patañjali guides man by using the contrary words as non-violence, truthfulness, non-covetousness, sensual control and non-possessiveness. He collectively terms these as *yama.* In Hindu mythology Yama is said to be the Lord of death. He is not a cruel personality. He is considered as a righteous person who unknowingly guides us not to do sinful actions so that death is not a curse but a guide to live cleanly. If the *sādhaka* gets induced and abets and falls in the trap of these defects, then it is indeed a path towards the death of the soul. Hence, he used the word – *Yama.* If man does not cultivate character to eradicate this instinctive nature of the mind, then it is a moral and spiritual death for him. The principles of *yama* uphold us from such death.

In order to minimise or to eradicate or to destroy these afflictive seeds, Patañjali suggests five constructive seeds in the form of *niyama.*

Please note that *niyama* is a means to establish a right order to follow that combats and destroys the *doṣabīja* – seed of afflictions. It is interesting to see how Patañjali covers each and every aspect of *niyama* that implicitly corresponds to the other petals of *aṣṭāṅga yoga,* namely *āsana, prāṇāyāma, pratyāhāra, dhāraṇā* and *dhyāna.*

a) *Śauca* or cleanliness is earned through the practice of *āsana* which cleanses the outer as well as the inner body and then takes further to conquer the dominant *tāmasic* and latent *rājasic* nature and takes the *sādhaka* towards the higher qualities of life.

b) *Santoṣa* or contentment is experienced through the practice of *prāṇāyāma* that conquers the active *rājasic* nature of the mind and leads one towards *tapas.*

Let me explain to you how this *santoṣa* is felt. If the vessel is filled with water, if one empties it, it gets filled with air. This analogy fits in well in *prāṇāyāma.* The torso is the vessel. If one inhales with *prāṇāyāmic* techniques, as the cosmic energy enters in the form of inhalation, one can feel something is giving room for the cosmic force to occupy the vessel – the torso. This is nothing but the *ātman* moving from the centre towards the outer body for the inbreath to cover the vessel.

Similarly as the outbreath is released, the vessel empties out but the *ātman* moves in.

From this you realise that through inbreath, the vessel is filled in with *prāṇa* and the core of the being moves out; while in outbreath, the energy moves out from the torso for the *ātman* to enter in.

In this observation of movement of *prāṇa* and *ātman* and *ātman* and *prāṇa,* the vibrative mind becomes quiet and nullifies fluctuations. Therefore contentment *(santoṣa)* is felt.

From this contented state of mind, the *sādhanā* for spiritual pursuit begins in the form of *tapas.*

c) *Tapas* is nothing but to follow the techniques of *pratyāhāra*, wherein the conative organs of actions and cognitive senses of perception divert their attention towards the inner space known as *cidākāśa* – the core of the being, establishing *sattvaguṇa* in *karmendriya*, *jñānendriya* and *manas*, and take one towards *svādhyāya*.

d) *Svādhyāya* is self-reading, self-enquiry and self-analysis, which is nothing but *dhāraṇā*, a path towards true *jñāna mārga*, which leads one towards *Īśvara praṇidhāna*.

e) *Īśvara praṇidhāna* is felt through *dhyāna* which takes one towards *viveka khyāti* – the crown of wisdom.

This crown of wisdom, which comes as the effect of *dhyāna*, culminates in *samādhi*, where *karma*, *jñāna* and *prajñā* become one due to the purification of *antaḥkaraṇa* – the conscience. The conscience matures with *saṁyak prajñā*, *saṁyak jñāna* and *saṁyak karma*. Hence, the seed of defective thinking and defective action gets totally destroyed. This state is nothing but the union of the individual consciousness with the cosmic consciousness.

Thus it is interesting to understand how *niyama* in a capsule covers the gamut of *aṣṭāṅga yoga* (from *āsana* to *samādhi*), and how Patañjali explicitly takes the practitioner from the ordinary weak mind to the state of an extraordinary exalted state of absolute mind.

THE JOURNEY FROM CONATIVE ACTION TO ALL-PERVASIVE AWARENESS*

Q.- Mr. Iyengar, you were mentioning about conative and cognitive actions in the class. Can you explain it? Does conative mean will?

No, conative does not mean will power in actions. Basically there are two ways of doing any action, namely conative and cognitive.

Conative means external action, physical action, and cognitive means the action done with knowledge by observation. When we do the *āsana* conatively, we are touching the exterior part of the body, the anatomical body, the bones and the muscles by motor nerves. This includes the movements of the body aiming at certain action such as stretching of the arms or bending of the knees. Such movements can happen mechanically or habitually where one does not find any involvement. While doing the *āsana* or being in the *āsana*, the observation and thoughtful application of the mind are required.

When we work conatively, first of all the senses of perception or the sensory nerves are supposed to cognise as feedback from physical action. For instance, if you smell the scent of the flower, the hand has to hold the flower and it has to take the flower to the nose. This is conative action. When you smell, the brain is involved in a different way, which makes you identify the flower because of its fragrance. You may see the flower with your eyes to appreciate its beauty, so on and so forth. This is called cognitive action since you cognise it. There is a specific reason behind that action in order to have the knowledge. In the same way we have to observe when we are doing the *āsana*, whether the senses of perception receives any message from the action of the flesh? In a way the flesh and bones are the organs of action – *karmendriya*, and cognitive nerves are the senses of perception – *jñānendriya*.

- In a way it's like a feedback system, we're feeding back the karmendriya *by* jñānendriya *and* jñānendriya *by* karmendriya *while performing an* āsana. –

---

* Interview from the *Iyengar Yoga Institute Review*, San Francisco, Winter 1992.

The conative organs have to supply the movements and actions to cognitive senses in order to get the feedback. Every conative action has to get converted into cognitive action. That is how the senses of perception receive the action from the muscles and the bones. However the senses of perception can only receive the action, they do not know how to correct, so they only send the message to the mind and brain, saying that they received the "done-action" from the body. There has to be the exchange of understanding between the spindles of the muscles and the spindles of the skin. When the spindles of muscles through their conative actions send messages to the cognitive spindles of the skin through nerve fibres, the mind is drawn there to interplay. The mind notifies the connection and communication between the spindles of the muscles and the spindles of the skin. But it cannot give a clear judgement whether the exchange of understanding is correct or incorrect. Therefore the mind appeals to intelligence, the superior friend. The power of its superior friend, the intelligence, is that it can dissect and analyse each action. The mind cannot dissect, analyse or judge the action.

- Is that the brain? -

Not exactly. The brain is a physiological organ. Neither brain nor the mind can dissect.

Brain undoubtedly is the seat of intellect and mind. But it is merely the seat. The mind, intelligence and I-consciousness as composition form the *citta* or consciousness, which is beyond the physiological body. Rather it is a mental body used as an instrument for spiritual progress. If the brain is the envelope, the *citta* is the content. the mind intelligence and consciousness run parallel to the body, but remain dormant. The sādhaka has to tap these to come out of the dormant state.

The discriminative intelligence comes to the rescue of the mind, the senses of perception and the organs of action. There happens to be a dialogue between the intelligence and the apparatus of "mind, organs of action and senses of perception". The intelligence explains, "I find this fault. You are overstretching, or you are understretching. Your conative action is strong or your cognitive action is strong. So can you dilate where they are too strong; can you concentrate or saturate a little more to get the feed-back?" When the correct adjustments take place and answers are given to the queries of intelligence, then the intelligence says, "That is the correct *āsana*".

Hope this clears your doubt.

Q.- So is it in a way correcting the relationship between the conative action of the body and the cognitive intelligence of the mind?

Yes! That is right. But then how do I introduce this? Suppose I'm doing *Paschimottānāsana*. If my right leg is straight and my left leg is not straight but tilted to one side, then, though I am doing *Paschimottānāsana*, I say the leg that is tilted is doing conatively and the leg that is straight is not only in conative action but also in cognitive observation. In *Paschimottānāsana*, it could also be that I stretch the right leg but the stretch is aggressive and therefore violent. The left is dropped, showing as though it is non-violent and non-aggressive. When I say violent, I am using the cells very strongly to act on the stronger leg, which means I am jamming the cells, the cellular system, by overstretching. And the left leg is not at all active. It's dull. It's not getting the feed properly and it is hampered due to lack of cognition. Though it seems to be non-aggressive, there is an unconscious wrong stretch which is harmful. Here comes your intelligence, which uses the power of judgement and corrects the wrong action as well as the aggressiveness in action.

My crude or clumsy explanation may be difficult for you people to understand, because nobody until now has thought over the overstretch and the understretch. One just thinks that this is done passively. But the passive way also can be harmful. Similarly the active way of doing can also prove to be harmful.

So, who has to judge these faulty actions? The watchful intelligence has to lead the body and mind to correct both the faulty actions and imbalances.

– I see, so one is too much one way and the other is too little the other way. –

Exactly! Unconsciously you are actively afflicting the cells on the one part while on the other you remain heedless. In one leg there is aggressiveness where consciously by overstretching we are drying out the cells; in the other leg, by not attending to that, you are allowing the cells to go towards an natural death. You learn here to balance non-violence in violence and violence in non-violence.

– Does it happen unconsciously? –

Yes, it may. Hence the yogi says, "Follow that *ahiṁsā*". That means, if this right leg is strong, and the left leg is not strong or not rightly attended to, then intelligence has to come to its rescue to adjust that correctly. There has to be evenness – *samatvam*. This means that the stronger, aggressive or active side has to contribute some energy to the weaker, non-aggressive or passive side. Therefore, stretching or extending, though seems to be something like violence, it is not the violence but a kind of balance between violence and non-violence. The leg which is weak draws the energy from the strong leg and tries to educate itself so that violence and non-violence or aggressiveness and non-aggressiveness are made to balance evenly so that the ideas of violence and non-violence disappear from the head and the heart.

– So there is a perfect balance. –

Perfect balance.

– No violence, no non-violence, just...... –

And because you have adjusted in a balanced way, you are moving towards the truth. It is a self-inquiry on the line of *pratipakṣa bhāvanam* such as what is the right way or the right approach towards the *āsana*. Am I getting that in *āsana* or not? So you cannot oscillate. Similarly, you have to compare each portion of the body such as hands and legs. Question yourself whether you are using your one hand more than the other. Why is one hand strong while the other hand is not?

Haṭha yoga also means to bring through communication, the rhythm on the right side and the left side of the body and vice versa towards the centre. The balancing of *iḍā*, *piṅgalā* and *suṣumṇa* is very important. *Iḍā* and *piṅgalā*, if imbalanced, create disparity between the right and the left. Realising that there is a disparity or duality between the right side of the body and the left side of the body, we see whether we can bring harmony and rhythm on both the sides so that there is no division, but a fine balance in each and every *āsana*.

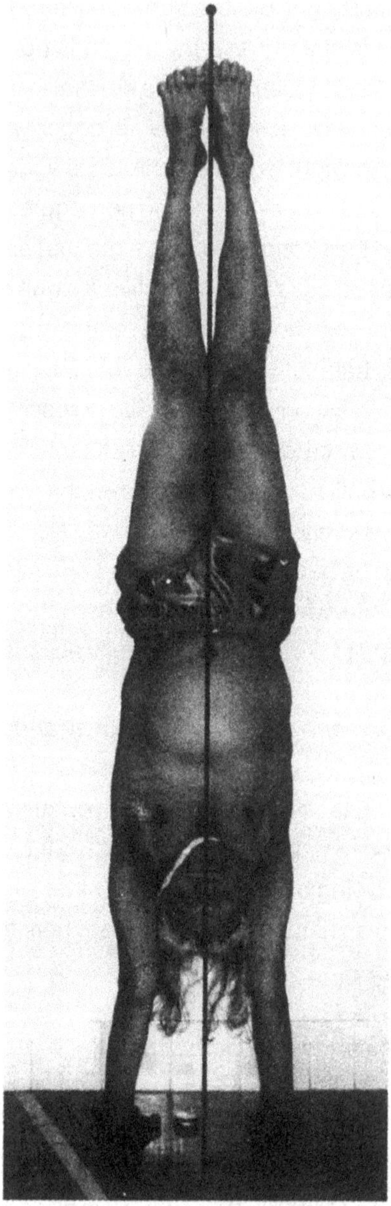

Plate n. 50 – Harmonious rhythm and balance; *Adho Mukha Vṛkṣāsana* (see also pl n. 27)

Q.- And does this awaken intelligence inside the body?

That's what I am coming to. Then in that state, there is a tremendous awareness of intelligence. The practitioner begins to feel that his intelligence is at one place and not at another place. He begins to feel whether his intelligence is extending and or expanding. Thus the *sādhaka*, the practitioner, has to go on observing and adjusting, he develops the quality of a *brahmacarya*. The self starts seeing its own coat, its own vestment, the body. It is celibacy in this sense. The Self begins to touch every nook and corner of the body. The person reaches the state where he is above all attachments and detachments. He feels the elevation.

You all know the movements of the body or elasticity of the muscles. You call somebody supple if there is a freedom in his movement. Do you know the suppleness or elasticity or freedom of the Self? The Self is a king and the body is its regime. The king reigns in the realm. Similarly the *sāshaka* has to reign and say, "I want to move as I am moving in this leg. I want to move myself as I am moving in this hand, please make me move freely in such a way that there is no hindrance. You adjust and also travel with me." This has to be a dialogue essentially between the Self and intelligence. That means the person who is doing forgets the body but makes the intelligence balance on the muscles, on the body, evenly so that he is one within himself.

- Then the body is forgotten for the moment. There is a unity. -

This is *dhyāna*. This means that the person, doing the *āsana*, retains the stretch, retains the contact, forgets or neglects no part of the body from one end to the other end, from the South to the North, East to the West, without deviation. The energy remains flowing uninterruptedly, and the intelligence also retained uninterruptedly as long as you are in that *āsana*, and that is *dhyāna*.

Q.- Or *samādhi*. Is it *samādhi* at the same time?

No, you cannot call this state a *samādhi*. You can reach up to meditation, with the seven steps of yoga. The eighth step is the fruit of the seventh step.

- Which one? -

Meditation – *dhyāna*.

So when we take the pupils to the state of meditation in *āsana*, they forget the sense of the body, the sense of the mind as well as the organs of action and senses of perception. Is it not then a spiritual *āsana?* All the limbs of yoga get involved. So *yama* and *niyama* are there. *Śauca* is there. The blood circulates. The cells are purified, sanctified and consecrated with energy. If you don't attend the way I have said then, the blood doesn't flow. The cells die soon. You give it an inner bath, just as you take an outer bath. This is the way to practise where you touch the intelligence everywhere.

Q.- Purification we might say, cleaning of the body, in preparation for *dhyāna*.

Again, you are limiting its scope. I just gave an example of *śauca*. In order to have a preparation, entry and establishment in *dhyāna*. This is how one has to proceed.

So *niyama* is introduced not only to cleanse the inner body but to prepare the mind and intelligence to have Self-realisation.[1]

- So that is the true sense of niyama. -

Yes, the cleanliness of *niyama* is sent in, the cleanliness in breath is set in. The energy then flows uninterruptedly without any impediments in the joints of the body. When this happens the senses are drawn inwards.

- *Pratyāhāra* is introduced. -

It is not introduced, rather it happens. When *pratyāhāra* happens, the senses move inwards. But they want some support, as they were used to being supported by external things earlier. Now they need some object to be drawn inwards and call out, "Let me look within." This makes the Self become the object.

There begins *dhāraṇā*, which means to focus on that intelligence as well as the source of the intelligence from where it sprouts.

Q.- Which is mind.

Please note that the miond is the cover of intelligence. Here, it is not the known mind, which communicates conative and cognitive actions, but the inner mind that takes the message to intelligence. You can call this mind the supermind or single mind. So the practitioner goes to the source of all intellectual actions and tries to remain there without allowing it to expand or contract. And that is meditation in *āsana*.

[1] *Sattvaśuddhi saumanasya aikāgra indriyajaya ātmadarśana yogyatvāni ca* (*Y.S.*, II.41). When the body is cleansed, the mind purified and the senses controlled, joyful awareness comes to realise the Self.

Q.- Then how do you move from *dhyāna* to *samādhi*?

Samādhi has to come on its own. Nobody can explain *samādhi*, don't ask that.

– It visits you. –

I say yes and no, as these words fade out in *samādhi*. But know that nobody can say, "I'm in *samādhi*". One cannot talk or communicate. *Samādhi* is a state of experience where even the existence of "I" disappears. That "I" is an experiencing state and cannot be explained. And again I tell you, *yama* and *niyama* can be explained so one can follow. By giving the ideas of how to live, one can make the practitioner to be in it and follow. You cannot teach *yama* and *niyama* through experiment. You cannot ask someone to experiment with *ahiṁsā* or *brahmacarya*. These principles have to be followed. They have to be carried out with full awareness, moment to moment in any situation, under any circumstances. So *yama* and *niyama* have to be learned by example. *Āsana, prāṇāyāma* and *pratyāhāra* are explanatory and can be experimented and therefore can be corrected. But *dhāraṇā*, *dhyāna* and *samādhi* are only experiencing states, not explanatory states. That is the end, you are already in *dhāraṇā*, *dhyāna* and *samādhi*. No one can explain. If anybody says, "I am teaching meditation", then as a student of yoga I say, "It is rubbish". Because meditation cannot be taught, it can only be experienced.

– So all the initial steps are preparation for that. –

Yes.

Q.- In order to understand *samādhi*, can you explain sleep to me?

Sleep and *samādhi* are not one. Sleep is the mental modification, the modification of *citta*, and *samādhi* is the transcendence of *citta*.

One does not witness the sleep while one is in the state of sleep. The experience of sleep is narrated only after waking up from sleep. In sleep you are nowhere and in *samādhi* you are all there. The simulation of sleep in a wakeful state with full awareness is *samādhi*.

Sleep does not enlighten but *samādhi* enlightens.

Sleep is not a direct experiencing state. The experience is shared after sleep whereas *samādhi* is an experiencing state, which cannot be shared. However both have to come on their own. You cannot say you can go to sleep. It has to come on its own. *Samādhi* has to come on its own.

Dreamless sleep is an inert state of consciousness. We forget our own existence in sleep, whereas *samādhi* is a complete wakeful state of consciousness in which our existence is felt totally, without any shadow.

Q.- What is the role then of seated meditation, especially sitting in *Padmāsana*. Is there a purpose for that?

For meditation one has to be essentially in a sitting *āsana*. Meditation is not possible in sleeping or standing *āsana*. In supine or *supta* position one is likely to go to sleep. In standing *āsana*, one cannot stand too long on the legs which causes strain. Meditation is done only in a sitting posture since one has to sit for a long time for the transformation of consciousness to occur.

Now, why *Padmāsana?* The reason simply is that you cannot stoop in *Padmāsana*. While sitting for meditation one should not drop the spine.

– Fall over. –

You cannot sink the spine. Some people cannot do *Padmāsana*. Therefore alternatives are required.

The best of all *āsana* is *Padmāsana* for meditation. In *Vīrāsana*, the lower lumbar moves deep into the frontal body so the spine can never be straight. In *Siddhāsana* the lower portions are completely inert, only the thoracic-dorsal spine will be active. Whereas in *Padmāsana* the entire spine from the tail bone to the brain is made to be kept alert and active. Only *Padmāsana* does this, no other *āsana*. That is why *Padmāsana* is considered the best of all *āsana*. Most people cannot do it, because they have lost the habit of sitting on the ground, which was there in the earlier days when chairs were not available. So one had to squat and sit on the ground. Because of squatting, people were getting the rotations in their groins, legs, and knees easily, so they could do *Padmāsana* easily. Now people have only restricted movements. They don't use their joints to the optimal level, therefore the joints are rusted. Hence I say that one can take any sitting *āsana* such as *Svastikāsana, Siddhāsana, Vīrāsana, Baddha Koṇāsana*, provided the sitting is correct.

– As you said, dhyāna *can happen in any* āsana, *it's just that* Padmāsana *is the best one. –*

Again I tell you, there is tremendous misconception when we think of the *sūtra – sthira sukham āsanam* (*Y.S.*, II.46)[1] as if it is said that any comfortable pose is an *āsana*.

[1] Perfection in *āsana* brings firmness in body and benevolence in mind.

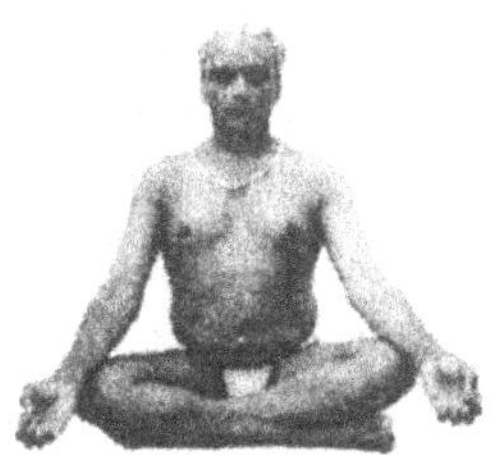

Svastikāsana

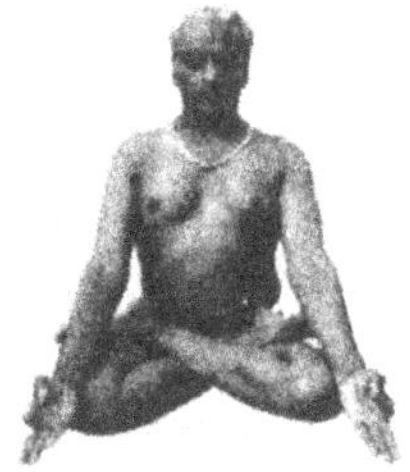

Padmāsana

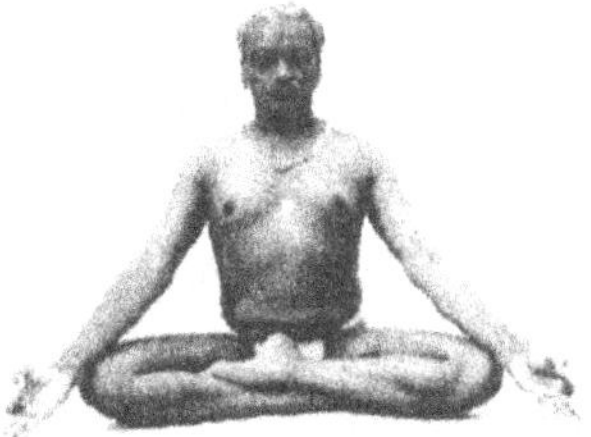

Siddhāsana

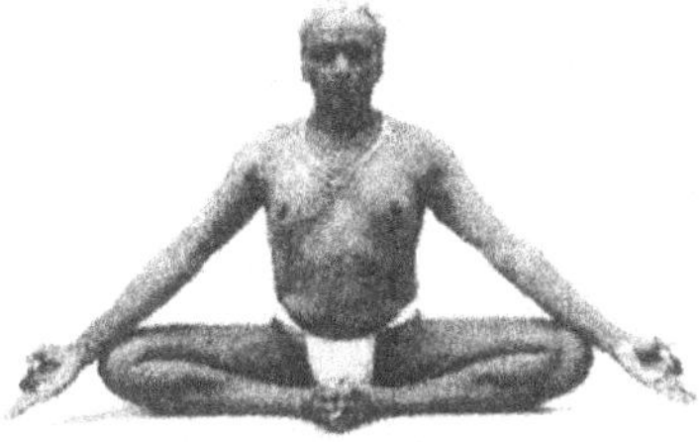

Baddhakoṇāsana

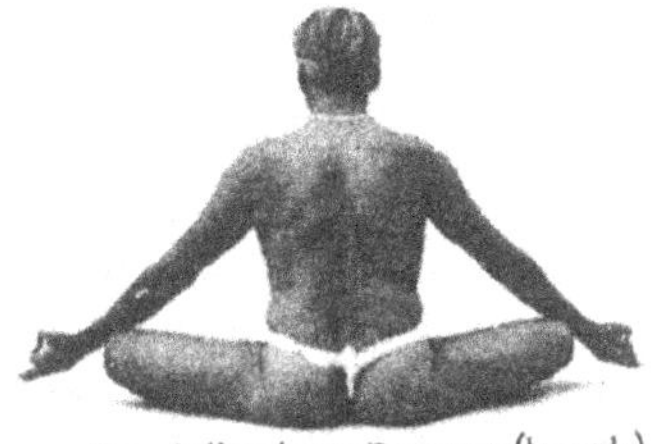

Baddhakoṇāsana (back)

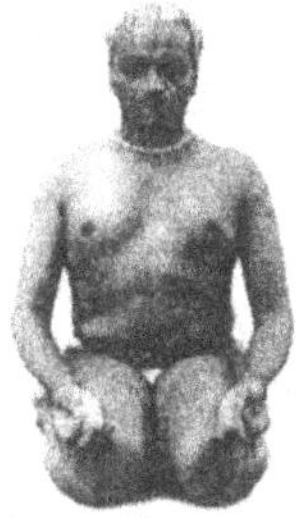

Vīrāsana

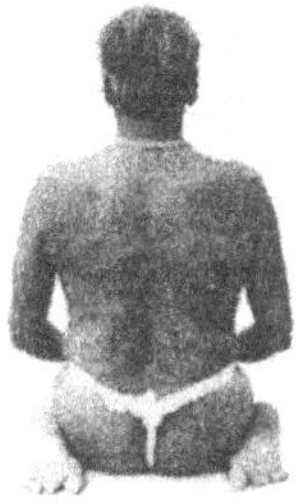

Vīrāsana (back)

Plate n. 51 – Sitting *āsana for Dhyānā (Svastikāsana, Padmasana, Siddhasana, Baddha Koṇāsana,* and *Vīrāsana)*

Suppose I put you this logic. You are sitting now. This is a comfortable pose for you. In a few minutes, what do you do?

– I change the position. –

You change. Then where is the comfort? In order to understand what Patañjali is saying, we have to take the next *sūtra* into consideration. He says, *prayatna śaithilya ananta samāpattibhyām* (*Y.S.*, II.47). When the effort becomes effortless, or when that effort ceases, you are a master of that *āsana*. He is referring to being in an *āsana*. This *sūtra*, nobody reads it. Only *sthira sukham āsanam* is known. But *prayatna śaithilya*, when the effort ceases, *ananta samāpattibhyām*, you and your *āsana* are one with the Universal. Your Self is one with the Universal. That is known as *sthira sukham āsanam*. It means that the body in *āsana* has to be firm and steady and you should be able to endure. Your intelligence should not waver. With all the correct efforts and right approach you establish yourself in *āsana*. A time has to come where your efforts convert to an effortless state and you feel that the efforts are ceasing. At that stage, when there is the absence of physical and mental efforts, you are easily turned towards the infinite within – the very soul. Again Patañjali says that at that moment the dualities within the body, mind and soul vanish. It is not the heat and cold as often explained. *Tataḥ dvandvāḥ anabhighātaḥ* (*Y.S.*, II.48). When you are one with the Self, where is the question of cold and heat? You have heard these explanations that the *dvandva* means dualities, such as heat and cold, honour and dishonour, success and failure. It is not these physical, psychological or mental dualities. They are objects, temperaments. But body, mind and soul are subjective, and even the subject is forgotten. Why think of honour and dishonour, which are all outside. Are they not objects? What is connected with yoga which is inside? It is the body, mind and intelligence that create dualities. They never give a clear picture and we get affected and caught.

And what is the effect of that *āsana?* Have you gone through that one, in *Patañjali's Yoga Sūtra? Rūpa lāvaṇya bala vajra saṁhananatvāni kāyasaṁapat* (*Y.S.*, III.47). *Kāya* means body. By the practice of *āsana* the wealth of the body has to be acquired. And what are those? Beauty *(rūpa)*, grace *(lāvaṇya)*, strength *(bala)*, and adamantine compactness *(vajra saṁhananatva)* (*Y.S.*, II.46). How many people understand and follow that? Patañjali has mentioned the effects of *āsana*, rather the result of *āsana*. Unfortunately, nobody quotes this *sūtra*. And people say Mr. Iyengar's yoga has nothing to do with Patañjali's. When I do the *āsana* or teach *āsana*, there is beauty, there is grace, there is strength, there is determination. According to Patañjali, I show it is there. I see essentially whether these qualities are brought in the practice. I do not say do as you like.

- So the effort is important. -

Patañjali uses the word *prayatna śaithilya*. *Prayatna* means efforts and *śaithilya* means laxity. The efforts are needed in the beginning in order to have laxity later. The effort has to terminate in laxity. It has to disappear. Now for instance, in the army there is military regimentation, but after ten years it becomes a natural thing for the soldiers, does it not? Similarly, while practising *āsana*, your body does not obey the orders, so you have to learn in order to get the proper movements, extensions, placements, etc. Every *āsana* demands discipline of the body, mind and intelligence. In the beginning the discipline has to be carried on. Eventually a forceful discipline becomes a natural discipline. When it turns into a natural discipline, you cannot say that it is a physical, forced or a false discipline, it's natural discipline. For me it is natural discipline. Because I have reached that level. But to reach that level I had to put extraordinary means to get it. So you can say it is a forceful discipline. But it has led me to natural discipline now.

Therefore the effort is important. It has to be in the right direction. Then the effort has to become so natural that it has to be an effortless effort.

Q.- Why then, if the goal of *āsana* practice is *dhyāna* and *samādhi*, then why must students learn so many different poses? Why not just learn a few poses?

Suppose this house had only one window. Would it ventilate the room? Would it illumine the room completely? Would it lighten the room, or would you want more light?

– *More windows, more air, more light.* –

When you have so many cells, muscles, bones, joints and organs in the body, how will you ventilate them? How will you energise or vitalise them? How will you supply blood everywhere? How will you keep the internal cleanliness? Patañjali uses the word *śauca* for cleanliness. You may have a bath to maintain external cleanliness. But how will you bring about internal cleanliness? In one pose do you mean to say that you are cleansing the entire body?

Suppose I've got an injury in my shoulder or sprain in the shoulder blades. What does *Padmāsana* have to do with this? If I've got arthritis in the shoulders, then how is *Padmāsana* going to help me there? Tell me.

– *So these are all part of the* niyama, *the cleansing.* –

Many *āsana* were taught in order to keep the millions and billions of cells in the body healthy. Not that they said that you have to do all the *āsana* in one day. They say you can divide. Today if you have done some *āsana*, you have trained certain cells. Tomorrow you do the other *āsana*, different types of cells will work. Therefore, you need to select the group of several *āsana*.

– *To enliven the body.* –

Yes! You enliven the body, that is the fact. For instance, Vyāsa in his commentary on *sūtra* on *āsana* gives a list of the *āsana*. He does not mention only one *āsana*. In *Haṭhayoga Pradīpikā* you hardly find fourteen or fifteen *āsana*, but the effects of *āsana* mentioned in the book indicate that even in those days, they were concerned about health – physical as well as mental. They too had to keep themselves free from diseases.

Why am I healthy even at this age? Tell me. Why is it that so many yogis cannot even walk straight at my age? Then they say that they are at a higher level. Why should they tell a lie, that they are at a higher level? If I can't do *āsana*, I say I am sorry, I am old, I'm injured, I can't do it. I tell the truth. Even now I am practising, in spite of having met with accidents and injuries. I have not stopped the practice. Whereas those who say that they are spiritual practitioners are not able to sit, stand or walk. Does any one question them why they are not practising *āsana?* Why don't you ask them the truth? The laziness, inertia, is the first enemy, which comes in the way, especially in the practice of *āsana*. One can sit and deliver a lecture for hours together, but one cannot practise *āsana* because it requires one's efforts. For me, the practice of *āsana* and *prāṇāyāma* comes under ethical discipline. I cannot break the ethics. Now if you ask me, I say that I don't care whether I experience spiritual knowledge or not. But I want to be ethical in my practice. So if I keep it up, say I've done wonderful service to my Self.

– Even if we don't move on to spiritual practice, these are the basics. –

Yes. In order to have the spiritual knowledge, these basics are a must. After having the spiritual knowledge, where has it been said that you forget the basics and stop the practice? It is the people who think that after having spiritual knowledge one can stop practising *āsana* or *prāṇāyāma*. It is a misunderstanding. Who has to judge whom? If somebody has realised the Self and stops the practice, does he not lose the fragrance of the self later.

I cannot lie. I will never say that practice is not required, even though I am at a spiritual level. I don't fool.

– So you don't bypass the important work. –

Mahatma Gandhi brought independence to India by following and applying two leaves of yoga, non-violence and truth. Did it not lead him to the highest level? Is there any other Mahatma Gandhi who can be compared to him? So why cannot the *āsana*, which is one leaf of yoga, give me a chance to challenge myself into the art of yoga and science of yoga. If it does not uplift me or take me to the highest level, then I say that it's not worth practising *āsana*. But it's given me all. As it has given me the feel, understanding and experience of all the aspects of yoga, why should I say that this is different and that is different and this is lower and higher? Why should I demarcate and differentiate when *āsana, prāṇāyāma, and pratyāhāra* are helping me in my evolution and involution.

My education was very poor. I was not cultured, but *āsana* educated me, taught me cultured me and elevated me to the spiritual level.

Q.- When you say "given me", what do you mean?

Āsana have given me the disciplines of *pratyāhāra*, *dhāraṇā* and *dhyāna*. Why should I do them separately when it is already there?

- A natural fruit -

Yes! So why should I say I teach only *āsana* and *prāṇāyāma?* I teach yoga. Like a musician who can play Beethoven or Bach or anything on one instrument and with his devotion reach God, can I not do the same? Why should I not play all the instruments of yoga on this body?

For instance, Saint Tyāgarāja[1] was a great musician who wrote songs in the praise of Rāma and framed them in South Indian classical music. He was a musician, poet and a devotee of Rāma as well. So my practice of *āsana* and *prāṇāyāma* is like devotional music. You may not understand my devotion and I too do not want to make it an issue for debate.

Q.- How about the role of *prāṇāyāma* in *āsana* practice? Is *prāṇāyāma* incorporated into *āsana* practice?

Prāṇāyāma can be incorporated with *āsana*, but *prāṇāyāma* essentially has to be practised separately in order to know its depth before one incorporates.

Patañjali and the commentator Vyāsa both clearly mention *prāṇāyāma* as a step after *āsana*. If one learns and does *prāṇāyāma* properly, one can introduce it in *āsana*. In fact, this needs not be introduced as it happens as a natural process.

Normally everybody says that *prāṇāyāma* should be followed with the *āsana*. I have also done this, I do it even now, not that I do not know it. Normally, the practitioners do the breathing and call it *prāṇāyāma*, which is not right. There is a difference between breathing and *prāṇāyāma*. While practising *āsana* undoubtedly one has to breathe. But that is not the point. The point is whether we are disturbing the right position of the *āsana* when we are doing breathing. Do you question this?[2] When I do *Paschimottānāsana* I go according to my optimum level. Retaining that optimum level, I find out while doing inhalations and exhalations, am I bringing disturbance in my body? Does my trunk go backward and forward with breath and so on? If so, then *prāṇāyāma* has no value at all

---

[1] Renowned saint musician (1757-1847) who through his songs made an outstanding contribution to *bhajana-paddhati* (path of adoring the Lord through songs) and provided a very rich musical medium for this method of worship, known as *Tyāgarāja kīrtana*

[2] See *Aṣṭadala Yogamālā*, vol. 4, plate n. 28.

because of the fluctuation of the breath and the fluctuation of the cells. In turn it causes the fluctuation of the mind too. So why should I fluctuate the cells in the breathing? Why should I fluctuate my mind? So I say, let me observe normal breathing what happens. In normal breathing it does not move.

In each *āsana* the dimension of normal breathing changes. The place, quantity and quality of breath changes. I observe these changes. The pattern of breath which remains suitable, adoptable and congenial in the *chosen āsana*, restrains the body and mind from their fluctuations. If this maturity comes in the practice, there is no question of introducing *prāṇāyāma* in *āsana*. The energy or *prāṇa* reaches everywhere and this is called *prāṇāyāma*. It is not at all breathing deeply or forcefully. It is the synchronisation of the movement of the breath with the spread of intelligence in the steady *āsana*.

Q.- Do you keep the normal breathing then because it doesn't disturb.

No, I'm not saying that. When I am doing deep breathing my motive is on deep breathing, my motive is not on the *āsana*. My major purpose of doing *āsana* is lost and only the minor issue, such as breathing, comes to the forefront. Then I say to myself, "Suppose I am doing the *āsana* in a very precise way, what type of breathing does the body adapt to? What type of inhalation, what type of exhalation?"

Q.- What does it adapt to actually?

Naturally it adapts. I catch that. In a correct positioned *āsana* the breathing occurs in a particular region according to the *āsana*, which keeps one in a comfortable position. One does not need to choose the region or area with one's will power. But it happens naturally. It is like a catchment area. I don't force my brain just because the teacher demands, that I do deep inhalation or deep exhalation.

I have already experimented and observed the results by doing the deep inhalation and exhalation. The induced breathing brings the strain on the brain cells. Instead of inducing the breath I see it the other way.

Then I say to myself, "Let me not do it, let me retain my optimum stretch and observe what type of breathing the body adapts or does."

– Naturally. –

Yes! It happens naturally on its own. So I catch that one, and from that I build up what type of breathing I should do in order to breathe without disturbing the body or the exhilaration I get in the stretch of the *āsana*.

- Rather than layering the prāṇāyāma *on top of the* āsana. -

Yes! I do not impose the *prāṇāyāma* on *āsana*. The imposed *prāṇāyāma* in *āsana* shakes not only the muscular or skeletal body but brain and nerves as well. Therefore, I take the precaution that I do not move my body like a turtle moving backward and forward with its limbs. The turtle takes its limbs in and out. So I observe whether I am doing my *āsana* like a turtle. Do my inhalations and exhalations disturb the shell of my body? As a turtle takes its limbs into the shell, I take my limbs in this *āsana* in a certain manner. The limbs, the cells, the body is placed in a certain manner. I watch and question myself, does my breathing disturb the limbs of this *āsana?* Can I do the *prāṇāyāma* or can I do the breathing without causing my body to go away from the shell of that *āsana*? And that is the *prāṇāyāma* in *āsana* for me.

- So it requires that we be attentive to our bodies, to really pay attention. -

True! That we have to pay attention to our body, is a fact. But what do you mean by paying attention? It does not mean paying attention to the body alone. Body is the instrument that seems to be performing the *āsana*. But the real fact is that the mind, intelligence and consciousness or *citta* are involved. The mind, intelligence and consciousness are not visible, non-perceivable instruments. These are conceivable instruments. As the body can cheat, these instruments also can cheat. I, while practising, do not allow any of these instruments to cheat me.

When I do *āsana*, for me the body is no more a *tāmasic* or lethargic instrument. It is charged with intelligence, consciousness and awareness.

The intelligence coming from the body is the factual knowledge, the factual intelligence. I am dictating from the brain, which means that the analytical knowledge derived from the brain is going into my body. Then how does the body receive it? It is the body that receives and says to me, "This is good" or "This is not good". I adjust because it gives me a feedback, saying, "Your analysis is wrong. Your analysis is right." In the *āsana*, when we use the brain and the body, then we have to find that there should be coordination between the body and brain. And I learn and I teach that. This coordination should be there.

Q.- You mentioned *yama* and *niyama*. Doing *yama* and *niyama* in the sense that you discussed, does this then lead to ethical action naturally?

Obviously.

- And if one then acts unethically, then . . . . -

First of all, understand the fact that the change or transformation occurs gradually. It is not instant or temporary. Only the fact is that it takes a long time to establish oneself in the practice of *āsana* and then understand and adapt *yama-niyama* in *āsana*. It takes time to utilise one's own mind, intelligence and consciousness or *citta* in order to adapt *yama* and *niyama* when one achieves in getting clarity, purity and sanctity.

You should know that to err is human. You and I or anybody else are not divine. Our aim is to go towards divinity, and we are struggling to experience the divinity little by little for this. We have to follow the discipline of *yama* and *niyama*.

As you asked me, suppose a person who is unethical comes to me and if I take him through a three hours class, I am sure that at least I have kept him in ethical disapline for three hours in my class. Like that, I build him up ethical and moral discipline. I would tempt him, "Why don't you come to the other classes?" This I say in order to keep him free from sensual thoughts for another few hours.

Unethical behaviour will not disturb on the physical level at all for a beginner but when one moves for further levels min yoga it will be affecting very badly. To build up for spiritual progress naturally it takes one a longer time. All are not fit to become spiritual people at once. For instance, you see a fruit on the tree. The fruit is not going to fall if you throw one stone, but if you go on throwing stones one after the other, perhaps one stone may hit the fruit and it may fall down. I use the same analogy. We are *yoga-sādhaka*, we are practitioners of yoga, we are not yogis. Do you understand the difference between these two levels? When I become a yogi then I am divine. I may have developed sensitivity, which keeps me in the ethical disciplines that guide me naturally. Because my *karmendriya*, the organs of action, and my *jñānendriya*, the senses of perception, do not drag me in a wrong direction. But those who are newcomers or neophytes on the yogic path have to learn the art of reflection by feeling the conjuction of motor nerves with the sensory nerves. It takes time to discipline these, hence, I cannot demand it either. But I keep on throwing the moral stones. I keep on giving them guidance, correcting them while teaching them *āsana*. Gradually, I awaken the cognitive intelligence in them. I introduce the principles of *yama* and *niyama* in *āsana*. I see how they lead towards *pratyāhāra*, *dhāraṇā* and *dhyāna*. All this does not happen instantly. The time factor is involved. But the self-discipline comes at one time or the other.

Let me tell you my experience. I had two pupils in the late 50's and 60's. One of them was a regular visitor to the house of prostitutes. He started doing yoga and initially the mind was cultured up to the level that whenever he did yoga he never felt like going to prostitutes. In those days, I was regularly going to Europe for three months to teach yoga. In my absence he used to fall back on his morals and used to confess on my return. With innocence he asked me, "How come I don't feel like going when I do yoga?" When I was out of India old temptation reappeared. Hence, I allowed him to come and practise in my house in my absence. He did so and got rid of his bad habits. In the second case too, I noticed that the practitioner, though he was going to a prostitute, realised that doing *Sālamba Śīrṣāsana* and *Sālamba Sarvāṅgāsana* was helping him a great lot to refrain himself from such temptation. The gradual change came and now he is leading an ascetic life.

In these circumstances I demand discipline, accuracy, precision which is far above the reasons to lift such people towards better thinking and living. The practice or *sādhanā* has to elevate the *sādhaka*. For example, today a reporter was in the class, watching the class in San Diego. He asked, "Is Mr. Iyengar always like that?" See the question: because I was correcting, I was guiding, he wondered why should I be so strict with everyone. Though I heard his question, I did not say anything. I'm a religious person, I'm not an irreligious person. I am a person who has realised the effect of the *āsana*, which I want to put in the heart of the students, so that they can also put that into the heart when they guide their students. So seriousness is involved; the spiritual life is a serious path, a sincere path. They say you have to walk on the sharp path which is like a razor blade for a spiritual life.[1] Often people say, "Oh, he should be soft!" They can't tell me what I should be. They cannot dictate the norms. So these doubts will always be in the minds of the people since they think that a spiritual person has to be a sweet talker. When I am religious, it is taken as seriousness. The religiosity in my teaching is *tapas*. *Tapas* means nothing but religiosity. True in its practice. But if you do not understand what "seriousness" is, how can I translate to those people?

Q.- So this reporter was suggesting that you were too serious?

That's what he was suggesting, "Is he always like that? Everybody says outside he is humorous but in the class he is serious." That's his opinion. He said, "He can see when people do wrong and he wants to guide them to come to the right method."

- You are somewhat well known for being a fiery teacher. -

[1] *Utthiṣṭhata jāgrata prāpya varān nibodhata: kṣurasya dhārā niśita duratyayā; durgam pathas tat kavayo vadanti* (*Kaṭha Upaniṣad*, I.3.14). Arise, awake, having attained thy boons, understand them. The wise ones describe that path to be as impassable as a razor's edge, which when sharpened, is difficult to tread on..

The reason why I am serious and sincere in the subject is such. What is yogic fire? What is the function of fire? – Burn or extinguish.

– To burn. –

So my practice of yoga is keeping the fire burning. What have I to do for that? And if I also practise or teach yoga like others, coolly, unenthusiastically, stupidly making people *mūḍha*, then what is the point? I do not want the fire to be extinguished. The mind of the people has to rise up. *Yogāgni*, means yogic fire. The quality of fire is to throw the light, heat and warmth. Fire spreads horizontally and vertically. It burns other matters and becomes strong itself. I have done yoga to such an extent that it has burnt the thought impurities in me and purified and refreshed. The *yogāgni* has spread in my body, in my cells, in my mind, in my heart. So how can it be extinguished?

*– So that fire (*yogāgni*) just comes out automatically. –*

It is there. It exists in a latent state in everyone. How can it be automatic? If I don't practise, if I do it casually, how can the fire remain burning? Then like a live coal, which slowly gets covered with ashes and fades away, my practice also fades away. Then you may say that Mr. Iyengar is a very silent man. I may fool the masses saying that I've mellowed, so I've become very silent. But that is not true. My fire, the *yogāgni*, "Don't do that." What is the job of the fire? It goes up. What does it do?

– It burns. –

For what purpose? It purifies. It sanctifies. So my *yogāgni* comes up to purify myself as well as the others. Therefore, my *yogāgni* is meant to ignite the fire in others. My fiery nature is meant to create enthusiasm, to encourage to practise, to make them courageous to take up *sādhanā*, to uplift them from falling from the chosen path.

Q.- Is this *yogāgni*, something that every *sādhaka* practises?

Yogāgni is there in everyone, but because of indulgence in sensual and worldly pleasures, the fire keeps on weakening. If one practises yoga honestly, devotedly, thoroughly, sincerely in the way I mentioned or the way I do, the *yogāgni* will remains burning.

Q.- So this is a positive thing, that should develop. Can this *yogāgni* get out of control?

Yes! when it gets out of control. Immediately it affects the mind. You should read *Patañjali's Yoga Sūtra* if you want to know how to control *yogāgni.* In the third chapter Patañjali has given lots of effects, what are called the supernatural powers. You know about the supernatural powers. They are guides to the sensitivity of the effect of your progress in the *sādhanā.* And Patañjali has given thirty-four to thirty-five various effects of the *sādhanā.* If any one effect is there, it indicates that you are on the right path, your *sādhanā* is ripe. If you don't experience any of these, effects, then your *sādhanā* is still raw. When the *sādhanā* is ripe, these powers or *siddhi* comes. However he warns in the third chapter that you should proceed further and purify the *sādhanā* and not get caught in the effects or *siddhi,* which come automatically from your *sādhanā.* And that is where the disturbances come.[1] Then the fire of yoga gets out of control.

- Oh! I got it. And that is a trap. -

Yes! That is a trap. The thought, "I don't want to do it because I have already seen" leads towards *anavasthitatva.* It is a failure to retain a level, rather a fall from the level. In the very first chapter, the 32nd *sūtra,*[2] Patañjali says that even if a person has reached *samādhi,* the impediments and obstacles may bring a fall, therefore he should not stop the *sādhanā.* Have you ever noticed it? But how many people follow? Often, the so-called yogis misguide and say, "It's not required." The man, the subject whom they follow, whom they quote, does not see it. *Avasthā* becomes *anavasthā. Avasthā* means you have reached a certain state, a qualitative state that Patañjali explains in the third chapter,[3] known as *avasthā pariṇāma.* In the third chapter he goes on explaining, that when the *sādhaka* gets the effect, he first gets the religiosity, the transformation takes a religious formation, that he wants to be ethical, he wants to be physically healthy, he wants to use his energy in the right direction. This is known as *dharma pariṇāma.* These things will come to him, who is determined in yoga. Then *lakṣaṇa pariṇāma,* where qualitative changes take place. Then when the qualitative changes take place, the person who is practising reaches the highest qualitative state, called

[1] Patañjali warns the practitioner against getting caught in *siddhi,* in three *sūtra: te samādhau upasargāḥ vyutthāne siddhayaḥ,* these attainments are impediments to *samādhi,* although they are powers in active life (III.38); *tadvairāgyāt api doṣabījakṣaye kaivalyam,* by destruction of the seeds of bondage and the renunciation of even these powers comes eternal emancipation (III.51); *sthānyupanimantraṇe saṅgasmayākaraṇaṁ punaraniṣṭa prasaṅgāt,* when approached by celestial beings, there should be neither attachment nor surprise, for undesirable connections can occur again (III.52).

[2] *Tatpratiṣedhārtham ekatattva abhyāsaḥ* (I.32). Adherence to single-minded effort prevents these impediments.

[3] *Etena bhūtendriyeṣu dharma lakṣaṇa avasthā pariṇāmā vyākhyātāḥ* (*Y.S,* III.13). Through these three phases, cultured consciousness is transformed from its potential state *(dharma)* towards further refinement *(lakṣaṇa)* and the zenith of refinement *(avasthā).* In this way, the transformation of elements, senses and mind takes place.

avasthā pariṇāma. He has to learn how to retain that state so that he may not fall back.

Now, this indicates that *sādhanā* cannot be stopped even though you are in the highest state of *samādhi.* See how clearly it is mentioned.

Q.- So you won't fall back, you have to maintain the level that you've achieved.

Yes. That's why *sādhanā* cannot be stopped. Ethical discipline, physical discipline, mental discipline, whatever its method, it cannot be stopped. You cannot say that this is not necessary, then I will say, have you demarcated the area between body and mind, mind and soul? Can anybody demarcate it?

– They're all interconnected, there's no separation. –

They are undoubtedly interconnected. But in normal course of life, the body pulls the person in one direction and the mind in another. The body and mind remain divorced from soul. The division is felt very clearly. Whereas in the case of a yogi, the body and mind become not only the servers but the listeners of the soul. One who has unity in these three is called a yogi. The one who practises yoga and brings union in these three is called a yogi.

Q.- Would you consider yourself a yogi?

Well, I don't say that I'm a yogi. It is not even right to declare that I am a yogi. I can only say that I am on the path and I'm very near. I can say I'm a forerunner, no doubt. I am near the goal, let it come on its own. I have no motive. I had lots of motives in the early days. I have no motive now. My motive is only to continue what I learned so that I may not lose. It's not an ambition, but I do not want to have a fall – *anavasthitatva.* And I do not want to develop the character of *tāmasic* nature in my system, that's all. You may ask, why do you practise then? I practise so that the *tāmasic* nature may not domineer over my *sāttvic* nature.

– So that's maintained, that level. You maintain a sāttvic level as much as possible. –

That's why I'm doing even now.

Q.- What about those students who become somehow preoccupied with the physical perfection of the pose? What would you say to such people? There seem to be quite a few in the yoga community.

Even if I take your conclusive views, I say a change has taken place in them. So your reading is inconclusive. Even if I agree with you I say never mind, at least they have become body conscious, which is the outer layer of the Self. After ten or fifteen years, if they go on, probably they may realise that this is not what they are hunting for, their thinking minds may change.

- So it's a stage. -

Just a stage. I remember the words of Buddha: If you can do good, if you can give them health, you have done the greatest service. So even making people to look at their own bodies is also, according to Buddha, a great service. One is great, and the other is greater. Even if they bring only this physical attention, we should say they are on the right path. Even the *Yoga Journal* need not worry at all. From body consciousness, they may go on towards mental consciousness. From mental consciousness, they may go to spiritual consciousness. Without any consciousness, where can they go? So at least they are focused on one side, what you call *dhāraṇā*. While doing *āsana*, even if they attend to an external *āsana*, externally representing, at least there is some concentration, there is some discipline, there is some *yama*. So let us appreciate that also. And then if they take it to a little higher state, it is well and good.

Q.- What about your own practice? What kind of problems do you face in your own practice?

Any problems that come, I know the remedy. Suppose my body says that it does not want to do *āsana*. I can tune the body in fifteen minutes and make it as fresh as it should be. If my brain refuses to do, whether it is *āsana* or *prāṇāyāma*, I know which ones to do, so that the brain gets refreshed. If my mind is dull, certainly I am not going to do *dhyāna* – meditation. Then what do you need to be explained? I will see first that my body, brain, mind, breath and intelligence are charged with the practice of *āsana* and *prāṇāyāma* so that I can do full justice to *dhyāna*.

You know people come to me with lots of problems. Because I have undergone these problems, I immediately give them the guidance – "Do this or do that and you will recover. And you are as fresh as you were before." I appreciate problems coming to me more and more so that I can work still with a greater humility than the natural one. I don't say that I will be unhappy if some problems come. I take it as God's gift for me to test on my own quality of faith in yoga. I was very good in my practice, my yoga *sādhanā,* till 1977. I was really on the top. After my sixtieth birthday I met with two severe accidents. You must have heard.

– *What happened?* –

My body spilled completely and my spine developed scoliosis. My shoulders were injured, I could not even control or lift my hand. I couldn't lift my spine upright at all. My shoulders were affected, my shoulder blades were affected, my hips were affected, and I could not do any *āsana,* not even *Utthita Trikoṇāsana.* I was struggling to do. And everybody in Pune knew how my practice was affected. Even my pupils thought that I may not be able to do anything from now onwards. It took ten years for me to come back to my original state. Now, if anyone comes with any of such problems, I can help and correct them very fast, since I have undergone all those problems. All those injuries have helped me to help people with arthritis, with scoliosis. What I could not do ten years ago to such affected people with that speed, today I've got speed to put them into a better line, faster than what I could do in the first fifty-sixty years.

Q.- What have you learned from your students? What have your students taught you?

My students have taught me a lot. They are my *guru.* I honestly tell you, my *guru* gave me only technique, beyond that nothing. But my pupils taught me the correct technique, because all their mistakes I could absorb. If there are fifty pupils in the class, I see all the fifty bodies very carefully as my *gurus.* The good points I take from them and I develop. So all my pupils were indirectly my *guru* to improve my subject.

I'm grateful to my pupils as I am grateful to my *guru.* My *guru* gave me technical points, my pupils gave me an emotional sense of how I should manage the techniques.

– *What do you mean by that?* –

I mean, I learnt how to go with the mind openly to help, to guide. As you all call me 'wild', but know in that wildness there is compassion in me to accept written-off cases and make them improve fast. I seem to be wild because I think why should they suffer so long when it is possible to bring them back to their joy of life fast. As if they cannot do it, on their own, they come to me. I want them to catch and learn quickly before the next mishap. This type of my expression seems to be wild. My quick decision and immediate approach seem to be wild. I do not want people to go slow cajoling themselves and fondling their problems. The compassion makes me wild. This is my attitude. If they do not do it as I want them to do, the fire in me raises up and makes me speak forcefully, and I make them do. And this attitude of mine makes people to mistake me. I have seen other yoga teachers, who go slow with those who are having pains, problems and injuries. Often, the teachers do not understand the problems of the pupils. They cannot put them in right position. They do not know the remedial methods in yoga. Therefore, if at all, they stop people from doing anything beyond their limmited knowledge. This seems to be a polite approach but basically it is carelessness or heedlessness or ignorance.

I was observing in some classes. When people were shaking and having tremors while in the *āsana*, I said, "Why are you keeping them in the *āsana* so long? First teach them where and how to relax the muscle so that the tremors stop and they can be in peace. But instead you are putting them into pieces. They are confused because they are tense. The tension is there in their body, therefore they are shaky. So learn."

The teachers should see why the pupils are shaky, why there is a tension in their muscles; which way and how they are using their nerves. The teachers are explaining but the pupils are unable to pay attention because they are shaking. They are unable to hear what the teachers say. They cannot even see anywhere, since they have to hold on the *āsana* full of tension in the mind. The teachers firstly have to make the brain and nerves of the pupils calm so that the pupils can listen to them properly.

Since I am a long time teacher, I have noticed all these problems of the pupils. I have studied their sufferings, that is why I am very fast adjusting them. I see quickly with one glance who can do and who cannot do. I catch their weak points and change my approach immediately so that they relax their nerves and do the *āsana* in a better way. I think quickly and see in what way I should help them to keep the same elixir of what they are just now getting. I am an advertant teacher, I am not a mild teacher. But many people have taken my advertance and seriousness as well as integrity as aggressive teaching. That is their way of thinking. That is how they apprehend my teaching. My intensive and quick adjustment is apprehended as violence and roughness. It does not affect me at all. I am not bothered about what people say about me. I am concerned with what the pupil feels when I touch and teach. My conscience is clear about my teaching.

I have been doing yoga since 1934, I have been teaching since 1935. I settled in 1937 in Pune as an independent yoga teacher. People have criticised me from the age of seventeen. I am now seventy-two. What I heard at the age of seventeen I am hearing the same words today about me and my teaching. Many of my pupils have passed away who have practised in my presence. They are gone. Now the new generations have come. They also say the same thing. But I have not changed. I did not change because I am not a teacher of the type to please the pupils. To please them one can do anything, there can be several paths. But to put them on the right path there is only one way – only the right way.

– So the wildness is compassion, an expression of compassion. –

If your son is not listening to you, don't you get wild? Why do you get wild? Do you abandon the child because it does not listen or do you go with the wildness so that the child may come around and grow better? What do you call it? Do you call such anger of parents as wildness?

– Well, some people are wilder than the others, some fathers are wilder than others. –

But tell me. What happens to their wildness? If they are very badly wild, then it breaks, is it not? Tell me, how many students have left me because of my wildness?

– Not many, really. –

You must be knowing, eh? If I am wild they would have abandoned me. Why did it not happen? Then what makes them stick to me?

It is others who are branding me as a wild teacher. The participants in the class never complain. It's the others, onlookers, who just see me while teaching. They of course appreciate the teaching and then they remark, "He is rough, he is wild." And that has stood out. But the real truth has not come out at all, truth is hidden. However, in India, after so many years at least one good change has taken place. The Indians have seen the consistency of my practice from the age of seventeen even up to now. Now I am commanding respect. They say, "This man is consistent, please go to him. He is more truthful than anybody else." So in India my wildness is accepted with respect. Even here in your country people have accepted my wildness. They know my sincerity and honesty. They know that I demand discipline. My anger or wildness sprouts from that sincere and honest approach..

– But you know Mr. Iyengar, you're not always wild. –

Not always. It comes in papers or magazines, and people read that and brand me as a wild teacher.

– But I have seen you with some people not be wild, but be absolutely the opposite. Why is that? –

I already told you. Those who appreciate my discipline and follow the instructions sincerely, putting their heart in it, why should I be wild? You do not know that sometimes my wildness makes the pupils to remove confusion and get clarity. The old, wrong ideas or the mistakes are cleared suddenly like a "brain wash". They become alert at once and follow correctly. Then I show my friendliness. Though I am very serious, often with humour I make them laugh. They do not know when I suddenly crack a joke. So that's the beauty of my teaching. That's also what is called knack of teaching. I am a natural teacher. Teaching has become a natural thing for me. Now you will be surprised if I tell you. As I went into the classes, I saw so many mistakes at once and all the senior teachers said, "How could you see quickly? You have not seen them before you walked in." I said, "Then what is my job? Why do you call me? That means my eyes should be a thousand times more aware than your eyes. That's why I am here. I look faster than you people so I get at once what is going on." Sometimes even as I'm walking or passing by, I hear the words and from the words used by the teacher I say, "The explanation is not correct."

– You did that this morning. –

You were there. You saw.

– I was there. You walked in commenting on what was going on in the room. You were just walking in talking about it. –

Yes! The teaching has gone deep into my system, in my blood.

Q.- How do you see your work, Mr. Iyengar, developing in the United States? How do you see the future of it?

It's really getting on very well. But at the same time I am afraid that it may lose the charm as time passes, though it may stay longer than any other method. My method may stay longer, but if our pupils search more, interweave their minds, it will stand for centuries to come. Otherwise maybe a hundred years, fifty years. It may survive longer than other yoga teachings of the world.

Q.- What do you mean by "interweave their minds"?

I mean intelligence. They have to go inwards, and penetrate with intelligence. They should not merely repeat the words like parrots. As a teacher, when I am teaching, I see if the sentence that I used, the words I have used have gone into the hearts of the students or not. If the words haven't gone into their hearts, then I have to think and change words so that it penetrates their heart. If I just keep on pouring the words, when nothing is expressed by their faces, then I am teaching from my head. That is an ego-trip. The teachers have to be humble. They should have humility so that they remain with the pupil. The teachers have to come to the level of the pupil. Then only can we make better students. And if the teachers learn that, I think the entire civilization of the world may change. When there is health in the body the fear of diseases goes away. The mind is always in contact with the external body in the form of diseases or pains. When the body pain is lessened, when the body is healthy, when it can take care of itself, naturally the mind comes closer to the Self. But for common man, the mind runs on the outer part of the body. And when I say outer part, it may be far away from the bones, even outside the bone. You have to go inside, that is known as interpenetration, interweaving the intelligence of the mind from outside to inside. Many people do *āsana* very well, but the question is whether they can draw the body towards the soul. If they do so, then they can build up very well.

Q.- If they do not take that step of turning inward, then, according to you, yoga won't last.

Yoga, basically, is a subject which demands "inward turning". All other subjects make us look outward. This is the only subject which makes us look within. Therefore, if practitioners fail to look inwards, they will lose track. Yoga can never get lost. It cannot diminish or die. But the practitioners will be the losers because of wrong adaptation. Therefore if they continue to practise without that interpenetration because of lack of interweaving, they mislead themselves.

Even if you see carefully, though the literature on yoga was available in *Veda* and *Upaniṣad*, there was a gap and Patañjali had to codify the subject. Svātmārāma wrote the *Haṭhayoga Pradīpikā* much later. And after that, I think there was no other book which has thrown light on the subject except *Light on Yoga*. Now all the books which are coming in the market, almost follow just *Light on Yoga*. They may use different names or change a bit here and there, but without using that book as the base they cannot write. I see the replica of my *Light on Yoga* words and positions of *āsana* in any book that I open. So it is the grace of God of yoga on me for this good work. I am quite happy about it, but it is for others now to build it up further. If they start from the point where I leave off, then a tremendous revolution may take place. That's why I'm trying my level best to build up the pupils of mine in this convention. I want to see whether they could build upon that, because that is the means to the end. So I'm trying to give the means to them. If they have the means, I do not think that there is any problem to spread yoga in the proper direction.

Yoga is spreading everywhere. Many people follow my books. Up to now I have not received even a single complaint from anyone saying that one has injured or ruined his or her health after reading or following my book. If at all there were any complaints, I wrote back and asked them,

"Have you done this without following the cycle?" They said, "Yes! How did you know we did not do it?" Then I said, "Go back to the cycle given in *Light on Yoga*, you will be corrected." And they were. Therefore, I can say emphatically that the given knowledge and methodology is correct. That is why people have benefited. Those who were callous, while reading and following the book casually had to face the problem but those who followed methodically, never had any problem.

But now, as I say, people have to be "inward looking". The practice that is done at the physical level, exhibitively, has to do be done inhibitively. Now, they have to be attentive internally and the practice has to be done contemplatively. To explain in practical language, it is the process, for instance, whereby while doing *āsana* the skin has to press and follow the flesh. The skin and the flesh together have to touch the bones. The skin, flesh and bones have to touch the intelligence. The intelligence has to feel where the source of it begins. This is known as interpenetration. From outer penetration they have to go towards interpenetration. That's why I use the word interpenetration very often. The practitioner, while practising *āsana*, has to connect the intelligence from the core of his being to the skin, again reverse it, from the skin towards the core. The thread of intelligence has to connect throughout the Self and the skin and the skin and the Self. The skin is the outermost layer of the body and Self is the inner most layer of the body. From the inner most layer of the being they come out, that is known as expansion or evolution of the Self. The expansion of the Self is exhibitionism. When they go in reverse from skin to the Self or from exhibitionism to inhibitionism, it is called involution, where everything merges into Self. The yogic terminology for evolution and involution is *prasava* and *pratiprasava*. This is what is needed for the practitioners of yoga.

Q.- I want to ask one more thing. I get questions a lot at *Yoga Journal*. People call me up and say, "What about the non-physical body, the subtle body, the causal body?"

Exactly! That is what I am explaining. We are wrapped and engulfed in five sheaths, namely *annamaya kośa, prāṇamaya kośa, manomaya kośa, vijñānamaya kośa* and *ānandamaya kośa*. Let me give the gross translation. These sheaths are namely, the physical body of bones and muscles, the physiological or organic body of vital organs, the psychological body of the nervous system and mind which includes senses of perception, the intellectual body of the mental faculty and the blissful body of the Self or *ātman*. The practice of yoga has to interpenetrate these five sheaths known as *pañcakośa*. In order to simplify it further, let me tell you this. The nervous system is the bridge between the subtle body and the external body, called the physiological body. Or *manomaya kośa* is the bridge between *prāṇamaya* and *vijñānamaya kośa*. If physical and physiological bodies are on one side, then intellectual and blissful bodies are on the other side. I address the nervous system as the psychological body or *manomaya kośa.* The nerves are like the bridge between the body and the mind. Therefore, for the practitioner it is very important to keep the nerves in a healthy condition. If the nerves are disturbed, they make the person completely dejected and depressed. The body, mind and intellectual faculty, all get affected. That's why I consider the nerves as the bridge between the external body and the inner body. And these *āsana* are meant to develop strength in the nervous system. When the strength develops, then the physical body is forgotten, but the physiological body is taught to bring the body nearer the mental body. Then from the mental action you try to develop, as I said, the oneness of your intelligence. Suppose I am doing *Vṛśchikāsana,* the scorpion pose. I watch how my intelligence is flowing from the bottom of the feet and bottom of the toes, up to the bottom of the middle of the fingers of my hands. Is it flowing crookedly in one arm and straight in the other arm? We don't look at the pose then. We see how the inner body is working, how the inner awareness is working. We adjust not the body but the awareness, because as the water finds its level, the awareness too finds the level. The intelligence flows according to the ways or paths we have created in our body. If the *āsana* is zigzag, the intelligence also flows zigzag. Awareness follows intelligence. Wherever you intelligise or energise, the awareness comes there. So if the awareness has to flow in the right channel and spread everywhere, then the *āsana* has to be in a correct position. When we use the word "consciousness" or *citta,* do you admit that consciousness does not exist everywhere?

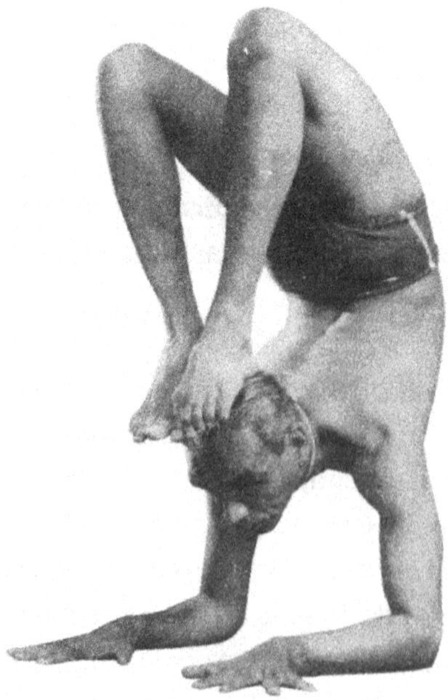

Plate n. 52 – *Vṛśchikāsana*

Secondly, man is made of three layers. These are *kāraṇa śarīra* (cause body), *sūkṣma śarīra* (subtle body)and *sthūla śarīra* (gross body – the external body, which easily sees and cognises). Practice of *āsana* takes the *sādhaka* from the external body to touch the subtle body and from there towards the causal body. Thus it connects and interweaves from the gross to the causal body and from the causal body to the gross body. This is how each *āsana* has to be done.

– I don't know but I'm sure it does. –

It is there but it does not exist everywhere. It remains in a dormant state. The *āsana,* when done accurately and precisely make the consciousness come out from the dormant state to a state of full awareness. Then it runs in the body without any divisions. And that comes in an advanced state of practice of *āsana,* when we go internally. The moment we move internally we see this conscious awareness on each and every part of the body. It is not the question of merely our muscles, ligaments or liver and spleen working. Rather we see the flow of intelligence and the spread of awareness. And that is spiritual presentation of the *āsana.*

Therefore, the question of demarcation between gross, subtle and causal body does not arise at all. The awareness ties all these three together and wraps it in consciousness. It is the pervasiveness of awareness.

www.ingramcontent.com/pod-product-compliance
Lightning Source LLC
Chambersburg PA
CBHW080414270326
41929CB00018B/3022
* 9 7 8 8 1 7 7 6 4 7 1 3 6 *